Pain and the Conscious Brain

Pain and the Conscious Brain

Luis Garcia-Larrea, MD, PhD
Research Director at the INSERM
Head
Central Integration of Pain—Lyon Centre for Neurosciences
Vice-Director
Human Biology Department
University Claude Bernard Lyon 1
University Hospitals of Lyon
Lyon, France

Philip L. Jackson, PhD
Full Professor
Social and Cognitive Neuroscience Lab
School of Psychology
Laval University
Quebec City, Canada

Wolters Kluwer
Philadelphia • Baltimore • New York • London
Buenos Aires • Hong Kong • Sydney • Tokyo

International Association for the Study of Pain
IASP®
Working together for pain relief

Acquisitions Editor: Keith Donnellan
Product Development Editor: Nicole Dernoski
Editorial Assistant: Kathryn Leyendecker
Senior Production Project Manager: Alicia Jackson
Design Coordinator: Joan Wendt
Manufacturing Coordinator: Beth Welsh
Marketing Manager: Dan Dressler
Prepress Vendor: S4Carlisle Publishing Services

9 8 7 6 5 4 3 2 1

Printed in China

Library of Congress Cataloging-in-Publication Data
Names: Garcia-Larrea, Luis, editor. | Jackson, Philip L. (Neuroscientist), editor.
Title: Pain and the conscious brain / [edited by] Luis Garcia-Larrea, Philip L. Jackson.
Description: First edition. | Philadelphia : Wolters Kluwer Health, 2016.
Identifiers: LCCN 2015051057 | ISBN 9781496333629 (paperback)
Subjects: | MESH: Pain Perception | Consciousness | Pain
Classification: LCC QP355.2 | NLM WL 704 | DDC 612.8--dc23 LC record available at http://lccn.loc.gov/2015051057

LWW.com

RRS1602

CONTRIBUTORS

Hélène Bastuji, MD, PhD
Tenured Neurologist - Neurophysiologist
Hypnology Section, Neurological Hospital of Lyon and NeuroPain Lab
Lyon Center for Neuroscience (CRNL)-Inserm U1028 & University Claude Bernard
Lyon, France

Camille Chatelle, PhD, MSc
Research Professor
Laboratory for NeuroImaging of Coma and Consciousness
Massachusetts General Hospital
Harvard Medical School
Boston, Massachusetts
Coma Science Group
GIGA-Research Center
University of Liege
Liege, Belgium

Luana Colloca, MD, PhD
Professor
Pain Translational Symptom Science
School of Nursing
Department of Anesthesiology
School of Medicine
Center to Advance Chronic Pain Research
University of Maryland
Baltimore, Maryland

Frederique de Vignemont, PhD
CNRS Researcher
Institut Jean Nicod
ENS-EHESS-CNRS
Paris, France

Athena Demertzi, PhD
Postdoctoral Researcher
Brain and Spine Institute (ICM)
Hôpital de la Pitié-Salpêtrière
Paris, France
Coma Science Group
GIGA Research University and University Hospital of Liège
Liege, Belgium

Marie-Elisabeth Faymonville MD, PhD
Professor
Algology-Palliative Care Department
University Hospital of Liege
University of Liege
Liege, Belgium

Luis Garcia-Larrea, MD, PhD
Research Director at the INSERM
Head
Central Integration of Pain Lab—Centre for Neuroscience of Lyon
Vice-Director
Human Biology Department
University Claude Bernard Lyon 1
University Hospitals of Lyon
Lyon, France

Aline Gillet, MSc
Researcher
Department of Work Psychology
University of Liege
Liege, Belgium

Joshua A. Grant, PhD
Postdoctoral Fellow
Department of Social Neuroscience
Max Planck Institute for Human Cognitive and Brain Sciences
Leipzig, Germany

Ruth E. Grunau PhD, RPsych
Senior Scientist/Professor
Pediatrics
University of British Columbia
Child and Family Research Institute
Vancouver, Canada

Thomas Hadjistavropoulos, PhD, ABPP, FCAHS
Professor/Research Chair in Aging and Health
Department of Psychology, and Centre on Aging and Health
University of Regina
Regina, Canada

Vanessa Harrar, PhD
Postdoctoral Fellow
Harl-Sanders Research Chair in Vision Sciences
School of Optometry
University of Montreal
Montreal, Canada

Philip L. Jackson, PhD
Full Professor
Social and Cognitive Neuroscience Lab
School of Psychology
Laval University
Quebec City, Canada

Ron Kupers, PhD
Professor
BRAINlab
Department of Neuroscience and Pharmacology
Panum Institute
Faculty of Health and Medical Sciences
University of Copenhagen
Copenhagen, Denmark

Hugo Lagercrantz, MD PhD
Senior Professor
Astrid Lindgren Children's Hospital
Karolinska Institute
Stockholm, Sweden

Steven Laureys, MD, PhD
Clinical Professor
Cyclotron Research Center
Coma Science Group
University of Liege
Liege, Belgium

Gilles Lavigne, MD PhD
Full Professor
Canada Research Chair in Pain, Sleep and Traumatology
Faculté de médecine dentaire
Université de Montréal
Surgery Department-Trauma Unit
Hopital Sacre Cœur de Montreal
Montreal, Canada

Anne-Claire Lukaszewicz, MD, PhD
Tenured Anesthesiologist
Department of Anesthesia-Reanimation
Neurological Hospital of Lyon and Lariboisière Hospital
Paris, France

Anne-Sophie Nyssen, PhD
Full Professor
Department of Work Psychology
University of Liege
Liege, Belgium

Jaak Panksepp, PhD
Professor
Department of Integrative Physiology and Neuroscience
College of Veterinary Medicine
Washington State University
Pullman, Washington

Pauline Perez, MD
Anesthesiologist
Department of Anesthesia-Reanimation
Neurological Hospital of Lyon and Lariboisière Hospital
Assistance Publique–Hôpitaux de Paris
Paris, France

Roland Peyron, MD, PhD
Professor
Central Integration of Pain (Neuropain)
Lyon Centre for Neurosciences
University and University Hospital of St Etienne
St Etienne, France

Maurice Ptito, PhD, DrMed, FRSC
Director
Harl-Sanders Research Chair in Visual Science
School of Optometry
University of Montreal
Montreal, Canada

Manon Ranger, RN, PhD
Professor
Pediatrics
University of British Columbia
Child and Family Research Institute
Vancouver, Canada

Claire Sergent, PhD
Assistant Professor
Laboratory of Psychology of Perception (UMR 8242)
CNRS / University Paris Descartes
Centre Biomédical des Saints-Pères
Paris, France

Hocine Slimani, MSc
Harl-Sanders Research Chair in Vision Sciences
School of Optometry
University of Montreal
Montreal, Canada
BRAINlab
Department of Neuroscience and Pharmacology
Panum Institute
Faculty of Health and Medical Sciences
University of Copenhagen
Copenhagen, Denmark

Carme Torras, PhD, MSc
CSIC Research Professor
Institute for Robotics and Industrial Informatics
Consejo Superior de Investigaciones Científicas (CSIC)
Polytechnic University of Catalonia(UPC)
Barcelona, Spain

Irene Tracey MA (Oxon), DPhil, FRCA, FMedSci
Nuffield Chair in Anaesthetic Science
Oxford Centre for Functional Magnetic Resonance Imaging of the Brain
Nuffield Division Anaesthetics
Nuffield Department Clinical Neurosciences
University of Oxford
Oxford, England

Sophie Vandenbroucke, PhD
Postdoctoral Researcher
Department of Experimental-Clinical and Health Psychology
Ghent University
Ghent, Belgium

Audrey Vanhaudenhuyse, PhD
Postdoctoral Researcher/Neuropsychologist
Algology-Palliative Care Department
University Hospital of Liege
University of Liege
Liege, Belgium

Katie Warnaby, MD, PhD
Researcher
Oxford Centre for Functional Magnetic Resonance Imaging of the Brain
Nuffield Division Anaesthetics
Nuffield Department Clinical Neurosciences
University of Oxford
Oxford, England

Fadel Zeidan, PhD
Assistant Professor
Department of Neurobiology and Anatomy
Wake Forest School of Medicine
Winston-Salem, North Carolina

FOREWORD

Consciousness is a unique achievement of the brain. Sensory receptors in the body convert physical stimuli into patterns of nerve impulses that are projected to specific areas of the brain. In those areas an extraordinary event occurs: The continuous flow of nerve impulses is transformed into our perception of our body and the environment we live in. We see, hear, smell, taste, and feel our body. These perceptions change from moment to moment. The transformation from nerve impulses into the visual, auditory, and other dimensions of our conscious world is an awesome challenge. One of the perceptions is pain. Some pains are generated by observable physical events that destroy body tissue. But other pains such as a phantom limb being crushed or burned are generated in the brain. Luis Garcia-Larrea and Philip L. Jackson have edited this unique book devoted to understanding the brain mechanisms that generate the conscious experience of pain.

Pain research and theories published during the 20th century have dealt primarily with acute pain that is evoked by injuries. However, the conscious brain also generates pains of far greater complexity than acute pains. These pains, such as phantom limb pain, and other chronic pains defy comprehension in terms of our current knowledge. Pick up almost any book or journal on clinical pain and you find descriptions of pain in viscera, muscles, and other body areas that have been treated with every pharmaceutical, surgical, psychological, and physical therapy yet fail to stop the pain.

This is the first book I have encountered that deals scientifically with consciousness as the salient feature of pains that persist despite all the knowledge and therapies that have accumulated for more than a century. It is devoted to understanding the brain mechanisms that generate the conscious experience of pain which often has no known physical cause. Pain research and theories published during the 20th century have dealt primarily with acute pain that has well-known stimuli and responses. However, the conscious brain also generates pains of greater complexity that defy comprehension in terms of our current theories that are based on known noxious stimuli.

Consciousness is the salient feature of pain but has often been ignored in the attempt to be "objective." However, consciousness is a scientific term, and this book is focused on the knowledge we have. Hopefully, it will stimulate research to illuminate the physiological substrates of consciousness. This book reveals a paradigm shift that has been evolving for half a century. In 1938, neurosurgeons began to question the belief that the cerebral cortex is the site that generates consciousness and shifted the location to the intralaminar thalamus. Classic experiments with cats and dogs after total cortical deafferentation revealed that the animals were conscious, but the "obvious" belief that the cortex generates consciousness persists. The chapters in this book reveal the complexity of the brain. They are a strong contrast to the theory that has dominated pain research during the past century. In 1895 von Frey discovered that sensitive “pain spots” in human skin have free nerve endings beneath them. This discovery led to a search for pathways from skin to the brain. Two spinothalamic tracts were designated as “pain pathways.” However, an ingenious experiment by Allan Basbaum revealed that sectioning the direct spinal pathways but leaving the short-fiber connections intact did not obliterate pain; the rats responded to painful stimulation. Nevertheless, the specificity theory of pain has persisted with a change in language. Pain receptors are now called “nociceptors,” and the pathways to the brain are “nociceptive pathways.” The end result is “nociception.” A recent experiment has revealed that the massive destruction of cutaneous nociceptors in mice did not abolish pain perception.

Pain is generated in the brain with or without cutaneous receptors, which makes this book particularly welcome. It adds to the accumulating evidence of the complexity of clinical chronic pain. It also adds to a gradual paradigm shift from peripheral receptors to the complexity of the brain.

Ronald Melzack
McGill University
Montreal, Canada

PREFACE

MODELING PAIN EXPERIENCES IN THE CONSCIOUS BRAIN: STILL NOT PERFECT BUT WE ARE GETTING CLOSER

Beyond what sounds like a simple title lies the project envisioned by two neuroscientists, from the neurophysiology and the neuropsychology realms, who succeeded in convincing international leaders in multiple fields to accept the challenge of tying the multifaceted concept of pain to the equally complex notion of consciousness.

As a function of the scientific (and philosophical!) background of the investigator, pain can be modeled in very different ways, from a response to excessive sensory input to a combination of sensoriality and emotion, an internal marker of alarm, the sign of some homeostatic deviance, and so forth—all of which will appear evident in the different chapters. Human pain, however, is not a sensation but a complex and multifaceted *experience*, which defies being modeled by such simple constructs. Not all excessive sensory inputs create pain; not all pains give rise to strong emotions, and contrary to homeostatic deviances (signalled by hunger, thirst, sensations from sodium or potassium excess), chronic pain, even extreme, does not kill. If modeling pain as a general capacity of living organisms is complex, trying to model *human* pain, and in particular clinical pain, becomes a gigantic task. The myriad of experiential nuances of human beings are inaccessible to other living organisms: while fear or anger may be at the reach of most mammal species, indignation and outrage, and guilt and remorse are clearly not. This singularity applies also to the pain experience, as shades of human suffering are at least as various as shades of human joy.

Bodily pain is intimately related to the experience of the physical self. Some 50 years ago, Ronald Melzack introduced the concept of the gating theory and the "neuromatrix" (a neural network extending throughout widespread areas of the brain) as a basis for the experience of self, and later explicitly stated that *"the neuromatrix for the physical self generates the neurosignature pattern for pain."*[*] This view has gained many adepts, and is supported by a bulk of data, from neuroimaging to electrophysiology to the pain clinics. Neuroscience has thus fueled the expansion of the study of consciousness, from theoretical and philosophical accounts to hypothesis-driven neuroimaging and neurostimulation experiments.

The first section of the book begins with introductions to consciousness from different domains, but always in the framework of pain experiences. The neurophysiologic substrate of consciousness, its connectivity and modulation, and its disruption in coma are

[*] Melzack R. Phantom limbs and the concept of a neuromatrix. Trends Neurosci 1990;13(3):88–92.

first detailed by Anne-Claire Lukaszewicz and Pauline Perez who also describe how understanding the imbrication of vigilance states is crucial to get the full picture and manage pain in such clinical settings. The chapter by Claire Sergent then explores the nonlinear mechanisms, giving access to consciousness, and posits that certain thresholds need to be reached for any experience to become "declarative." Drawing inspiration from pain as another subjective process, she presents the notion of connectivity between different brain areas and systems, including "long-distance" communication and synchrony in the brain. Frédérique De Vignemont follows by exposing how awareness of one's body is related to pain, and explores the boundaries of this specific aspect of self-awareness. She brings the reader to the conclusion that pain does contribute to establish the boundaries of the body and, mostly, may be necessary to attribute positive valences to it. This section ends with a presentation by Luis Garcia-Larrea, Philip L. Jackson and Roland Peyron on the different neural substrate of pain, organized in functional and interacting matrices processing nociception, attention-perceptual and affective information that yield the full experience of pain.

The second section regroups work on the many ways, natural or experimental, by which it is possible to modulate the level of consciousness of healthy individuals, and how this affects the pain experience. Hélène Bastuji and Gilles Lavigne start by showing how sleep, its distinct stages and cerebral signatures can affect pain processing, how pain disrupts sleep, and how access to consciousness and memory during sleep is superior than previously believed. Irene Tracey and Katie Warnaby then move on to discuss the recent advances of pharmacological imaging to probe the cerebral circuits involved in changes in brain states. They show that subcortical changes in brain activity during anesthesia, such as those within the thalamus, can be understood as a *consequence* of a broad reduction of cortical activity, rather than the opposite. Pharmacologically induced changes in consciousness appear, therefore, distinct from natural changes like sleep, where the thalamus is leading. Another powerful means by which to modulate consciousness and pain is hypnosis. Audrey Vanhaudenhuyse, Aline Gillet, Anne-Sophie Nyssen, and Marie-Elisabeth Faymonville discuss how hypnosis changes brain activity, how this can be related to both internal and external awareness, and how hypnosis can contribute to the clinical management of pain syndromes. Mindfulness-based meditation, which is now known to alter brain function and brain structure, is thought to act, according to Joshua A. Grant and Fadel Zeidan, not on the pain sensation per se but rather on the interpretation and affect about the pain. Mindfulness meditation could thus favor a decoupling of the different dimensions of pain, raising the intriguing question whether "a fully mindful experience of noxious stimulation still fits the definition of pain." Luana Colloca then tackles the placebo and nocebo effects—well documented in phenomenology but still elusive in terms of neurobiological mechanisms. She not only discloses some of them, but also shows evidence that placebo and nocebo are present under different states of consciousness, including those without declarative awareness.

The third section of the book addresses pain from the perspective of specific clinical populations in whom both pain and conscious awareness are systematically modified. Pain assessment in noncommunicating patients in vegetative state, "unresponsive wakefulness syndrome" (VS/UWS) or minimally conscious state (MCS), poses of number of clinical, neurobiological, and ethical challenges discussed by Camille Chatelle, Steven Laureys, and Athena Demertzi. Although nociceptive stimuli can lead to changes in somatosensory cortex activity in all these patients, brain imaging suggests that these modifications often fail to trigger changes in higher-order associative cortical regions in VS/UWS patients, while they do in MCS. It remains to be confirmed whether this activity is related to a "pain experience" in these patients.

The level at which infants, including the very premature, can experience pain compared to older children and adults is not fully understood, but accumulating data shows that unmanaged pain during some of the early stages of development can have detrimental and far-reaching consequences. Ruth E. Grunau, Manon Ranger, and Hugo Lagercrantz discuss infant pain and consciousness within the framework of the developing brain; they show that an aversive emotional response is tied to nociception in infants, and that premature newborns show cortical responses to nociceptive stimulations. How much of a full conscious pain experience such pattern of cortical activity reflects needs further testing, but raises alertness about the emergence of pain perception and some primal form of consciousness from the earliest stages of human viability, at 24–25 weeks' gestational age. Rather than an "all-or-non" phenomenon, consciousness likely emerges gradually in the human neonate outside the protective intrauterine environment.

At the other end of the age continuum, patients suffering from dementia constitute another population historically "neglected" with regard to questioning their level of pain or consciousness. As dementia impairs communication, the need to develop means to assess pain other than the clinical gold standard of the verbal report has become urgent, and is summarised comprehensively by Thomas Hadjistavropoulos. He describes how cumulative reports on pain processing in dementia yield somewhat contrasting results: although clinically suffering does not appear to diminish in dementing illness, changes in threshold and autonomic responses indicate that the neurobiological changes that accompany dementia *do* affect some aspects of pain perception. Increased training of health care professionals and adoption of a person-centered patient care framework are essential to improve the detection of pain in such vulnerable population.

Taking as standpoint that our perception of the world is multisensory, and that information from individual senses is most often combined before reaching awareness, the chapter by Vanessa Harrar, Sophie Vandenbroucke, Hocine Slimani, Maurice Ptito, and Ron Kupers first explores the interactions of vision and somatoperception in sighted individuals, then introduces the emerging field of pain perception is the absence of vision. They also explore the complex and intriguing world of the vision-based treatment of chronic pain conditions, including neuropathic pain.

The fourth section of the book starts by addressing the complexity of human pain arising from the continuous interplay between low-level sensory and high-level cognitive and emotional systems: attention, memory, beliefs, and values. Beyond the interaction between cognition, emotion, and pain, the chapter by Luis Garcia-Larrea and Philip L. Jackson discusses how contextual and social factors can influence the pain experience and how such complexity offers additional clinical challenges. This is followed by the neuroevolutionary perspective of Jaak Panksepp who presents data from brain function and chemistry in animals, supporting the notion that feeling physical pain and feeling emotional/psychological pain stem from common evolutionary origins. This chapter offers corollary evidence that animals experience states very much alike the physiological core pain, and discusses the much debated possibility of their access to some forms of psychological pains too. To finish this book on a futuristic note, the systematic and provocative inquiry proposed by Carme Torras about what it would take for a robot to experience acute pain provides an insightful framework to study consciousness. By using concepts like occurrent pain as reinforcement in learning routines, pain expertise as a form of memory that can influence decision-making in the face of threat, and body schema in robots (resonating with De Vignemont's introduction), Torras brings the reader to the conclusion that robot pain is to some extent possible. However, to be analogous to human pain robots would have to develop some form of self-knowledge, through which consciousness might arise—a very hot and much-debated topic at this very moment.

Thanks to the quality of these contributions from our colleagues, we believe this book succeeds in gathering compelling evidence that pain (and pain-related suffering) cannot be adequately understood without considering simultaneously (a) the neural substrates of nociception, which imply a diversity of cortical and subcortical targets activated in parallel; (b) the neural substrates of consciousness and self-consciousness, whose development was intimately related to the aversion–attraction axis; (c) the interactions between these systems and those supporting emotional drives; and (d) the continuing action of higher cognition systems, which render sensory inputs and basic emotions meaningful, context-dependent, and modulated by past experience. We hope that the readers of this book will acknowledge the complexity of the pain experience, while appreciating how the last 50 years have produced lines of research bringing us closer to the understanding of its underlying processes, and to multimodal means of managing and alleviating this "aversive experience of the self."

Luis Garcia-Larrea
Philip L. Jackson

CONTENTS

SECTION 1

An Introduction to Consciousness and Pain

From Being Awake to Being Aware

CHAPTER 1

Neurobiological Bases of Coma, Vegetative, and Minimal Conscious States

Anne-Claire Lukaszewicz and Pauline Perez

Brain injuries result in variable clinical presentations, including disorders of consciousness, that are related to the location and characteristics of the brain lesions (e.g., localized or diffuse). Consciousness is altered when lesions either interfere with arousal mechanisms in the brain stem and diencephalon or disrupt broad regions in bilateral hemispheres. Arousal occurs when pathways originating in the brain stem activate the cerebral cortex through the thalamus and basal forebrain or through direct innervation of the cortex. Awareness and the neural processes underlying consciousness do not occur in a specific pathway or cerebral area; they result from complex neuronal architecture and connections.

Beginning in the 20th century with Bremer [11] and Moruzzi and Magoun [36], neurophysiological and anatomical studies have established a link between the necessary integrity of certain brainstem structures and the level of arousal or consciousness. The integrity of the ascending reticular activating system (ARAS) activation in particular is necessary for conscious perception of external sensory stimuli. However, different hemispheric lesions, such as diffuse axonal injury (DAI), a brain injury involving extensive white matter damage, may also result in severe consciousness disorders [1, 50]. Some recent studies of reversible unconsciousness, such as anesthesia or seizures, have brought new insight into the mechanisms underlying consciousness [10].

Patients with alterations of consciousness are classically categorized according to deficits of arousal (e.g., coma) or deficits of awareness (e.g., vegetative state [VS] and minimal conscious state [MCS]), which are primarily clinically distinguished by a patient's response to the environment and to different intensities of stimulation or nociception. Noxious stimulation is a routine clinical procedure for bedside assessment of consciousness because acute pain travels via spinothalamic tract and terminates on several thalamic nuclei, including the ventrobasal complex, from where the information is transmitted to various cortical areas. This clinical classification reflects the impact of lesions on information and task processing. Coma is defined by a complete failure of the arousal system, with no spontaneous eye opening and the inability to be awakened with vigorous sensory stimulation. VS is characterized by a complete absence of behavioral evidence for self- or environmental awareness but with a preserved capacity for spontaneous or stimulus-induced arousal (eye opening), movements, and evidence of sleep–wake cycles [46]. MCS is characterized by a partial preservation of conscious awareness and behavioral evidence of adaptation to the environment but the inability to consistently reproduce this behavior [25]. Note that these different statuses result from varying levels of brain lesion severity and are also associated with patient outcomes.

Not all coma patients experience all these clinical steps, and some will unpredictably demonstrate good recovery. Notably, patients who remain unresponsive for more than 12 months following a traumatic brain injury would be considered to have a poor outcome, with a small chance of recovery (if any), but some patients demonstrate late recovery after 1 year, particularly the youngest patients. In some studies, MCS patients have demonstrated better outcomes than persistent VS patients, maintaining improvement more than 1 year after the injury onset [31]. Such different outcomes indicate the need for a clearer distinction between the two types of patients. Of notice, the clinical presentation of some MCS patients is very similar to that of VS patients in terms of the absence of communication, including speech, notably due to the lack of motor function. In this context, the differences between the clinical presentations of VS versus MCS were debatable until recent advanced brain-imaging studies suggested the presence of consciousness in patients who clinically appear unconscious [12]. Functional imaging is a promising complement to clinical bedside assessment for distinction among states of VS versus MCS. However, such exploration of unconscious patients in clinical practice remains challenging and is limited by the difficulty of performing behavioral tests.

DISORDERS OF CONSCIOUSNESS RELATED TO ALTERATIONS OF SUBCORTICAL STRUCTURES

Lesion studies have revealed key mechanisms of arousal, which implicate brain stem, thalami, and subcortical networks. Basilar territory infarction or cerebral posterior vascular deficiency provoke a sudden loss of consciousness related to focal lesions in the upper brain stem including the ARAS, although arousal and consciousness remain present when the ARAS is preserved, as is the case of the locked-in syndrome due to infarcts of the ventral pons. In patients with multiple sclerosis, attentional deficits and impairment of consciousness have also been associated with ARAS impairment. The brainstem reticular formation consists of many different nuclei and fiber bundles. Complex anatomical connections with diencephalic and cortical structures in humans have been recently unveiled by neuroimaging studies [21]. These nuclei are located in the core of the brainstem and distinguished according to their histochemical features, functions, and anatomical connections. The extensive connectivity between brainstem monoaminergic-, cholinergic-, and glutamatergic-related nuclei and the hypothalamus, thalamic nuclei, or basal forebrain supports different aspects of the human arousal system and circadian sleep–wake cycles.

Severe alterations of consciousness have also been related to focal thalamic lesions; usually both thalami must be injured. One of the main thalamic functions is to integrate and modulate interactions between the brainstem arousal network and cortical awareness network as a critical juncture in the inflow of sensory information. Isolated thalamic lesions leading to alteration of consciousness are mainly related to stroke affecting vessels supplying the midline nuclei. This may obey to uncommon vascular variations (i.e., the artery of Percheron, a solitary arterial trunk branching from the posterior cerebral artery and supplying blood to both paramedian thalami) or deep venous thrombosis. The clinical presentation is dominated by somnolence and disorientation of time and place, which demonstrate the cardinal implications of these subcortical structures in information processing. Delayed deficits related to bithalamic insufficiency has also been observed in patients with persistent hypokinesia and loss of psychic self-activation. The different clinical manifestations of bithalamic lesions may result from slight variations in the anatomy of thalamic nuclei and their vascular supply and may be related to disruptions of the connections with striatal and cortical structures. Midline and internuclear nuclei are classically involved in this type of lesion; they are a critical relay for cortical arousal because of their extensive input from the nuclei of brainstem reticular formation and their prominent output to the striatum and cortical areas [4, 52]. The midline thalamic nuclei can be predominantly affected after a brain injury, and the degree of postlesional neuronal loss relates to patient outcomes [33]. The paraventricular nucleus of the thalamus has strong reciprocal connections with the prefrontal cortex, nucleus accumbens, and amygdala, and it is involved in the awareness of viscerosensory stimuli and stress responses. Intralaminar nuclei, including the central lateral nucleus, are the principal target of the midbrain reticular formation and receive projections from the spinothalamic and cerebellar tracts and are strongly connected to the medial prefrontal and anterior cingulate cortical areas. Via reciprocal connections, the thalamo–cortico–thalamic network constitutes an integrated functional unit, and synchronization between these structures determines the state of arousal, allowing perceptual awareness and cognition. A recent study or functional magnetic resonance imaging (fMRI) in VS and MCS patients demonstrated a correlation between the responsiveness to a word-detection task and the intensity of thalamofrontal functional connectivity as a marker of willful behavior [34]. The central thalamus is closely linked to the frontal lobe area, including the supplementary motor, anterior cingulate, premotor, and prefrontal cortices; it is also indirectly linked to cortical areas through the cortical–striatopallidal–thalamocortical loop systems [52]. After experiencing a brain injury, the more severely disabled patients presented midthalamic lesions including the parafascicular and central medial nucleus [33], both sustaining prominent connections to the basal ganglia. These thalamostriatal projections are associated with excitatory corticostriatal inputs and seem to play a key role in maintaining activity in the anterior forebrain, particularly through the inhibitory projections from medium spiny neurons in the striatum to the internal globus pallidus, a structure that can inhibit the central thalamus. Diffuse disturbance of this network, such as that which occurs from diffuse axonal injury, vasospasm, or hypoxia–ischemia, can sharply reduce the medium spiny neuron output controlling globus pallidus inhibitory activity in the thalamus [23], thus lending support to the "mesocircuit" hypothesis of disorders of consciousness (Fig. 1-1). This hypothesis, which has received increasing attention for innovative therapy for recovery of awareness after severe brain injury, states that (i) disorders of consciousness after diffuse brain injury may stem from functional release of globus pallidus, entailing reduced central thalamus activity, and (ii) selective metabolic depression of the anterior forebrain could provide a target for treatment. For example, the behavioral results of severely disabled patients administered dopaminergic agents suggest the facilitation of striatal and frontal functions or the paradoxical effect of zolpidem on the inhibitory output of the internal globus pallidus to the thalamus. The improved behavioral responsiveness of MCS patients undergoing deep brain stimulation of the anterior intralaminar nuclei is another example that supports this hypothesis.

The effect of subcortical structures on arousal and awareness is also illustrated by the evolution of complex partial seizures. Because sudden alteration of consciousness is dangerous for patients with seizures, the mechanism underlying its occurrence has attracted much attention, and one prevalent hypothesis is that the development of seizures involves subcortical structures. Complex partial seizures are defined as a partial seizure with alteration of consciousness, during which simple response can be preserved although tasks requiring higher-order processing or decision making are profoundly impaired [5]. A recent study revealed slow-wave electroencephalographic (EEG) activity in the bilateral frontal and parietal neocortices during complex partial seizures, compared with simple partial seizures, and this extended depression of activity was inversely correlated with fast seizure activity in the temporal lobe. The

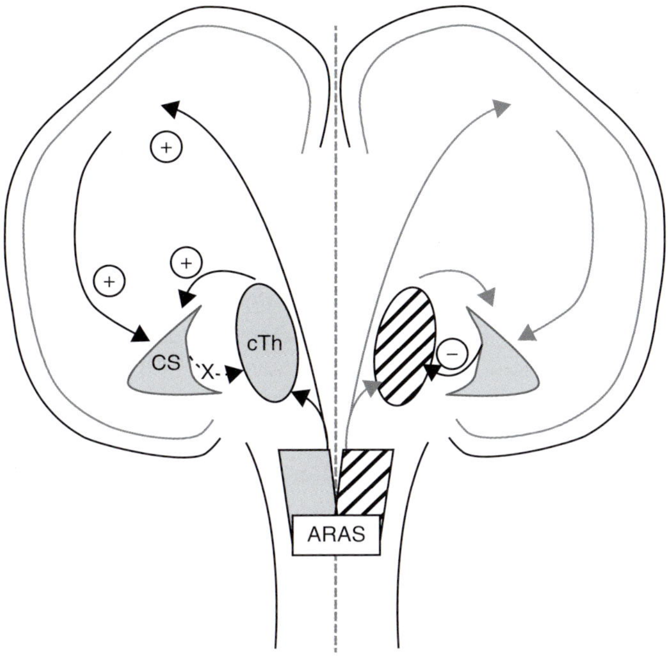

FIGURE 1-1 Subcortical and cortical connections implicated in arousal **(left)**. These mechanisms are impaired in unconscious patients **(right)** in relation to ascending reticular activating system (ARAS) or thalamic lesions or deafferentation of these structures and inhibition by globus pallidus interna.

reversibility of these results provided the opportunity to investigate the neural correlates of awareness. A "network inhibition hypothesis" suggests that temporal lobe complex partial seizures disrupt brainstem and diencephalic arousal systems, indirectly leading to depressed cortical function and impaired consciousness. Slow-wave EEG activity was accompanied by decreased cerebral blood flow in the same frontoparietal neocortical regions, which contrasted with increased regional blood flow in the midline subcortical structures. Frontoparietal and subcortical blood flow were inversely correlated, and the authors suggested that seizures arising in the temporal lobe propagate to the medial thalamus, disrupting their normal activating functions and leading secondarily to functional inactivation of widespread regions of frontal and parietal association cortex. These investigations have been reinforced by intracranial EEG studies demonstrating slow activity in the medial and lateral frontoparietal regions instead of the fast activity typically seen in seizures. Another approach suggests that thalamocortical over synchrony may contribute to impaired consciousness in patients with partial seizures (for review, see reference [2]).

ALTERATIONS OF CONSCIOUSNESS RELATED TO ALTERED CONNECTIVITY BETWEEN CORTICAL AREAS

The impairment of consciousness most often alters tasks requiring complex information processing for high-order cognitive functions, such as writing logic, working memory, and judgment, relative to simple sensory tasks. Conscious effortful tasks and responses to complex stimuli require more cortical processing than do elementary sensory-motor tasks, suggesting the importance of connectivity between areas through the thalamus (via the medial pulvinar essentially) [13]. Over the last few decades, the concept of "global neuronal workspace" has been progressively developed: this concept is based on complex architecture of distributed neurons with long-distance corticocortical connectivity [18]. This model implies that workspace neurons are in dense cortical layers 2 and 3 but are also differentially distributed across the cortical areas, ensuring interconnections and coordination between specialized brain areas. Unconscious processing by these "workspace neurons" distributed throughout the brain and their long-distance connectivity make the incoming information available to a variety of brain processes and would be necessary to access consciousness (see Chapter 2). Neurophysiological, anatomical, and brain-imaging data strongly support a major contribution of the prefrontal cortex (especially anterior cingulate regions) and the parietal cortex to the workspace [18]. Accordingly, the effort engaged in a complex task (as compared with an automatized task) is associated with specific brain activation, as in the dorsolateral prefrontal cortex and anterior cingulate, but declines with routinization of the process [18]. Lesion studies have reinforced this concept and, as an example, linked the prefrontal cortex with decision making and reward-based learning in dynamic environment. Recently, a variation on the "global work space" hypothesis was applied to seizures in terms of alteration of consciousness [2], and it stresses the importance of long-distance corticocortical synchronization between distant brain areas in a perioperative context. Intracerebral EEG patient data provided important information suggesting an excess of synchronization ("oversynchronization") within corticothalamic networks associated with conscious impairment after temporal and parietal seizures.

Another example of diffuse alteration of connectivity between cortical areas would be anesthesia administration, which commonly involves functional impairment of the thalamus and frontoparietal areas. Most general anesthetics are GABAergic agents that decrease spontaneous neuronal firing in the cerebral cortex and slow cortical activity independently of subcortical structures. Conversely, ketamine induces unconsciousness in concomitance with active enhancement of EEG activity. These differences in the process of reaching unconsciousness suggest that different anesthetics interfere with, rather than inhibit, cortical activity. Moreover, depending on the dose, the sedative–hypnotic effects of different anesthetics may not affect the connections between the thalamus and primary sensory areas but may alter the functional connections between higher-level cortical areas. Positron emission tomography revealed that anesthesia-induced unconsciousness was associated with global reduction of regional cerebral blood flow, particularly with deactivation of the mesial parietal cortex, posterior cingulate cortex, and precuneus (PCC/C). The exploration of emergence from deep anesthesia to recovery of consciousness showed the temporal activation sequence in the subcortical and limbic structures before the frontal area and then the parietal area [28]. On the basis of such data, some authors have proposed the disruption of "top–down" functional connectivity from the frontal area to more posterior sensory areas as a mechanistic approach for the effects of general anesthetics [10]. It might be worth to note that, contrary to anesthesia, natural sleep induces first a thalamic deactivation, followed by cortical deactivation only minutes later [32].

Posterior parietal areas were also deactivated in VS and were the first areas to reactivate with recovery [29]. As a central hub of human brain anatomical connectivity, the integrity of the frontoparietal network may be necessary for consciousness to occur [19]. Interestingly, theses cortical areas are part of the "default mode network" (DMN) of brain function, which encompasses areas that were shown to be more active at rest compared with when the subjects were involved in cognitive tasks demanding attention. The potential major result of using this approach to study the default network in patients is that patient collaboration is not required. Functional magnetic resonance imaging (fMRI) resting state investigations have demonstrated that decreases in functional connectivity in patients, particularly in the posterior cingulate cortex and precuneus (PCC/C), are a function of the level of consciousness [53], which may differentiate MCS from unconscious patients. From a functional viewpoint, most recent investigations have suggested that alterations to the effective connectivity between DMN nodes, particularly precuneus and its inhibitory or excitatory influences, control the process of attention and efficient information integration [14, 30]. The functionality of DMN in MCS suggests the preservation of self-related processes and, among them, perception of pain (Chapter 10). Conversely, in unresponsive/VS patients the internal self-related mentation is disrupted. However, the anticorrelated pattern or switch between external awareness system (related to "global workspace") and internal awareness system (DMN) seems to be of critical importance for conscious cognition [19].

Among the EEG signals, event-related potentials (ERPs) have been extensively applied to assess information-processing ability, with the interest to be interpretable in absence of explicit behavior from patient [22]. In particular, long-latency components of ERPs (recorded while healthy subjects perform cognitive tasks) have been described as a reliable marker of neuronal conscious perception involving fronto–temporo–parietal cortices and backward connection between these areas. The top–down process or late cortical interconnections might be reflected by the occurrence of a long-latency period as a reliable marker of conscious perception. Disruption of these task-related electrophysiological elements was observed in VS patient in comparison with MCS patients and healthy controls [9]. Some of these components may demonstrate a long-term prognostic value [49]. Those long-latency ERPs result from the synchronized activity of multiple brain regions and reflect the integrity of multiple brain connections. In patients, the persistence of these signals may indicate that these regions and connections are not too badly injured or that there may be a chance of recovery.

The anatomical correlates of impairment in functional connection between high-level associative structures have been documented recently. Historically, examinations of the brains of patients who died after prolonged coma secondary to closed head injury have reported diffuse degeneration of white matter and marked loss of nerve fibers unrelated to cortical cell loss [50]. Axonal injury is the most common consequence of diffuse traumatic brain injury, secondary to axonal disconnection and degradation, particularly for more vulnerable fine-caliber fibers [1]. The determinants of recovery for cell-soma and terminals are unclear, but the mechanism of the disease (i.e., traumatic or nontraumatic) appears to be important [16]. Clinical practice requires that unresponsive patients be evaluated using simple noninvasive techniques. "Conventional" computed tomography (CT) and magnetic resonance imaging (MRI) failed to accurately detect white matter alterations [37]. However, fiber-tracking techniques, noninvasive techniques implemented in MRI, may help to detect microstructural brain damage. Several studies have investigated the altered diffusion parameters with many regions of interest of bundles and tracts in association with cognitive status and outcomes. Such DTI was performed over a period of months in an unresponsive patient after cardiac arrest, and it was compared with classical T2-weighted FLAIR imaging and postmortem neuropathological findings [24]. This example suggests that DTI can be used to predict patient outcomes after cardiac arrest, and the approach was applied to test the hypothesis of alteration in the DMN and if the functional disconnections were predominantly between the main DMN nodes. Impairments in network and corticocortical pathways were clearly demonstrated, including pathways connecting the posterior cingulate cortex and precuneus, in patients compared with healthy controls. This structural connectivity deficit correlated to the clinical severity and could be an indicator of nonrecovery. Furthermore, an early DTI-based fractional anisotropy map demonstrated diffuse alterations before evidence from conventional MRI and late microscopic findings [24]. A recent study has suggested that there are differences in the localizations of abnormalities on DTI, depending on the mechanism of axonal injury (e.g., after cardiac arrest or traumatic brain injury and axonal or myelin damage) [37, 51]. In particular, this study observed brainstem lesions after a traumatic brain injury, and the lesions were essentially hemispheric ischemia/anoxia, indicating significant heterogeneity of neuroanatomical substrates. In addition to clinical and functional studies, this approach could be a promising tool to better characterize patients, particularly in terms of their brainstem lesions and prognoses, according to the etiology of disorders of consciousness.

ADVANCES IN THE DIFFERENTIAL DIAGNOSIS OF VS VERSUS MCS

Clinically, patients in VS or with unresponsive wakefulness syndrome are characterized by the absence of response to commands in the presence of wakefulness (showing eye opening). MCS patients differ from VS patients by their ability to integrate external stimuli with an adapted response. Recent progress in neuroimaging has permitted the visual depiction of brain activity in terms of the severity of consciousness disorders (Table 1-1). Better characterization of the level of consciousness has resulted in the risk of misclassification and inappropriate management of these patients.

Functional imaging by PET confirmed that alteration of consciousness in VS might not be related to ARAS inactivation because the regional blood flow was increased in the midbrain tegmentum and, under stimulated conditions, in sensorimotor cortex [45]. Conversely, posterior medial associative cortices (precuneus) demonstrated reduced regional cerebral blood flow, which was not correlated to ARAS metabolism as it was in healthy subjects [45]. The recovery of the activity in this area was linked with functional recovery [29]. These results align with other functional impairments of precuneus that have been described in reversible unconscious states, such as general anesthesia.

Unlike VS, MCS patients are capable of much more complicated and sustained responses defined by functional communication or functional use of objects [25]. Recently it was proposed to categorize MCS patients as minimally conscious PLUS (+) or MINUS (−), on the basis of the complexity level of behavioral responses observed in MCS+ [12], such as being able to follow commands with gestual or minimal verbal responses, as against minimal interaction, some nonreflex movements, and limited cognitive capacities observed in MSC−.

The limitation of such clinical evaluation has been highlighted by recent advances in neuroimaging. Neuroimaging studies using external stimulation or active cognitive paradigm [39] followed by EEG equivalent studies [15, 35] have revealed the ability of such disabled patients to respond to command in an intentional manner in the absence of explicit behavior. The impact of the accurate diagnosis of patient disorder is also related to better outcome of MCS in comparison with VS patients and the follow-up of patient recovery.

MCS tend to show preserved functional temporal correlations (spectral coherence) between cortical areas compared with VS, as illustrated in EEG studies [9, 26], with much more complicated and sustained responses in MCS patients than in VS patients. Metabolic studies revealed a significant correlation between whole-brain energy metabolism and level of consciousness [48], with a lower cerebral metabolic rate of glucose in patients with disorders of consciousness compared with healthy individuals, even lower in VS compared with MCS. The difference of metabolic rate was more pronounced in the frontoparietal cortex.

TABLE 1-1 **Different Techniques for Multimodal Approach on Neural Correlates in VS and MCS**

Technique	Findings	Passive/Active Paradigm	References
DTI	Structural white matter damage Differences related to etiology of injury Correlated to 1-y functional outcome	Passive	[37, 51]
PET FDG	Correlated to CRS-R, level of consciousness Decrease in brain metabolic activity in lateral and medial frontoparietal associative cortices in VS Predominant dysfunction in the dominant left-hemispheric language network in MCS–	Passive or active	[12, 23, 47, 48]
H_2O PET	Cerebral blood flow Awareness network functionally disconnected from primary cortical area in VS	Passive	[7, 8, 45]
fMRI	Cerebral blood flow. Low level of cortical activation in VS	Passive using auditory, tactile, or visual stimuli, or active paradigms	[3, 6, 20, 39, 53]
BOLD fMRI	Spontaneous fluctuation related to DMN? Reduced interhemispheric connectivity	Passive	[38]
EEG	Periodic activity	Passive	[15, 16, 46]
ERP	Long-latency electrophysiological response related to top–down process involved in conscious perception	Passive or active auditory oddball paradigm, response to patient's own name, motor imagery	[9, 17, 27, 40, 41, 44, 49]
TMS	Local EEG response in VS Complex activation in MCS	Passive	[42, 43]

Abbreviations: DTI, quantitative diffusion tensor imaging; PET, positron emission tomography; FDG, fluorodeoxyglucose; CRS-R, coma recovery scale–revised; fMRI, functional magnetic resonance imaging; BOLD, blood oxygen level-dependent; DMN, default mode network; EEG, electroencephalography; ERP, event-related potentials; TMS, transcranial magnetic stimulation; VS, vegetative state; MCS, minimal conscious state.

The EEG has been used to detect awareness in terms of responses to commands in clinically unresponsive patients who showed appropriate EEG signals over the same region of the head where this activity is known to occur in healthy individuals [15, 16]. Event-related potential or electromyography active paradigms have been developed to detect possible motor-independent signs of command-following with markers such as the amplitude of the P3 potential to oddball stimuli [9, 26]. Even clinically unresponsive patients could react to hearing their own name spoken, especially by a familiar voice, or repeatedly perform mental imagery tasks as shown by fMRI [20]. In one study, when patients were asked to imagine playing tennis, robust activation was observed in the supplementary motor area [39] similarly to that observed in healthy volunteers [6]. It should be stressed, however, that some MCS+ patients failed to show a response to active fMRI tests. This approach depends probably on the adequate processing and performance of cognitive task, and we cannot ignore the limitation of such functional evaluation that results from the fluctuation of arousal, perceptual sensory and cognitive insufficiencies.

CONCLUSION

The clinical characterization of brain-injured patients with disorders of consciousness remains limited compared with the diversity of related brain lesions and etiologies. Alteration of consciousness may result from lesions focused in cerebral core arousal (i.e., subcortical structures) or awareness areas (i.e., frontoparietal cortex), and other diffuse lesions may produce neurological impairment by disconnecting large brain networks (i.e., global space and DMNs). Clinically, patients with disorders of consciousness show restricted self- and environmental awareness but such statement is limited by undetected fluctuations of arousal, and/or perceptual sensory and cognitive insufficiencies. A multimodal approach with electrophysiological, metabolic, and structural investigations of the patients' brains should better characterize their consciousness status and improve clinical management. A significant risk of misdiagnosis remains for conscious patients who are unable to communicate. Advances of knowledge in the underlying mechanisms of disorders of consciousness may result in new therapeutic options for improving outcomes.

REFERENCES

1. Andriessen TM, Jacobs B, Vos PE. Clinical characteristics and pathophysiological mechanisms of focal and diffuse traumatic brain injury. J Cell Mol Med 2010; 14:2381–2392.
2. Bartolomei F, McGonigal A, Naccache L. Alteration of consciousness in focal epilepsy: the global workspace alteration theory. Epilepsy Behav 2014;30:17–23.

3. Bekinschtein TA, Manes FF, Villarreal M, Owen AM, Della-Maggiore V. Functional imaging reveals movement preparatory activity in the vegetative state. Front Hum Neurosci 2011;5:5.
4. Benarroch EE. The midline and intralaminar thalamic nuclei: anatomic and functional specificity and implications in neurologic disease. Neurology 2008;71:944–9.
5. Blumenfeld H. Impaired consciousness in epilepsy. Lancet Neurol 2012;11:814–26.
6. Boly M, Coleman MR, Davis MH, Hampshire A, Bor D, Moonen G, Maquet PA, Pickard JD, Laureys S, Owen AM. When thoughts become action: an fMRI paradigm to study volitional brain activity in non-communicative brain injured patients. Neuroimage 2007;36:979–92.
7. Boly M, Faymonville ME, Peigneux P, Lambermont B, Damas P, Del Fiore G, Degueldre C, Franck G, Luxen A, Lamy M. Auditory processing in severely brain injured patients: differences between the minimally conscious state and the persistent vegetative state. Arch Neurol 2004;61:233–8.
8. Boly M, Faymonville ME, Schnakers C, Peigneux P, Lambermont B, Phillips C, Lancellotti P, Luxen A, Lamy M, Moonen G. Perception of pain in the minimally conscious state with PET activation: an observational study. Lancet Neurol 2008;7:1013–20.
9. Boly M, Garrido MI, Gosseries O, Bruno MA, Boveroux P, Schnakers C, Massimini M, Litvak V, Laureys S, Friston K. Preserved feedforward but impaired top–down processes in the vegetative state. Science 2011;332:858–62.
10. Boly M, Seth AK, Wilke M, Ingmundson P, Baars B, Laureys S, Edelman DB, Tsuchiya N. Consciousness in humans and non-human animals: recent advances and future directions. Front Psychol 2013;4:625.
11. Bremer F. Cerveau "isolé" et physiologie du sommeil. C R Soc Biol 1935;118:1235–41.
12. Bruno MA, Majerus S, Boly M, Vanhaudenhuyse A, Schnakers C, Gosseries O, Boveroux P, Kirsch M, Demertzi A, Bernard C. Functional neuroanatomy underlying the clinical subcategorization of minimally conscious state patients. J Neurol 2012;259:1087–98.
13. Cappe C, Morel A, Barone P, Rouiller EM. The thalamocortical projection systems in primate: an anatomical support for multisensory and sensorimotor interplay. Cereb Cortex 2009;19:2025–37.
14. Crone JS, Schurz M, Holler Y, Bergmann J, Monti M, Schmid E, Trinka E, Kronbichler M. Impaired consciousness is linked to changes in effective connectivity of the posterior cingulate cortex within the default mode network. Neuroimage 2015;110:101–9.
15. Cruse D, Chennu S, Chatelle C, Bekinschtein TA, Fernández-Espejo D, Pickard JD, Laureys S, Owen AM. Bedside detection of awareness in the vegetative state: a cohort study. Lancet 2011;378:2088–94.

16. Cruse D, Chennu S, Chatelle C, Fernández-Espejo D, Bekinschtein TA, Pickard JD, Laureys S, Owen AM. Relationship between etiology and covert cognition in the minimally conscious state. Neurology 2012;78:816–22.

17. Cruse D, Wilding EL. Temporally and functionally dissociable retrieval processing operations revealed by event-related potentials. Neuropsychologia 2011;49:1751–60.

18. Dehaene S, Kerszberg M, Changeux JP. A neuronal model of a global workspace in effortful cognitive tasks. Proc Natl Acad Sci U S A 1998;95:14529–34.

19. Demertzi A, Soddu A, Laureys S. Consciousness supporting networks. Curr Opin Neurobiol 2013;23:239–44.

20. Di HB, Yu SM, Weng XC, Laureys S, Yu D, Li JQ, Qin PM, Zhu YH, Zhang SZ, Chen YZ. Cerebral response to patient's own name in the vegetative and minimally conscious states. Neurology 2007;68:895–9.

21. Edlow BL, Takahashi E, Wu O, Benner T, Dai G, Bu L, Grant PE, Greer DM, Greenberg SM, Kinney HC, et al. Neuroanatomic connectivity of the human ascending arousal system critical to consciousness and its disorders. J Neuropathol Exp Neurol 2012;71:531–46.

22. Fischer C, Luaute J, Nemoz C, Morlet D, Kirkorian G, Mauguière F. Improved prediction of awakening or nonawakening from severe anoxic coma using tree-based classification analysis. Crit Care Med 2006;34:1520–4.

23. Fridman EA, Beattie BJ, Broft A, Laureys S, Schiff ND. Regional cerebral metabolic patterns demonstrate the role of anterior forebrain mesocircuit dysfunction in the severely injured brain. Proc Natl Acad Sci U S A 2014;111:6473–8.

24. Gerdes JS, Walther EU, Jaganjac S, Makrigeorgi-Butera M, Meuth SG, Deppe M. Early detection of widespread progressive brain injury after cardiac arrest: a single case DTI and post-mortem histology study. PLoS One 2014;9:e92103.

25. Giacino JT, Ashwal S, Childs N, Cranford R, Jennett B, Katz DI, Kelly JP, Rosenberg JH, Whyte J, Zafonte RD, et al. The minimally conscious state: definition and diagnostic criteria. Neurology 2002;58:349–53.

26. King JR, Bekinschtein T, Dehaene S. Comment on "preserved feedforward but impaired top–down processes in the vegetative state." Science 2011;334:1203; author reply 1203.

27. King JR, Faugeras F, Gramfort A, Schurger A, El Karoui I, Sitt JD, Rohaut B, Wacongne C, Labyt E, Bekinschtein T, et al. Single-trial decoding of auditory novelty responses facilitates the detection of residual consciousness. Neuroimage 2013;83:726–38.

28. Langsjo JW, Alkire MT, Kaskinoro K, Hayama H, Maksimow A, Kaisti KK, Aalto S, Aantaa R, Jääskeläinen SK, Revonsuo A, et al. Returning from oblivion: imaging the neural core of consciousness. J Neurosci 2012;32:4935–43.

29. Laureys S, Boly M, Maquet P. Tracking the recovery of consciousness from coma. J Clin Invest 2006;116:1823–5.
30. Leech R, Sharp DJ. The role of the posterior cingulate cortex in cognition and disease. Brain 2014;137:12–32.
31. Luaute J, Maucort-Boulch D, Tell L, Quelard F, Sarraf T, Iwaz J, Boisson D, Fischer C. Long-term outcomes of chronic minimally conscious and vegetative states. Neurology 2010;75:246–52.
32. Magnin M, Rey M, Bastuji H, Guillemant P, Mauguière F, Garcia-Larrea L. Thalamic deactivation at sleep onset precedes that of the cerebral cortex in humans. Proc Natl Acad Sci U S A 2010;107:3829–33.
33. Maxwell WL, MacKinnon MA, Smith DH, McIntosh TK, Graham DI. Thalamic nuclei after human blunt head injury. J Neuropathol Exp Neurol 2006;65:478–88.
34. Monti MM, Rosenberg M, Finoia P, Kamau E, Pickard JD, Owen AM. Thalamo-frontal connectivity mediates top–down cognitive functions in disorders of consciousness. Neurology 2015;84:167–73.
35. Monti MM, Vanhaudenhuyse A, Coleman MR, Boly M, Pickard JD, Tshibanda L, Owen AM, Laureys S. Willful modulation of brain activity in disorders of consciousness. N Engl J Med 2010;362:579–89.
36. Moruzzi G, Magoun HW. Brain stem reticular formation and activation of the EEG. Electroencephalogr Clin Neurophysiol 1949;1(4):455–73.
37. Newcombe VF, Williams GB, Scoffings D, Cross J, Carpenter TA, Pickard JD, Menon DK. Aetiological differences in neuroanatomy of the vegetative state: insights from diffusion tensor imaging and functional implications. J Neurol Neurosurg Psychiatry 2010;81:552–61.
38. Ovadia-Caro S, Nir Y, Soddu A, Ramot M, Hesselmann G, Vanhaudenhuyse A, Dinstein I, Tshibanda JF, Boly M, Harel M, et al. Reduction in inter-hemispheric connectivity in disorders of consciousness. PLoS One 2012;7:e37238.
39. Owen AM, Coleman MR, Boly M, Davis MH, Laureys S, Pickard JD. Detecting awareness in the vegetative state. Science 2006;313:1402.
40. Perrin F, Schnakers C, Schabus M, Degueldre C, Goldman S, Brédart S, Faymonville ME, Lamy M, Moonen G, Luxen A, et al. Brain response to one's own name in vegetative state, minimally conscious state, and locked-in syndrome. Arch Neurol 2006;63:562–9.
41. Qin P, Di H, Yan X, Yu S, Yu D, Laureys S, Weng X. Mismatch negativity to the patient's own name in chronic disorders of consciousness. Neurosci Lett 2008;448:24–8.
42. Ragazzoni A, Pirulli C, Veniero D, Feurra M, Cincotta M, Giovannelli F, Chiaramonti R, Lino M, Rossi S, Miniussi C. Vegetative versus minimally conscious states: a study using TMS-EEG, sensory and event-related potentials. PLoS One 2013;8:e57069.

43. Rosanova M, Gosseries O, Casarotto S, Boly M, Casali AG, Bruno MA, Mariotti M, Boveroux P, Tononi G, Laureys S, et al. Recovery of cortical effective connectivity and recovery of consciousness in vegetative patients. Brain 2012;135:1308–20.

44. Schnakers C, Perrin F, Schabus M, Majerus S, Ledoux D, Damas P, Boly M, Vanhaudenhuyse A, Bruno MA, Moonen G, et al. Voluntary brain processing in disorders of consciousness. Neurology 2008;71:1614–20.

45. Silva S, Alacoque X, Fourcade O, Samii K, Marque P, Woods R, Mazziotta J, Chollet F, Loubinoux I. Wakefulness and loss of awareness: brain and brainstem interaction in the vegetative state. Neurology 2010;74:313–20.

46. Sitt JD, King JR, El Karoui I, Rohaut B, Faugeras F, Gramfort A, Cohen L, Sigman M, Dehaene S, Naccache L. Large scale screening of neural signatures of consciousness in patients in a vegetative or minimally conscious state. Brain 2014;137:2258–70.

47. Stender J, Gosseries O, Bruno MA, Charland-Verville V, Vanhaudenhuyse A, Demertzi A, Chatelle C, Thonnard M, Thibaut A, Heine L, et al. Diagnostic precision of PET imaging and functional MRI in disorders of consciousness: a clinical validation study. Lancet 2014;384:514–22.

48. Stender J, Kupers R, Rodell A, Thibaut A, Chatelle C, Bruno MA, Gejl M, Bernard C, Hustinx R, Laureys S, et al. Quantitative rates of brain glucose metabolism distinguish minimally conscious from vegetative state patients. J Cereb Blood Flow Metab 2015;35:58–65.

49. Steppacher I, Eickhoff S, Jordanov T, Kaps M, Witzke W, Kissler J. N400 predicts recovery from disorders of consciousness. Ann Neurol 2013;73:594–602.

50. Strich SJ. Diffuse degeneration of the cerebral white matter in severe dementia following head injury. J Neurol Neurosurg Psychiatry 1956;19:163–85.

51. van der Eerden AW, Khalilzadeh O, Perlbarg V, Dinkel J, Sanchez P, Vos PE, Luyt CE, Stevens RD, Menjot de Champfleur N, Delmaire C, et al. White matter changes in comatose survivors of anoxic ischemic encephalopathy and traumatic brain injury: comparative diffusion-tensor imaging study. Radiology 2014;270:506–16.

52. Van der Werf YD, Witter MP, Groenewegen HJ. The intralaminar and midline nuclei of the thalamus. Anatomical and functional evidence for participation in processes of arousal and awareness. Brain Res Brain Res Rev 2002;39:107–40.

53. Vanhaudenhuyse A, Noirhomme Q, Tshibanda LJ, Bruno MA, Boveroux P, Schnakers C, Soddu A, Perlbarg V, Ledoux D, Brichant JF, et al. Default network connectivity reflects the level of consciousness in non-communicative brain-damaged patients. Brain 2010;133:161–71.

CHAPTER 2

Neurobiological Mechanisms of Conscious Access and Implications for Pain Perception

Claire Sergent

WHAT IS "CONSCIOUS ACCESS?"

Can "consciousness" be an object of science? In the early days of experimental psychology and cognitive sciences, the general consensus was that it could not: indeed, how can you build objective knowledge about the workings of subjective experience? But, as is often the case in science, strange discoveries have compelled researchers to venture into this initially disreputable zone, with good success, as we will see in this chapter. One such major discovery relates to patients with partial or total cortical blindness following lesions to the primary visual cortex. Researchers such as Larry Weiskrantz [56] have observed that some of these patients display preserved visual abilities within their "blind" visual field [53]. For example, if you present a square or a rectangle to their blind field, they claim not to be aware of the stimulus, but if you ask them to guess anyway whether it is a square or a rectangle, they can be correct more than 80% of the time, much better than chance [53] (Fig. 2-1). Their good performance comes as a complete surprise to them. If the patient is also asked to report their subjective sensation of having seen the stimulus or not on each trial, results confirm a complete dissociation between the two measures, with excellent objective recognition performance in the absence of subjective awareness (Fig. 2-1). Such preserved objective performance despite V1 lesion can be attributed to alternative pathways between the retina and intermediate visual areas, bypassing V1 [56]. Strikingly, these alternative visual pathways seem to work efficiently with no associated conscious experience.

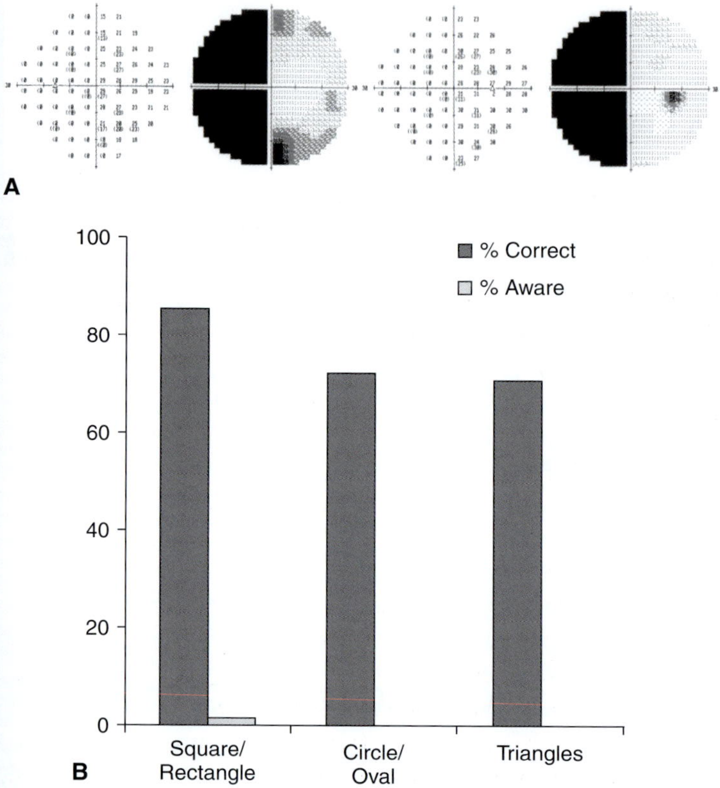

FIGURE 2-1 Blindsight. **A:** Patient DB's field defect, a left hemianopia, measured prior to testing in 2003, on Humphreys Visual Field Analyser, 30-2 Full Threshold program. Locations marked as "<0" represent locations where the brightest stimulus (10,000 cd/m^2) did not elicit a response. Areas in which the brightest stimulus failed to evoke any response are marked in black. Areas marked in gray represent amblyopic vision. **B:** Dissociation between objective performance (% correct) and subjective report (% aware) for three discrimination tasks in DB's blind field: discriminating a square from a rectangle, a circle from an oval, a straight triangle from a curved triangle. Note that objective performance for all discriminations is well above chance (50%), while the patient reported to be aware of the stimuli only on 1% of the trials. (Adapted from Trevethan et al. [53].)

The discovery that a high level of cognitive analysis can be accomplished in the absence of conscious access to the analyzed representations marks the entry into scientific investigation of consciousness. Although "consciousness" is a multiform concept of naïve psychology, this initial observation offers a well-circumscribed and empirically tractable question that seems relevant for starting to understand consciousness in general: since it appears that information processing in the brain can occur with or without subjective access to this information, what are the "added" neural mechanisms that allow this conscious access?

MEASURING CONSCIOUS ACCESS: LESSONS FROM MEASURING PAIN

This foundational case of blindsight shows that scientific investigation of conscious access inherently requires collecting subjective reports in a way that allows objective analysis [19]. Most studies probe subjective conscious access with a straightforward two-alternative forced choice: did you detect the stimulus or not? As we will see, even this very simple procedure has proved fruitful for unveiling the neural basis of conscious access.

At the beginning of my PhD thesis, I also wondered whether we could collect more than just a binary choice to further interrogate the psychological properties of conscious perception. In this search for a measure that would be richer but still easy to use, I remembered a very striking conference of clinicians in a "center for pain management." Although pain is difficult to describe, complex, and multidimensional, I had been surprised to learn that having people rate their pain on a one-dimensional scale was immensely helpful and was routinely used by clinicians to orient pain management and assess the efficiency of treatments. This was an encouragement to use a similar procedure for studying conscious perception: if pain scales produced reliable, reproducible results, we might be equally successful in using subjective visibility scales to assess consciousness of visual stimuli. And indeed, it turned out that volunteers can use such scales reliably and reproducibly [17, 18, 46, 47, 49]: visibility rating correlated finely with objective performance measures; fine increase in stimulus strength was associated with reproducible increase in visibility rating; and behavior on the scale was reproducible both within and across subjects. Beyond its validation as a reliable measure, the use of a consciousness scale proved useful in revealing dynamical properties of conscious perception that could not have been captured by binary choice, notably the existence of a nonlinear threshold for conscious access, as will be detailed later in this chapter [47]. So, as much as consciousness and pain are intricate and complex subjective phenomena, simple robust methods can still be found to collect subjective reports in an analyzable way in both domains. Since they share this particularity of dealing with subjective phenomena, there can be clear benefits in methodological cross talks between them.

NEURAL CORRELATES OF CONSCIOUS ACCESS

Starting in the 1990s, several scientists and philosophers showed the way for investigating the neurophysiology of conscious access [10, 13, 19]. This has led to extremely fruitful and diverse studies in fMRI (functional magnetic resonance imaging), EEG/MEG (electroencephalogram/magnetoencephalography), intracranial recordings, etc., all aiming at finding the neural correlates of conscious access. Although these studies use a broad range of experimental paradigms, they obey a common general principle: they contrast brain activity evoked by the same external stimulus in a situation where it is reported as "seen" (or "felt" or "heard") and in a situation where it is reported as "unseen" (or "unfelt" or "unheard") despite minimal or no change in the external stimulation.

This famous contrastive method has revealed a set of neural events that consistently correlate with conscious access (Fig. 2-2):

1. Increased activity in sensory areas that specifically process the stimulus
2. Involvement of a network of higher order areas, typically frontal and parietal areas
3. Increased long-distance connectivity within a broad network, including both frontoparietal areas and sensory areas

We will examine each of them in turn.

A nice demonstration of increased stimulus-specific activity with conscious awareness can be found in "binocular rivalry": when two very different images are shown to the two eyes (e.g., a face to the left eye and a house to the right eye), we subjectively perceive an alternation between the two images. In fMRI, this spontaneous alternation between two conscious percepts despite no change in external stimulation is reflected by changes of activity in the ventral part of the temporal cortex, which

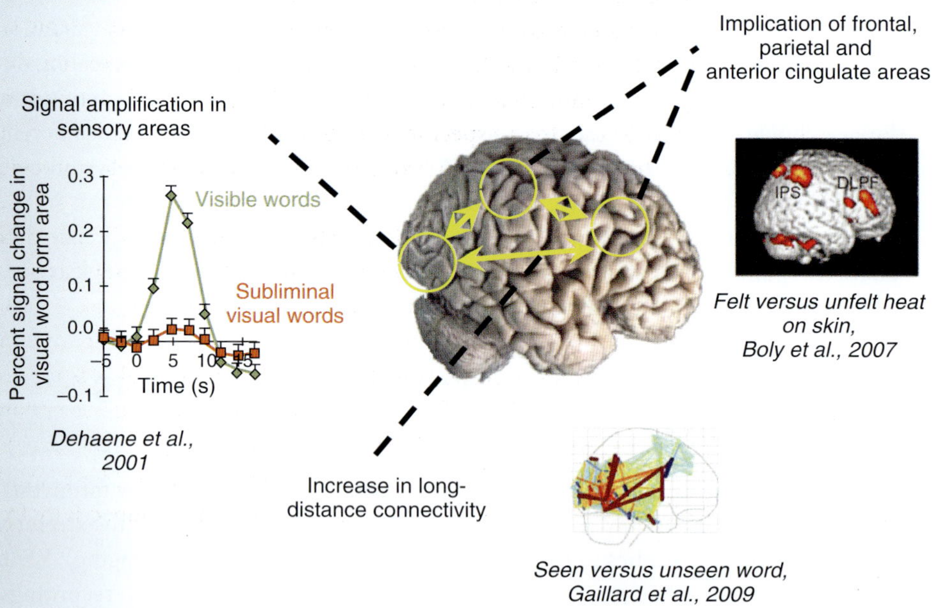

FIGURE 2-2 Summary of the neural correlates of conscious perception.

encodes different integrated aspects of vision. During the periods where subjects report seeing the face, activity rises in the fusiform face area, which typically encodes faces, and drops to almost baseline in the parahippocampal place area, which typically responds to houses, and conversely when the opposite percept is reported [52]. Such modulation of sensory activity with conscious access in the absence of physical change can be found at every level of visual analysis in the cortex, including primary visual cortex [44], and with many different types of protocols, including stimulation at threshold [44] or visual masking [14]. This observation also extends to other sensory modalities, notably audition [45] and touch [26].

Beyond this modulation of stimulus-specific activity, conscious access is also systematically accompanied by much more widespread activations than unconscious processing. While unconscious processing seems restricted to stimulus-specific sensory areas, with isolated frontal activation in some very specific cases [54, 55], conscious access consistently involves a distributed network including sensory areas and frontoparietal areas [5, 14, 21, 24, 43] (Fig. 2-3). In most studies, this frontoparietal network encompasses the "executive network": dorsolateral prefrontal cortex, anterior cingulate, and intraparietal sulcus [20]. This specific set of areas consistently increases its activity when people have to work harder on a given stimulus [20]. Conversely, this fronto-parieto-cingulate "executive network" shows a strong reduction in metabolism in different situations with loss of consciousness, such as slow-wave sleep [40] or general anesthesia in healthy individuals [27], or the vegetative state that follows coma in some patients [36]. These observations provide strong support to the idea that these areas collectively constitute an essential network for conscious access. However, it is important to emphasize that there is an important flexibility in which precise regions take part in the "conscious" network at any given time, notably depending on the type of stimuli that are employed and the type of task that is performed on these stimuli. Rather than a specific set of activations, what seems inherent to conscious access is the involvement of a broad network beyond stimulus-specific regions.

This leads us to the final essential ingredient, which is the establishment of a strong functional connectivity within this network. The importance of long-distance communication for conscious access has been demonstrated many times [4, 21, 23, 24, 28, 41]. One pioneer study used MEG and an "attentional blink" procedure, in which a visual target is sometimes seen and sometimes missed across trials despite no change in the external stimulation [23]. The study showed that conscious detection of the target was accompanied by increased long-distance synchrony, notably across frontal, parietal, and temporal sites, in the beta band (around 20 Hz). Many other studies have confirmed this pivotal role of long-distance functional connectivity for conscious access [21, 28, 41].

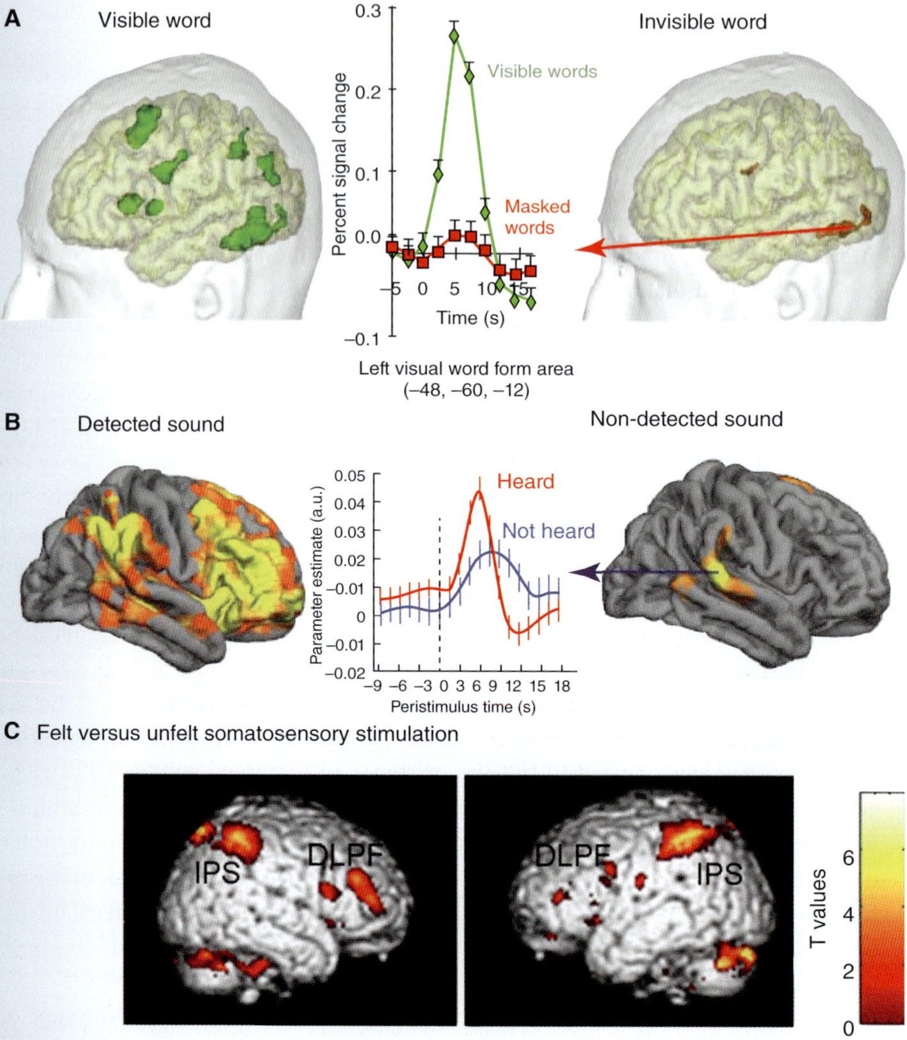

FIGURE 2-3 The neural correlates of conscious access are similar across different modalities. **A:** Brain areas activated in fMRI when a visible word is presented **(left)** and when a masked, invisible, word is presented **(right)**. Visible words activate a much wider network of areas, including parietal and prefrontal cortex. Activation in stimulus-specific areas such as the visual word form area **(middle)** increases for visible versus invisible words (Dehaene et al. [14], redrawn in Dehaene and Changeux [16]). **B:** Similarly detected sounds evoked stronger activity in the auditory cortex than nondetected sounds of the same physical amplitude. Furthermore, detected sounds also activated frontal and parietal areas (Sadaghiani et al. [45], redrawn in Dehaene and Changeux [16]). **C:** The difference map between detected and undetected somatosensory stimulation similarly reveals increased frontoparietal activations for conscious stimuli as compared to identical stimuli that went undetected (Boly et al. [7]).

GENERALIZATION TO SOMATOSENSORY AND PAINFUL STIMULATIONS

These neural correlates of conscious access have essentially been established in vision, which is currently the most studied sensory modality. However, they generalize to other types of inputs, notably auditory and tactile [7, 9, 45]. Regarding painful stimulations, two very interesting fMRI studies used laser stimulation on the back of the hand at different temperatures, going from nondetectable to painful stimulations [7, 9]. They showed that, for identical low levels of stimulation (nonpainful), conscious detection of the stimulation was associated with increased activations in bilateral, middle, and inferior frontal gyri, intraparietal sulci, posterior parietal cortices, and the anterior cingulate cortex [7] (Fig. 2-3C), in other words, a network that is very similar to the one described for conscious vision. As the stimulation became more painful, this conscious access network maintained its activity, but also extended to additional activations, typical of pain processing, in the bilateral insula and the posterior part of the anterior cingulate cortex, not overlapping with the anterior part associated with conscious access proper [7, 9]. These studies suggest that, as for other sensory modalities, conscious access to somatosensory stimulation relies on the sharing of the somatosensory representations across a network of fronto-parieto-cingulate areas. The additional painful character of the stimulation relates to the probable interaction of this conscious access network with the network encoding the different dimensions of pain, notably anterior cingulate cortex and insula. However, to further validate this last point, one would need to test the existence of increased connectivity between "pain" and "conscious access" networks, an aspect that has not yet been investigated.

MAKING SENSE OF THESE NEURAL CORRELATES: THE GLOBAL NEURONAL WORKSPACE MODEL OF CONSCIOUSNESS

The description of the neural correlates of conscious access still leaves us with a relatively static and incomplete view of the phenomenon. Can we provide a more specific model of how a stimulus becomes conscious through this pattern of brain activity? This is what we attempt to do with the "global neuronal workspace model" of conscious access [11, 12, 15], which uses the metaphor of a global workspace, borrowed from Bernard Baars [1–3], to describe the collaborative work among distant areas that seems to be typical of conscious processing. Importantly, the global neuronal workspace model (GNW) is sufficiently detailed to allow simulations in biologically realistic neural networks [15]. The three main objectives of this model are to

- account for the known psychological properties of conscious access,
- account for the known neural correlates of conscious access, and
- produce empirically testable and falsifiable predictions.

The GNW model proposes that at any given time, many modular cerebral networks are active in parallel and process information in an unconscious manner. Information becomes conscious, however, if the corresponding neural population is mobilized by top–down attentional amplification into a self-sustained brain-scale state of coherent activity that involves many neurons distributed throughout the brain. The long-distance connectivity of these "workspace neurons" can, when they are active for a minimal duration, make the information available to a variety of processes including perceptual categorization, long-term memorization, evaluation, and intentional action.

We postulate that this global availability of information through the workspace is what we subjectively experience as a conscious state. Indeed, broadcasting a selected sensory representation to high-level executive systems such as language areas or motor planning areas appears as a straightforward neurophysiological counterpart of reportability—either verbal or motor—which is a defining behavioral feature of conscious access. Through the GNW, a consciously accessed stimulus gets the chance to be integrated in current plans through its broadcast to executive systems in the frontal lobe [20, 29], probably bringing more control or "intentionality" to the actions performed toward this stimulus. Finally, through the GNW, current stimulations also get the opportunity to be compared with stored memories, allowing a more flexible and informed processing of information, which is also typical of conscious processing.

So the GNW model can provide a fair account of the behavioral, introspective properties of conscious access. It also proposes a neural mechanism that unifies the diverse neural correlates of conscious access revealed by neuroimaging studies. Within the GNW, a specific (sensory) representation gets amplified and maintained through reciprocal connections with frontal and parietal areas. Frontal and parietal areas are important nodes in the GNW because of their particularly dense long-distance connectivity that confers them an advantage in enforcing brain-wide stabilization. Finally, long-distance communication is the key feature allowing the GNW to emerge.

The structural properties of the GNW model imply very specific dynamics, as can be observed in simulations of the model [15]. In the next section, we will confront these predictions to the empirical findings on the neural dynamics of conscious access.

CONSCIOUS ACCESS AT WORK

In this section, we will focus on empirical work that has got us closer to the dynamics of conscious access, notably through the use of time-resolved techniques such as EEG, MEG, or intracranial electrophysiology in humans. These studies allow a more and more precise understanding of the scenario of neural events leading to conscious access, and several original dynamic predictions of the GNW model find a confirmation in these findings.

The most original and "surprising" dynamic prediction of the GNW model is that conscious access should be characterized by a sharp nonlinear transition in brain-scale activity [15]. Indeed, conscious access arises through synchronization and reciprocal amplification between different distant areas. In any type of dynamic system, reciprocal amplification leads to nonlinear dynamics, and simulations of the GNW model clearly confirm this aspect [15]. So, subjective conscious access itself should display a sharp threshold. This is what we set out to test by using a subjective visibility scale inspired from clinical pain scales (see section "Measuring Conscious Access: Lessons From Measuring Pain" above). We first used this scale in a paradigm called the attentional blink in which the perception of a visual target (for example a written word) is hindered when the participant is also asked to pay attention to a preceding item presented 200–500 ms before this target. Remarkably, in this paradigm, the target's duration and contrast are such that it is easily seen when there is no attentional requirement on the preceding item. On the subjective visibility scale, this "decreased perception" caused by the attentional blink was not manifested by a gradual displacement from high visibility to lower visibility ratings. Instead, it resulted in a dissociation between two groups of responses on the scale: for exactly the same external stimulation, on some trials participants reported high visibility, and on some trials they reported a visibility of zero, as if no target had been presented [46, 47]. In other words, the attentional blink does not gradually worsen target perception; it increases the number of trials in which the target is not consciously accessed. These studies offer clear evidence for the existence of nonlinear dynamics in subjective report. Importantly, this observation is not restricted to the attentional blink: similar results were obtained using this visibility scale in other paradigms such as masking [17, 18, 22] and simple stimulation at threshold contrast [49].

These nonlinear dynamics can also been observed in brain activations. We recorded EEG in an attentional blink paradigm and separated the two groups of responses obtained on the scale for the same external stimulation: "not seen at all" versus "seen." The initial neural events evoked by the visual target word were exactly the same for "seen" and "not seen," up until 250 ms; then, a sharp transition occurred only in "seen" trials leading to sustained brain events up until 800 ms poststimulus [46]. These "late" brain events were "all-or-none": they were completely absent in "not seen" trials. A similar study varying the strength of masking of target words confirmed that the sharp transition in conscious visibility observed around threshold levels of masking was not reflected in the first 200 ms of processing, but in a secondary phase of late and sustained waveforms [17]. Intracranial recordings in humans confirmed this observation and further showed that this late "all-or-none" phase typical of conscious processing was accompanied by increased communication between visual sensory areas in the occipital lobe and frontal areas [21]. Recently, Kouider et al. [30] recorded EEG in infants (12–15 months old) viewing pictures of faces presented at different levels of masking. Remarkably, although this study only involved spontaneous viewing, with no task or no report of the stimuli, Kouider et al. [30] found the previously described dichotomy between early neural events showing a gradual increase with increased stimulation strength and later neural events showing a sharp transition, presumably marking the entry into conscious perception. This sharp transition occurred later in infants than in adults, starting around 800 ms post-stimulus, suggesting that the maturation of the nervous system during development shapes the temporal dynamics of conscious processing.

In our model, only a specific set of representations can be amplified, maintained, and broadcasted through the GNW at any given time, with the exclusion of all the other representations that are active in parallel in sensory systems [15]. Many empirical studies also point to the fact that conscious access is selective and serial. This competition is ubiquitous in cognitive psychology, notably in the above-mentioned attentional blink, whereby asking participants to pay attention to a stimulus hinders detection of a following target within a time window of 200–500 ms, which seems to match with the typical time window for conscious processing. And the EEG results confirm that the attentional blink phenomenon arises precisely from the fact that while the GNW is occupied with the processing of the first target, it remains unavailable for processing the second one, which thus remains "preconscious" and can eventually be erased from sensory buffers by subsequent masks and be lost for consciousness [46].

In summary, it seems that the initial phases of sensory processing, including the feed-forward sweep of information from primary sensory areas (e.g., V1) to higher level sensory areas (e.g., V2, 3, 4, 5, IT) within 100 ms after stimulus presentation [33, 34], as well as local recurrent loops, operate preconsciously and in parallel for many representations (Fig. 2-4). Conscious access seems to occur when a specific representation reaches the threshold for triggering the "ignition" of the GNW, thus locking the activity of this broad network onto this specific representation or set of representations (Fig. 2-4). This metastable "locking" of brain-wide activity displays sharp dynamics that are characteristic of auto-amplified systems.

So finally, what triggers conscious access? In the GNW model, the attentional system plays this key role of selecting a specific sensory representation, sending top–down amplification that can spark the broadcasting of this representation through the workspace. This last point is the most disputed at the moment among different models of consciousness [6, 11, 31, 32, 48]. Recent findings provide a strong argument in favor of a causal role of attention in conscious access. In a series of behavioral experiments, we showed that visual stimuli at threshold contrast that failed to trigger conscious perception by themselves could nevertheless become conscious if spatial attention was later directed to the location where they had been presented. This retrospective effect of attention on conscious perception, which we called retroperception, could occur as late as half a second after the disappearance of the stimulus. This suggests that, as long as a sensory representation remains within sensory buffers—visual representations typically remain in iconic memory for 1 second or even more—if we manage to target top-down amplification on this specific representation, this can trigger the entry of this representation within the GNW and thus conscious access. This newly described retroperception phenomenon thus confirms that the attentional system plays a key role in conscious access. It also suggests that, contrary to the initial preconscious phases of sensory processing that are sharply time-locked to the stimulation [50, 51], the moment we become conscious of this stimulation can be extremely flexible relative to its actual timing, at least within a second—thanks to sensory buffers and the possibility to trigger top-down amplification in retrospect.

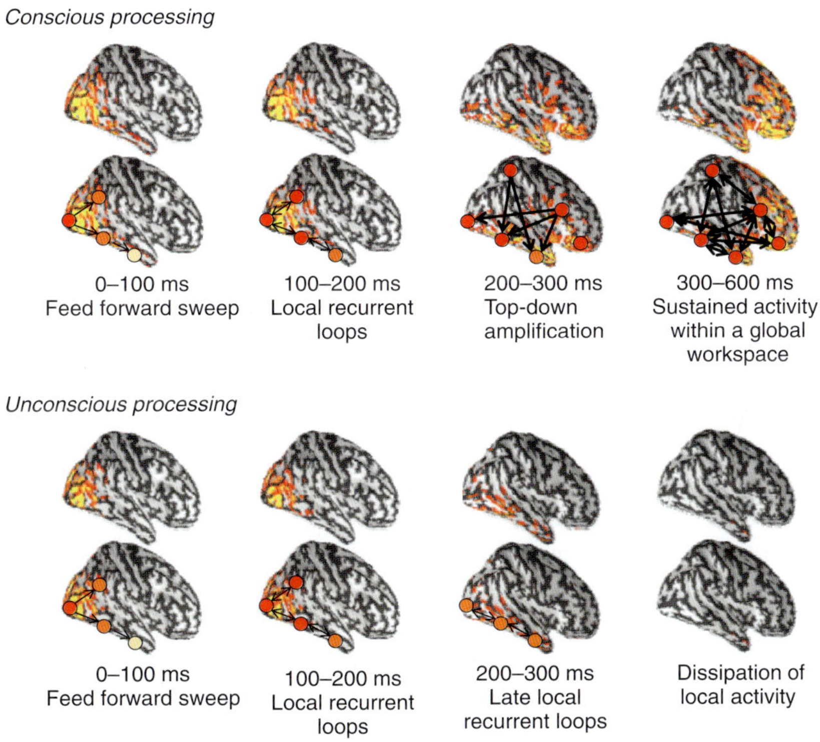

FIGURE 2-4 The neural scenario of conscious and unconscious processing. For conscious **(top)** and unconscious **(bottom)** processing, the top rows represent reconstructed brain sources of EEG activity evoked by seen words and unseen words in an attentional blink experiment (Sergent et al. [46]). Note that in both cases, external stimulation is identical and trials are just sorted based on subjects report of having seen the stimulus or not. The bottom rows represent the corresponding interpretation of the observed different stages of brain activity within the global neuronal workspace model.

IMPLICATIONS FOR PAIN PERCEPTION

So, what are the implications of the above-mentioned mechanisms of conscious access for the perception of pain in particular? And first, can there be unconscious pain? According to the mechanism described above, in principle there can be unconscious pain if the representation of pain relies on modules or circuits of modules that can function independently of typical nodes of the global workspace in frontal and parietal areas. Conscious pain is known to be a complex, multicomponent sensation that can be described as having somatosensory, affective, and cognitive dimensions [42]. Accordingly, it relies on the activation of a complex circuit involving several areas, notably somatosensory areas, insula, and anterior cingulate cortex [42]. It is clear that there can be unconscious somatosensory activations: an fMRI study has shown that threshold stimulation of the hand with a laser evoked isolated activations in the somatosensory cortex even when subjects report not feeling the stimulation [7]. In another study [35], while painful above-threshold stimulation in healthy controls produced activations in the full network of areas usually associated with pain, patients in a vegetative state only showed activations in the somatosensory subset of such areas. Finally, other studies using PET have shown insular activations in response to noxious thermal stimulation under general anesthesia [25]. So, clearly some elements of pain representation, notably in somatosensory and insular cortex, can occur in the absence of conscious access, sometimes leading to autonomic responses and motor reflex, such as withdrawal reflex, bypassing the "central executive" circuits [8]. However, as is the case for other types of representations, it is highly probable that conscious access, when it occurs, does not simply operate passive broadcasting of these various pain-related representations: in return, it shapes and transforms them. Notably, broadcasting during conscious access is expected to allow confrontation of current representations with the general context and with long-term memories. For example, similar noxious stimulations will be interpreted differently and will trigger different subsequent planning if you are being vaccinated or if a bee is stinging you. Through conscious access, pain-related activations can be integrated with other sensory entries such as the visual perception of your own body, which has been shown to modify the perception of pain, a phenomenon called "visually induced analgesia" [37, 38]. More generally, conscious access allows self-regulation of pain [57]. So the more "cognitive" aspect of pain seems to fit with the properties of conscious access as described in this chapter.

Finally, what we know about the dynamics of conscious access can help understand how pain perception in particular affects the conscious stream. We have seen that conscious access implies a competition among different representations or sets of representations that cannot be processed within the same conscious episode. It is highly probable that painful stimulations have a very special status in this competition, with a higher priority than other types of stimuli. Indeed, painful stimulations are often signs that urgent reaction is required. We could propose that the anterior cingulate activations that are often associated with pain perception reflect its privileged connection with the global neuronal workspace, potentially bypassing more standard attentional competitions through frontoparietal networks. If the proposition of a privileged access to consciousness remains to be explored empirically for pain perception, it has been quite well investigated with related stimuli, such as emotional stimuli. Indeed, it is well established that the threshold for conscious detection of emotional words or self-related words is lower than for neutral words [22]. The competition for conscious access and the relative priority of pain representations would explain the disruptive nature of medium to strong pain on any other types of conscious processing, notably reasoning. This really confirms that the central executive system is involved in conscious perception in general, and thus cannot pursue complex reasoning when busy processing pain signals. Conversely, if the pain is mild, keeping the global workspace busy with demanding computations should logically block conscious perception of pain in a similar way that a difficult task will make us miss an obvious visual stimulation [39]. And indeed that is what we observe in daily life: we will forget about a small pain if taking a difficult exam.

REFERENCES

1. Baars BJ. A cognitive theory of consciousness. Cambridge, MA: Cambridge University Press; 1989.
2. Baars BJ. The conscious access hypothesis: origins and recent evidence. Trends Cogn Sci 2002;6(1):47–52.
3. Baars BJ. In the theater of consciousness. New York, NY: Oxford University Press; 2007.
4. Barttfeld P, Uhrig L, Sitt JD, Sigman M, Jarraya B, Dehaene S. Signature of consciousness in the dynamics of resting-state brain activity. Proc Natl Acad Sci U S A 2015;112(3):887–92.
5. Beck DM, Rees G, Frith CD, Lavie N. Neural correlates of change detection and change blindness. Nat Neurosci 2001;4(6):645–50.
6. Block N. Consciousness, accessibility, and the mesh between psychology and neuroscience. Behav Brain Sci 2007;30(5/6):481–99; discussion 499–548.
7. Boly M, Balteau E, Schnakers C, Degueldre C, Moonen G, Luxen A, Phillips C, Peigneux P, Maquet P, Laureys S. Baseline brain activity fluctuations predict somatosensory perception in humans. Proc Natl Acad Sci U S A 2007;104(29):12187–92.
8. Boly M, Faymonville ME, Schnakers C, Peigneux P, Lambermont B, Phillips C, Lancellotti P, Luxen A, Lamy M, Moonen G, et al. Perception of pain in the minimally conscious state with PET activation: an observational study. Lancet Neurol 2008;7(11):1013–20.

9. Buchel C, Bornhovd K, Quante M, Glauche V, Bromm B, Weiller C. Dissociable neural responses related to pain intensity, stimulus intensity, and stimulus awareness within the anterior cingulate cortex: a parametric single-trial laser functional magnetic resonance imaging study. J Neurosci 2002;22(3):970–76.
10. Crick F, Koch C. A framework for consciousness. Nat Neurosci 2003;6(2):119–26.
11. Dehaene S, Changeux JP, Naccache L, Sackur J, Sergent C. Conscious, preconscious, and subliminal processing: a testable taxonomy. Trends Cogn Sci 2006;10(5):204–11.
12. Dehaene S, Kerszberg M, Changeux JP. A neuronal model of a global workspace in effortful cognitive tasks. Proc Natl Acad Sci U S A 1998;95(24):14529–34.
13. Dehaene S, Naccache L. Towards a cognitive neuroscience of consciousness: basic evidence and a workspace framework. Cognition 2001;79(1–2):1–37.
14. Dehaene S, Naccache L, Cohen L, Bihan DL, Mangin JF, Poline JB, Rivière D. Cerebral mechanisms of word masking and unconscious repetition priming. Nat Neurosci 2001;4(7):752–58.
15. Dehaene S, Sergent C, Changeux JP. A neuronal network model linking subjective reports and objective physiological data during conscious perception. Proc Natl Acad Sci U S A 2003;100:8520–25.
16. Dehaene S, Changeux JP. Experimental and theoretical approaches to conscious processing. Neuron 2011;70(2):200–227. doi: 10.1016/j.neuron.2011.03.018
17. Del Cul A, Baillet S, Dehaene S. Brain dynamics underlying the nonlinear threshold for access to consciousness. PLoS Biol 2007;5(10):e260.
18. Del Cul A, Dehaene S, Leboyer M. Preserved subliminal processing and impaired conscious access in schizophrenia. Arch Gen Psychiatry 2006;63(12):1313–23.
19. Dennett DC. Consciousness explained. London: Penguin; 1992.
20. Duncan J. The structure of cognition: attentional episodes in mind and brain. Neuron 2013;80(1):35–50.
21. Gaillard R, Dehaene S, Adam C, Clémenceau S, Hasboun D, Baulac M, Cohen L, Naccache L. Converging intracranial markers of conscious access. PLoS Biol 2009;7(3):e61.
22. Gaillard R, Del Cul A, Naccache L, Vinckier F, Cohen L, Dehaene S. Nonconscious semantic processing of emotional words modulates conscious access. Proc Natl Acad Sci U S A 2006;103(19):7524–9.
23. Gross J, Schmitz F, Schnitzler I, Kessler K, Shapiro K, Hommel B, Schnitzler A. Modulation of long-range neural synchrony reflects temporal limitations of visual attention in humans. Proc Natl Acad Sci U S A 2004;101(35):13050–5.
24. Haynes JD, Driver J, Rees G. Visibility reflects dynamic changes of effective connectivity between V1 and fusiform cortex. Neuron 2005;46(5):811–21.

25. Hofbauer RK, Fiset P, Plourde G, Backman SB, Bushnell MC. Dose-dependent effects of propofol on the central processing of thermal pain. Anesthesiology 2004;100(2):386–94.

26. Jones SR, Pritchett DL, Stufflebeam SM, Hamalainen M, Moore CI. Neural correlates of tactile detection: a combined magnetoencephalography and biophysically based computational modeling study. J Neurosci 2007;27(40):10751–64.

27. Kaisti KK, Metsähonkala L, Teräs M, Oikonen V, Aalto S, Jääskeläinen S, Hinkka S, Scheinin H. Effects of surgical levels of propofol and sevoflurane anesthesia on cerebral blood flow in healthy subjects studied with positron emission tomography. Anesthesiology 2002;96(6):1358–70.

28. King JR, Sitt JD, Faugeras F, Rohaut B, El Karoui I, Cohen L, Naccache L, Dehaene S. Information sharing in the brain indexes consciousness in noncommunicative patients. Curr Biol 2013;23(19):1914–9.

29. Koechlin E, Ody C, Kouneiher F. The architecture of cognitive control in the human prefrontal cortex. Science 2003;302(5648):1181–5.

30. Kouider S, Stahlhut C, Gelskov SV, Barbosa LS, Dutat M, de Gardelle V, Christophe A, Dehaene S, Dehaene-Lambertz G. A neural marker of perceptual consciousness in infants. Science 2013;340(6130):376–80.

31. Lamme VA. Why visual attention and awareness are different. Trends Cogn Sci 2003;7(1):12–8.

32. Lamme VA. Towards a true neural stance on consciousness. Trends Cogn Sci 2006;10(11):494–501.

33. Lamme VA, Roelfsema PR. The distinct modes of vision offered by feedforward and recurrent processing. Trends Neurosci 2000;23(11):571–9.

34. Lamme VA, Zipser K, Spekreijse H. Masking interrupts figure-ground signals in V1. J Cogn Neurosci 2002;14(7):1044–53.

35. Laureys S, Faymonville ME, Peigneux P, Damas P, Lambermont B, Del Fiore G, Degueldre C, Aerts J, Luxen A, Franck G, et al. Cortical processing of noxious somatosensory stimuli in the persistent vegetative state. Neuroimage 2002;17(2):732–41.

36. Laureys S, Owen AM, Schiff ND. Brain function in coma, vegetative state, and related disorders. Lancet Neurol 2004;3(9):537–46.

37. Longo MR, Betti V, Aglioti SM, Haggard P. Visually induced analgesia: seeing the body reduces pain. J Neurosci 2009;29(39):12125–30.

38. Longo MR, Iannetti GD, Mancini F, Driver J, Haggard P. Linking pain and the body: neural correlates of visually induced analgesia. J Neurosci 2012;32(8):2601–7.

39. Mack A, Rock I. Inattentional blindness. Cambridge, MA: MIT Press, 1998.

40. Maquet P, Degueldre C, Delfiore G, Aerts J, Péters JM, Luxen A, Franck G. Functional neuroanatomy of human slow wave sleep. J Neurosci 1997;17(8):2807–12.

41. Melloni L, Molina C, Pena M, Torres D, Singer W, Rodriguez E. Synchronization of neural activity across cortical areas correlates with conscious perception. J Neurosci 2007;27(11):2858–65.
42. Peyron R, Laurent B, Garcia-Larrea L. Functional imaging of brain responses to pain. A review and meta-analysis. Neurophysiol Clin 2000;30(5):263–88.
43. Rees G, Russell C, Frith CD, Driver J. Inattentional blindness versus inattentional amnesia for fixated but ignored words. Science 1999;286(5449):2504–7.
44. Ress D, Heeger DJ. Neuronal correlates of perception in early visual cortex. Nat Neurosci 2003;6(4):414–20.
45. Sadaghiani S, Hesselmann G, Kleinschmidt A. Distributed and antagonistic contributions of ongoing activity fluctuations to auditory stimulus detection. J Neurosci 2009;29(42):13410–7.
46. Sergent C, Baillet S, Dehaene S. Timing of the brain events underlying access to consciousness during the attentional blink. Nat Neurosci 2005;8(10):1391–400.
47. Sergent C, Dehaene S. Is consciousness a gradual phenomenon? Evidence for an all-or-none bifurcation during the attentional blink. Psychol Sci 2004;15(11):720–28.
48. Sergent C, Naccache L. Imaging neural signatures of consciousness: "what," "when," "where," and "how" does it work. Arch Ital Biole 2012;150(2/3):91–106.
49. Sergent C, Wyart V, Babo-Rebelo M, Cohen L, Naccache L, Tallon-Baudry C. Cueing attention after the stimulus is gone can retrospectively trigger conscious perception. Curr Biol 2013;23(2):150–5.
50. Super H, Spekreijse H, Lamme VA. Two distinct modes of sensory processing observed in monkey primary visual cortex (V1). Nat Neurosci 2001;4(3):304–10.
51. Thorpe S, Fize D, Marlot C. Speed of processing in the human visual system. Nature 1996;381(6582):520–2.
52. Tong F, Nakayama K, Vaughan JT, Kanwisher N. Binocular rivalry and visual awareness in human extrastriate cortex. Neuron 1998;21(4):753–9.
53. Trevethan CT, Sahraie A, Weiskrantz L. Form discrimination in a case of blindsight. Neuropsychologia 2007;45(9):2092–103.
54. van Gaal S, Ridderinkhof KR, Scholte HS, Lamme VA. Unconscious activation of the prefrontal no-go network. J Neurosci 2010;30(11):4143–50.
55. van Gaal S, Ridderinkhof KR, van den Wildenberg WP, Lamme VA. Dissociating consciousness from inhibitory control: evidence for unconsciously triggered response inhibition in the stop-signal task. J Exp Psychol Hum Percept Perform 2009;35(4):1129–39.
56. Weiskrantz L. Consciousness lost and found: a neuropsychological exploration. New York, NY: Oxford University Press; 1997.
57. Woo CW, Roy M, Buhle JT, Wager TD. Distinct brain systems mediate the effects of nociceptive input and self-regulation on pain. PLoS Biol 2015;13(1):e1002036.

CHAPTER 3

Pain and the Spatial Boundaries of the Bodily Self

Frédérique de Vignemont

Many discussions have been had about the relationship between pain and consciousness. Can humans be unaware of their pains? Can only animals that are fully conscious be said to be in pain? These questions, among others, are still a matter of controversies. Surprisingly, however, most of these discussions left untouched the issue of self-consciousness, although there is a sense in which it seems to be intimately connected with pain. One might report, for instance, how one feels extremely self-aware when one is in deep pain, as if the rest of the world ceased to exist. One of the main features of pain is indeed that it can grab our attention far more than any other bodily experiences. One may then say that by attracting attention to the body, pain enhances our sense of the bodily self, which otherwise remains recessive and elusive. However, one faces many difficulties if one wants to account for the relationship between pain and self-consciousness. For one thing, the notion of self-consciousness is a ragbag of various concepts of the self, from the embodied sensorimotor self to the disembodied mental and narrative self. Here, I shall exclusively focus on the former. In particular, I will investigate how the awareness of one's body as one's own (hereafter, sense of bodily ownership) is related to pain. An intuitive sense is that one feels pain only in parts of the body that one feels as one's own. Pain can be experienced in phantom limbs, but they are experienced as parts of one's own body. The challenge then is to understand the nature of the relationship between pain and the sense of bodily ownership. It can be conceived at least from the following two angles. To what extent does pain require self-consciousness, and more specifically the sense of bodily ownership? Conversely, to what extent does self-consciousness, and more specifically the sense of bodily ownership, require pain? Offering the beginning of an answer to this last question shall be my main objective in this chapter.

How am I aware that this specific body is my own? One strategy to answer this question consists in rephrasing it in spatial terms. The question then is how I am aware of the spatial boundaries of my body. Many factors can come into play. One may note, for instance, that tactile, thermal, proprioceptive, and interoceptive signals carry information exclusively about one's own body. One may then conclude that through bodily sensations, where one can or cannot feel oneself, one can draw the boundaries of one's body. On this view, the body that I feel as mine is the body that I feel from the inside. More recently, it has been suggested that vision, the sense of space *par excellence*, plays a crucial role and that multisensory correspondence allows distinguishing self from nonself. In this view, the body that I feel as mine is the body common to various sources of sensory information. Another proposal puts emphasis on efferent rather than afferent information. In this view, the body that I feel as mine is the body that I can directly control. In this manifold of factors, how does pain contribute to the sense of bodily ownership? Does it play any specific role or is it just one type of bodily sensation among others?

AN APPARENT PARADOX

> When in pain, I experience disorder as located within a boundary of whose exterior I can have no similar awareness; I am aware that a part of my body—not just of that body—is disordered.
>
> (Bain [2], p. 523)

Seeing injuries and feeling pain have a different phenomenology. It is not only that the latter is more unpleasant than the former. They seem to have a different relationship to the sense of bodily ownership. When I see a blow on a face, I can remain unaware that this is actually my face that I see injured in the mirror. By contrast, when I feel the blow, I cannot help but feel that this is my own face that hurts. Consequently, one cannot conceive feeling pain in a part of the body that feels as alien [2, 6, 16]. Or so it seems. The limits of the philosophers' imagination do not always match what can actually be found in the neurologic literature. We know that some patients do not feel parts of their body as belonging to them and feel them as alien. This is the case in somatoparaphrenia after parietal lesions. Patients then deny ownership of parts of their body to such an extent that they can attribute their so-called alien limb to another individual or that they ask to be amputated of it. Yet some clinical reports indicate that some—but not all—patients with somatoparaphrenia are able to feel pain in their "alien" limb:

> Patient: I still have the acute pain where the prosthesis is. Examiner: Which prosthesis? P: Don't you see? This thing here (indicating his left arm). The doctors have attached this tool to my body in order to help me to move. But it's completely useless and very painful (...) Once home could I ask my wife, from time to time, to remove this left arm and put it in the cupboard for a few hours in order to have some relief from pain? [14]

Another patient whose "alien" hand was pinched winced and cried out, but still denied that the hand was his own [17]. Hence, pain and the sense of bodily ownership can come apart. More precisely, one can be in pain in a body part that one does not feel as one's own. It is not because I feel pain in a specific part of the body that I will experience this body part as mine. To feel pain is not sufficient for the sense of bodily ownership.

The question I asked in the introduction, however, was not whether pain could be sufficient, but whether it was necessary for the sense of bodily ownership. In order to answer this question, one needs to analyze the consequences of pain deprivation. What happens when one has never been in pain? This has been tested in animals. For instance, some terrier dogs were raised in isolation preserved from pain. They required more intense electric shocks to learn avoidance responses, and they spent more time near the experimenter after he burnt their noses with a flame [18]. Another pain deprivation study was done with infant monkeys that were raised preserved from all threats, in the absence of potentially damaging objects and of elders who could slap or bite them. Still they could hear, see, and touch themselves. When released, these monkeys viciously bit their own limbs and torn their flesh [13]. Thus, if one has not been hurt before, pain partly loses its unpleasantness, or at least its motivational force. Since these animals were also in social deprivation, one might say that they could not learn from others what were bad for them or how to react to it. However, the social explanation does not suffice to explain why they also engaged in acts of self-destruction. Interestingly, self-inflicted injuries can also be found in patients with congenital pain insensitivity [4, 9, 10, 23]. These patients are characterized by dramatic impairment of pain sensation since birth, caused by a hereditary neuropathy or channelopathy. They show a complete lack of discomfort, grimacing, or withdrawal reaction to prolonged pinpricks, strong pressure, soft tissue pinching, and noxious thermal stimuli. Like the animals raised in isolation, they can sometimes have endogenous pain (stomachache, for instance), but no exogenous pain. Like them also, they often engage in self-mutilation, including burns and self-amputations of fingertips and tongues.

Not to avoid pain is one thing, but to voluntarily injure oneself is another thing. The former can be explained by abnormality of nociceptive processing. But the latter requires further explanation. The hypothesis that I want to suggest is that self-injuries after pain deprivation are caused by the failure to recognize that this body that one injures is to be protected because it is one's own body. In this view, past pain experiences contribute to the development of the representation of the boundaries of one's own body and in their absence, one may lose track of what belongs to oneself and what does not. In other words, when patients bite their fingertips, they are not aware that they are biting their *own* fingertips. Failing to feel one's limb as one's own leads to a failure to protect it from harm. Unfortunately, no experimental study on body representations and the sense of bodily ownership has been done yet in congenital pain insensitivity. However, patients have described that their body feels like an external object, a kind of tool. For instance, an eighteen-year-old boy with congenital insensitivity to pain reported, "A body is like a car, it can be dented but it pops out again and can be fixed like a car. Someone can get in and use it but the body isn't you, you just inhabit it" [9]. In addition, patients with disownership syndrome also display aggressive behavior toward the limb they feel as alien. For instance, many patients with somatoparaphrenia and xenomelia regularly hit their "alien" limb, scorched it, pricked it with pointed objects such as needles, and burned it with a cigarette [5]. Without always going as far as self-inflicted injuries, they display misoplegia, trying quite often to get rid of their "alien" limb by pulling their leg out of their bed, giving it to the doctor, putting it in the garbage, and so forth. Their subjective reports are confirmed by their attitude when their "alien" limb is threatened [24, 25]. For instance, in one study, patients with somatoparaphrenia saw either a Q-tip or a syringe approaching either their right hand, which they felt as their own, or their left hand, which they felt as alien. Their skin conductance response (SCR) was measured. When the syringe approached the right hand, the SCR increased, as expected. But when the syringe approached the left "alien" hand, there was no modification of the SCR. This lack of effect could not be explained by the inability of anticipating the pain because of anesthesia or neglect. When the experimenters tested another population of right hemisphere lesions patients, with anesthesia and neglect but without disownership, they found that these patients reacted normally when their left hand was threatened.

Self-injuries can thus be partially understood in relation to the disruption of the sense of bodily ownership, although there may be other explanations in other disorders. They can be explained at least in two ways depending on the clinical condition and the extent of the disruption of bodily ownership. On the one hand, patients who are not aware of the boundaries of their body are not voluntarily injuring themselves, but rather they are injuring *a body*, which happens to be their own. On the other hand, in other patients who have some awareness of bodily boundaries but disturbed to some extent, injuring this specific body may be a way to test whether it is their own or not. Feeling something can then strengthen a fading feeling of confidence in their sense of bodily ownership, whereas feeling nothing can confirm that this body has nothing to do with them. This may be the case in patients with anorexia nervosa, who display self-injurious behaviors, and who have been shown to have a stronger sensitivity to ownership illusions and disturbed cortical processing of painful stimuli [7, 30]. This may also be the case in patients with depersonalization syndrome, who feel detached from their body and react to pain as if they were not concerned. A patient with depersonalization reports, "it is as if I don't care, as if it was somebody else's pain" [28]. They also report a sense of disownership of their own body. Another patient reports, "I can sit looking at my foot or my hand and not feel like they are mine" [28]. Consequently, they often feel the urge to touch their body, to pour hot water on it, or even to hurt it to reassure themselves of its existence [11, 29].

To recap, we seem to face an apparent paradox. On the one hand, contrary to what one might have expected, one can feel pain in parts of the body that do not feel as one's own. It may then seem that pain plays only a minimal role for the sense of bodily ownership. On the other hand, if one is raised deprived of exogenous pain, then one may lose track of the boundaries of one's own body. It may then seem that pain plays a crucial role for the sense of bodily ownership. In the next section, I will analyze what pain can and cannot offer to bodily self-awareness.

GIVING SIGNIFICANCE TO BODILY BOUNDARIES

We have seen that pain deprivation can suffice to alter the representation of one's own bodily boundaries. This is especially puzzling insofar as both the monkeys raised in isolation and the patients with congenital pain insensitivity can experience other types of bodily sensations. For example, monkeys were not deprived of tactile experiences and patients with congenital pain insensitivity often show no abnormality in tactile processing. Yet it seems that touch, and even self-touch, cannot suffice to compensate for pain deprivation in the drawing of one's own bodily boundaries. That indicates that pain does not play the same role as touch for the development of the sense of bodily ownership. We shall now see what the difference may be.

The sense of bodily ownership requires drawing the distinction between what is inside and what is outside of bodily boundaries. This can be given by tactile experiences, for instance, because they have both an exteroceptive component (a pen, for instance) and a bodily component (the hand that holds the pen). Through touch, one is aware of external objects in contact with one's body. One can thus contrast what is inside from what is outside and become aware of the boundaries of the body [16]. Pain, however, differs from touch. It has only a bodily component (the hand in pain, for instance). Even when our painful experience is caused by an external painful stimulus, it represents the body part in pain, and not the stimulus that caused the pain. Many factors can intervene to modulate the pain, including factors that concern the stimulus and the environment. Still the content of our experience is filled in by the body. As defined by IASP, pain can be described in terms of bodily damage. It is not described in terms of whatever external caused the damage. Consequently, pain by itself cannot suffice to draw the boundaries of the body. It is too embodied, so to speak. It leaves no space for what is beyond the body. There is only an inside. This explains why one can simultaneously feel pain and *not* feel ownership in a body part. The consequence of this conception is that if the representation of bodily boundaries is already destroyed or altered for one reason or another, like in somatoparaphrenia and in xenomelia, then there is little that pain could do to re-establish it.

Why is pain then so important and why does its deprivation lead to such devastating consequences? I will now argue that the awareness of bodily boundaries, given by tactile experiences, does not suffice for the sense of bodily ownership, or more precisely for the first personal content of the sense of ownership. One can draw a parallel here with nationalism. To be aware of the boundaries of a country does not necessarily entail that you feel that this is your own country. You know that this is where you can vote and that beyond the boundaries you cannot, but this is different from patriotic feelings. How can you then appropriate the country in which you live and vote as your own? A classic conception in social psychology is that the awareness of external threats reinforces the feeling of national identity. One does not feel especially patriotic when one is merely aware of the boundaries of one's country; one feels patriotic when these boundaries are in danger. I propose here that something similar applies for the sense of bodily ownership.

The awareness of the boundaries of the body is not self-referential. It is simply spatial with no reference to the subject. How can one then inject some first-personal character into the spatial awareness of the body? How can bodily awareness become bodily *self*-awareness? Pain does not draw bodily boundaries. Rather, pain gives a valence to these boundaries. It indicates that these boundaries are the ones to care about and to protect if one wants to survive. It vividly highlights for the subject that what is inside bodily boundaries matters for the self, for its needs, its comfort, and its preservation. Pain teaches that it is important to keep track of the boundaries and to be able to act quickly. Without pain, without even pain expectation, bodily boundaries are just spatial boundaries. Hence, it is not simply in virtue of the awareness of the boundaries of one's body that one is aware of one's body as one's own. It is in virtue of the awareness of the boundaries as having *a major import for the self* that one is aware of one's body as one's own. This is possibly the reason why pain can play such a crucial role for the sense of bodily ownership. This does not mean that it is only when the body is in danger that we feel our body as our own. I defend a weaker conception, according to which it suffices that it has been in danger at some point to set up a specific valence to the boundaries of the body. All I am proposing is that there is a stage in development in which it is important, possibly even necessary, to experience exogenous pain in order to give affective and motor significance to the boundaries of the body, a significance that is at the origin of the sense of bodily ownership. In short, past experiences that the boundaries of the body could be at risk make these boundaries the boundaries of the body that we experience as our own now.

DENYING THE BOUNDARIES OF ONE'S BODY

I have argued that pain contributes to establishing a meaning to the boundaries of the body, a meaning that is essential to feel those boundaries as boundaries of one's own body. I will now consider one possible objection against this view on the basis of the analysis of complex regional pain syndrome (CRPS). In this syndrome indeed, it seems that pain can induce a sense of *disownership*. I will then explain how this is compatible with our leading hypothesis.

CRPS is a chronic pain condition, which often happens after an injury like a broken arm or nerve lesions, and which causes intense burning pain, associated with a decreased ability to move the affected body part with swelling and stiffness in affected joints. It has been described as a kind of motor neglect because patients need to focus specifically on the limb in order to move it and experience a sense of disconnection from the affected limb [8]: "It was just like this foreign body you were carrying around with you cause it didn't feel like it was part of you" [12]. In addition to CRPS, when individuals are in extreme pain, like burn patients and war prisoners, they no longer refer to the body part in pain by using the first-person pronoun and they disconnect themselves from their body [20]. For instance, a prisoner reported, "It's like the torture starts and as it gets stronger I just get further away from the body" [1].

Do CRPS and other related cases give us new insight into the relationship between pain and the sense of ownership? Like in somatoparaphrenia, CRPS shows that a sense of disownership can be concomitant to pain and thus, that pain does not suffice to induce a sense of ownership. However, unlike somatoparaphrenia, in which pain is most of the time anecdotal, pain is the primary clinical sign of CRPS. Another possibly interesting feature of CRPS is that it shows that pain is not only compatible with disownership, but that it can actually cause it. In line with this hypothesis, it has been shown that pain can disrupt the representation of the body [3, 21, 27].

It may thus seem that with or without pain, one can feel one's body as alien. In what sense is pain then so essentially related to the sense of ownership? We need to refine our leading hypothesis. So far I have referred to pain as if it were a homogenous phenomenon. However, this is far from being the case and there are many different types of pain, which may explain the puzzling conclusion that I have just reached. One must first distinguish between what we may call pain expertise based on prior experiences of pain, occurrent pains, and chronic pains. One can also distinguish between endogenous (toothache, for instance) and exogenous pains (a cut, for instance). Finally, one can distinguish between painful experiences that are unpleasant but tolerable and those that are excruciating so that one can no longer tolerate them. The relationship to the sense of bodily ownership may then vary depending on the type of pain.

One must also be careful when describing the sense of disownership. It is interesting to note that when asked, patients with CRPS still rated their sense of ownership of the affected hand on average at 5.9 on a scale for 0–10, with 10 corresponding to "It feels like I own it completely" [22]. Interestingly, as far as I know, they display no aggressive behavior toward their "alien" limb. Their sense of disownership thus seems to be different from the one displayed by patients with somatoparaphrenia, who have an unshakable confidence that this body part does not belong to them. At the physiological level, there are also differences between these two types of patients. In both types of patients, the temperature of the affected hand was cooler than of the healthy one. However, in patients with CRPS, the temperature, as well as their rating of ownership, increased when their affected limb was moved to the other side of their body beyond their body midline (for instance, left hand on the right) [22]. On the contrary, somatoparaphrenic patients do not recover from their disownership syndrome when they move their "alien" hand to their contralateral side [19]. The interpretation of CRPS in terms of disownership is thus still controversial. In particular, one should avoid confusing a disruption of the sense of ownership and a low feeling of confidence associated with a preserved sense of ownership. One can also wonder whether patients with CRPS do not feel their limb as their own or whether they do not desire their limb to be their own:

> It really was very, very hard to do it. When I touched it, in lots of ways it actually reinforced the idea that it wasn't mine at all because it didn't feel like it and I couldn't make it feel like mine and *I didn't want to make it feel like mine* in a lot of ways because it hurt so much. [12]

Disownership can then be conceived as a defense mechanism against intense pains (see, for instance, [15] for a similar view on anosognosia for hemiplegia). Roughly speaking, a little bit of pain may be good to strengthen fading confidence in bodily ownership, but too much pain (because of its intensity and/or its duration) is bad, and by detaching oneself from one's body, one is hoping to detach oneself from the pain. This coping strategy, however, does not work since the average pain at rest was rated higher in patients with CRPS who reported finding their hand "foreign" or "strange" [8]. As said earlier in our description of somatoparaphrenia, one can still feel pain in a body part that feels alien. Pain is necessary but not sufficient to induce a sense of ownership. Neither is the sense of disownership sufficient to relieve pain. As Schilder claims in his monograph *The Image and Appearance of the Human Body*, "When the whole body is filled with pain, we try to get rid of the whole body" [26]. But does it work? It does not seem so.

CONCLUSION

To conclude, it is important to distinguish between the mechanisms used to fix the boundaries of the body (i.e., distinguishing what is inside and what is outside of the body) and the mechanisms used to give a positive valence to these boundaries (i.e., being aware that these boundaries matter for the self and must be protected). I have argued that both types of mechanisms are necessary for the sense of bodily ownership. I have further argued that pain is just one factor among many for the first type of mechanisms. This explains why feeling pain does not suffice to reintegrate a body part that has been excluded outside bodily boundaries. However, I have argued that pain, or more precisely pain expertise, plays a crucial role for the second type of mechanisms. This explains why if you have never been in pain, your body is just the body that happens to be your own instead of the body that you *feel* as your own.

REFERENCES

1. Ataria Y. Sense of ownership and sense of agency during trauma. Phenom Cogn Sci 2015;14:199–212.
2. Bain D. Intentionalism and pain. Philos Q 2003;53(213):502–23.
3. Bank PJ, Peper CL, Marinus J, Beek PJ, van Hilten JJ. Motor dysfunction of complex regional pain syndrome is related to impaired central processing of proprioceptive information. J Pain 2013;14(11):1460–74.
4. Danziger N, Willer JC. Congenital insensitivity to pain. Rev Neurol (Paris) 2009; 165(2):129–36.
5. Dieguez S, Annoni IM. Asomatognosia: disorders of the bodily self. In: Godefroy O, editor. The behavioral and cognitive neurology of stroke. 2nd ed. New York, NY: Cambridge University Press; 2013. pp. 170–92.
6. Dokic J. The sense of ownership: an analogy between sensation and action. In: Roessler J, Eilan N, editors. Agency and self-awareness: issues in philosophy and psychology. Oxford: Oxford University Press; 2003. pp. 329–44.
7. Eshkevari E, Rieger E, Longo MR, Haggard P, Treasure J. Increased plasticity of the bodily self in eating disorders. Psychol Med 2012;42(4):819–28.
8. Förderreuther S, Sailer U, Straube A. Impaired self-perception of the hand in complex regional pain syndrome (CRPS). Pain 2004;110(3):756–61.
9. Frances A, Gale L. The proprioceptive body image in self-object differentiation—a case of congenital indifference to pain and head-banging. Psychoanal Q 1975;44:107–26.
10. Jewbury EC. Insensitivity to pain. Brain 1951;74(3):336–53.
11. Klonsky ED, Muehlenkamp JJ. Self-injury: a research review for the practitioner. J Clin Psychol 2007;63(11):1045–56.
12. Lewis JS, Kersten P, McCabe CS, McPherson KM, Blake DR. Body perception disturbance: a contribution to pain in complex regional pain syndrome (CRPS). Pain 2007; 133(1):111–9.
13. Lichstein L, Sackett GP. Reactions by differentially raised rhesus monkeys to noxious stimulation. Dev Psychobiol 1971;4(4):339–52.
14. Maravita A. Spatial disorders. In: Cappa SF, Abutalebi J, Demonet JF, Fletcher PC, Garrard P, editors. Cognitive neurology: a clinical textbook. New York, NY: Oxford University Press; 2008. pp. 89–118.
15. Marcel AJ, Tegnér R, Nimmo-Smith I. Anosognosia for plegia: specificity, extension, partiality and disunity of bodily unawareness. Cortex 2004;40(1):19–40.
16. Martin MGF. Bodily awareness: a sense of ownership. In: Bermudez JL, Marcel T, Eilan N, editors. The body and the self. Cambridge, MA: MIT Press; 1995. pp. 276–90.

17. Melzack R. Phantom limbs and the concept of a neuromatrix. Trends Neurosci 1990;13(3):88–92.

18. Melzack R, Scott, TH. The effects of early experience on the response to pain. J Comp Physiol Psychol 1957;50(2):155–61.

19. Moro V, Zampini M, Aglioti SM. Changes in spatial position of hands modify tactile extinction but not disownership of contralesional hand in two right brain-damaged patients. Neurocase 2004;10(6):437–43.

20. Morse JM, Mitcham C. The experience of agonizing pain and signals of disembodiment. J Psychosom Res 1998;44(6):667–80.

21. Moseley GL. Why do people with complex regional pain syndrome take longer to recognize their affected hand? Neurology 2004;62(12):2182–6.

22. Moseley GL, Gallace A, Iannetti GD. Spatially defined modulation of skin temperature and hand ownership of both hands in patients with unilateral complex regional pain syndrome. Brain 2012;135(12):3676–86.

23. Nagasako EM, Oaklander AL, Dworkin RH. Congenital insensitivity to pain: an update. Pain 2003;101(3):213–9.

24. Romano D, Gandola M, Bottini G, Maravita A. Arousal responses to noxious stimuli in somatoparaphrenia and anosognosia: clues to body awareness. Brain 2014;137(Pt 4): 1213–23.

25. Romano D, Sedda A, Brugger P, Bottini G. Body ownership: when feeling and knowing diverge. Conscious Cogn 2015;34:140–8.

26. Schilder P. The image and appearance of the human body. New York, NY: International Universities Press; 1935.

27. Schwoebel J, Coslett HB, Bradt J, Friedman R, Dileo C. Pain and the body schema: effects of pain severity on mental representations of movement. Neurology 2002;59(5):775–7.

28. Sierra M. Depersonalization: a new look at a neglected syndrome. Cambridge: Cambridge University Press; 2009.

29. Simeon D, Stein DJ, Hollander E. Depersonalization disorder and self-injurious behavior. J Clin Psychiatry 1995;56(suppl 4):36–9.

30. Strigo IA, Matthews SC, Simmons AN, Oberndorfer T, Klabunde M, Reinhardt LE, Kaye WH. Altered insula activation during pain anticipation in individuals recovered from anorexia nervosa: evidence of interoceptive dysregulation. Int J Eat Disord 2013;46(1):23–33.

CHAPTER 4

Cortical Imaging of Pain in Humans: A Journey from Nociception to Compassion

Luis Garcia-Larrea, Philip L. Jackson, and Roland Peyron

Constructing a model is making a bet.

—Anonymous

It is now clear that there is no such thing as a "pain center" in the brain. Nociceptive stimuli activate multiple subcortical and cortical areas, the pain experience being the result of their joint and coordinated activation in time and space. The group of brain structures jointly activated by painful stimuli is commonly described as "the pain matrix" (PM). This concept owes a great deal to notions developed in the 1980s by Ronald Melzack, who conceived the anatomical substratum of the physical self as a "neuromatrix," that is, a network of neurons extending throughout widespread areas of the brain, and generating characteristic patterns of neural impulses distinguishing each bodily sensation. In his own words, "the neuromatrix for the physical self (…) generates the neurosignature pattern for pain" [40].

In the trail of Head and Holmes [22], the first half of the 20th century was dominated by the idea of pain being limited to subcortical structures, not extending beyond the thalamus. The importance of the cerebral cortex for pain perception was not clearly acknowledged until the 1950s, thanks to clinicians studying patients with cerebral lesions [8], and in 1968 Melzack and Casey [41] suggested that the pain experience reflected *interacting sensory, affective, and cognitive dimensions* that could influence each other. This view implied that there was no "brain pain center": pain was considered multidimensional and produced by distributed and interacting neural patterns, usually triggered by sensory inputs but modulated by and even generated independently of them. The notion of a PM was almost born.

The conceptual advance represented by the PM notion over many prevailing concepts was clearly supported by functional imaging studies; in 1991 positron-emission tomography (PET) showed for the first time a distributed pattern of brain structures activated by noxious heat [54]. A bulk of consistent data rapidly accumulated, showing positive correlations between energy of the stimulus, subjective perception, and PM responses, but it became also clear that *most of the areas showing changes in activity levels were not specific for pain*. In particular, PM regions such as the anterior cingulate cortex (ACC), the anterior insula (AI), and the prefrontal and posterior parietal areas (PFC, PPC) showed enhanced activity in a wide range of nonpain experiments, especially in emotionally or cognitively laden contexts. By opposition, the sensory encoding of noxious intensity was typically reflected by spatially limited brain activations (reviews in references [2, 47, 56]).

While data on activated PM areas are consistent across most pain studies, their interpretation has led to contrasting conceptual positions. Some authors posit that functional imaging and the PM may contain a genuine and objective "signature" of the painful experience [60], which could even be used to derive an "individual pain phenotype" [1]. Pushing this logic further, activation of PM subsets (essentially anterior insular and cingulate cortices) has been sometimes *equated* with physical pain, leading to questionable conclusions such as that social rejection [physically] hurts [14, 37]. In robust rebuttal to this, other investigators have assailed the very concept of a specific pain network, claiming that most, if not all the regions present in the PM represent a nonspecific salience-detection system for the body activated by relevant events "regardless of the sensory channel through which these events are conveyed" [24, 30]. Between these extreme positions, a few investigators have put forward the idea that the so-called PM should not be seen as a stable construct unequivocally defined, but rather as a combination of nociceptive-specific components and nonspecific, context-dependent activations, whose ever-changing interaction determines the pain experience (see references [47, 56]).

Because spinothalamic projections inform brain networks on the bodily nature of the input, the healthy brain recognizes at once whether a menacing signal arrives through a somatosensory channel. Information on the somatic origin is likely to be transferred to PM regions secondarily involved, thus giving to perceptive networks a stable reference to its own body. In this chapter, the neural substrate of the pain experience will be conceptualized at different levels of progressively higher-order cortical networks, from cortical nociception to the conscious experience we call "pain"—which can still be subject to reappraisal by internal states, feelings and beliefs, as well as the physical and social environment, prior to stabilization into memory stores.

A NOCICEPTIVE CORTICAL MATRIX

The primate spinothalamic system (STS) chiefly originates from neurons in spinal laminae I, V, and VII, whose axons terminate in multiple nuclei of the posterior thalamus, essentially the ventral posterior, central lateral, mediodorsal, and posterior group nuclei [3, 39]. The main spinothalamic cortical targets in primates have been defined using trans-synaptic viral transport, and established in the posterior insula (~40%), medial parietal operculum (~30%), and midcingulate cortex (~24%), with a tiny projection of ~6% to the primary sensory-motor cortex [13]. Not surprisingly, these receiving regions are the source of the earliest responses to noxious stimuli recorded in the human brain [17, 33, 44] and therefore contain a "nociceptive matrix" specific for spinothalamic projections.* Within this matrix, midcingulate sections are likely to support orienting to, and withdrawal from, noxious stimuli, while the posterior insular and opercular regions subserve their earliest sensory processing. The functional relevance of operculoinsular areas as a funnel for nociceptive input is supported by a bulk of experimental data: the posterior insula and inner operculum are *the only regions* in the human brain where direct stimulation (i.e., with intracortical electrodes during the investigation of intractable epilepsy) can trigger acute pain [38]), where focal lesions entail selective pain deficits [8, 21], and where cortical injury gives rise to neuropathic pain (review reference [18]). Lenz et al. [32] informed of "full pain experiences" when stimulating thalamic regions projecting to the posterior insula and operculum. Focal epileptic activity in the posterior insula can trigger painful seizures by igniting other PM areas in less than 100 ms, and painful seizures have been blocked up by millimetric thermocoagulation of posterior insular foci [43].

While this "nociceptive matrix" appears as an essential entry to generate physiological pain experiences attributed to the body, it cannot provide the countless nuances that characterize human pain. Furthermore, the nociceptive matrix by itself is unable to sustain consciousness, since its activation has been shown to persist during sleep or vegetative state ([6, 27]; see also Chapter 5). The transition from cortical nociception to conscious pain and its multiple attentional-cognitive modulations needs therefore the recruitment of a second set of cortical networks (Fig. 4-1).

FROM NOCICEPTION TO PAIN: A SECOND-ORDER PERCEPTUAL MATRIX

The "classical" PM encompasses activity in many areas distinct from the nociceptive network described above, the most consistent being the mid- and anterior insulae, the anterior cingulate, prefrontal and posterior parietal areas. Although with lesser consistency, activations are also often described within the striatum, supplementary

*These regions are said to "contain" rather than "represent" a nociceptive matrix, since in all of them nociceptive-specific units coexist with other wide dynamic or multisensory networks processing non-nociceptive information. For instance, at macroscopic (millimetric) level, the operculoinsular regions responding to nociceptive-specific laser pulses are also activated (at different latencies) by non-noxious somatosensory inputs (Frot et al., 2001;94:65–73).

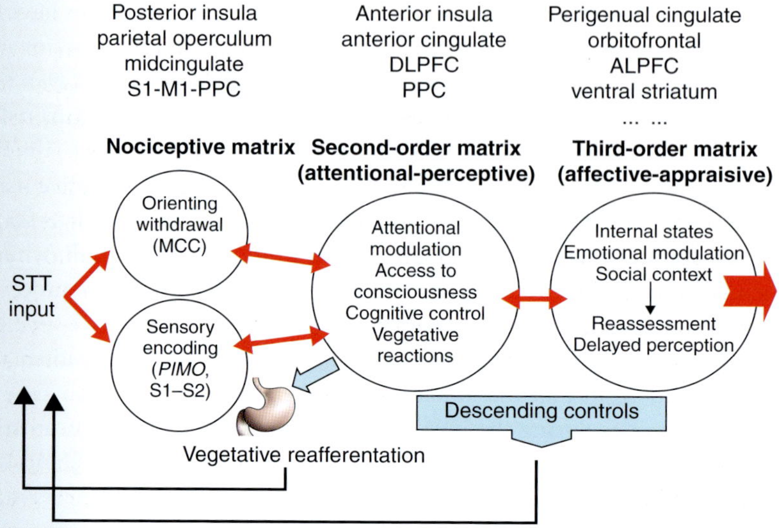

FIGURE 4-1 Interacting "pain matrices" activated following a noxious somatic stimulus. Distribution of regions of the "full pain matrix" according to their putative functional role in pain perception and memory. Note that although the flux of information tends to be from left to right, continuous interaction among matrices exists, creating dynamic and continuously reconstructing patterns. Although not indicated with further arrows, pain memories at the far right can also change pain perception by affecting both internal affective states (third-order matrix) and attentional modulation (second-order matrix). STT, spinothalamic tract; PIMO, posterior insula–medial operculum; PPC, posterior parietal cortex; ACC, anterior cingulate cortex; MCC, midcingulate cortex; DLPFC, dorsolateral prefrontal cortex; ALPFC, anterolateral prefronta cortex.

motor area, hippocampus, cerebellum, and temporoparietal junction. All these areas, which we will term "second order," share a number of important features which differentiate them from the nociceptive-specific matrix:

1. None of them is a direct main target of the STS.
2. Their direct stimulation does *not* evoke pain.
3. Their selective destruction does *not* induce analgesia.
4. They can all be also activated in contexts not involving pain.
5. Their contribution to the PM, from nil to predominant, depends on the context where noxious stimuli are applied.

Two of these second-order areas participate almost constantly to the PM, namely the anterior insula (AI) and the dorsal anterior cingulate (ACC). Mid- and anterior insular activation probably reflects the posterior-to-anterior information flux within this structure [16], supporting the transformation of sensory events into internal feelings and vegetative reactions [9, 61]. The "cognitive section" of the anterior cingulate (rostral to the anterior commissure) is also consistently activated by painful stimuli [23, 59], and together with prefrontal and posterior parietal areas is thought to sustain attentional and evaluative processes of anticipation, learning, and cognitive control. The contribution of these areas to the PM varies enormously with contextual factors, and their activation can be dissociated from actual stimulus intensity (reviews in references [2, 56]). This second-order contextual network receives input from the nociceptive matrix, but can also greatly influence the nociceptive areas via top–down projections. For instance, attending actively to noxious stimuli enhances activity in areas receiving spinothalamic tract (STT) afferents, such as the posterior insula, S1, and midcingulate, whereas distraction tends to suppress such activities ([5, 44, 46, 58]; review reference [63] and see Chapter 14). Such top–down influences modify perception by changing the sensory gain "at the source," that is, in cortical receiving areas, thalamus, and even at brain stem and spinal cord [53, 57, 64]. Further, vegetative peripheral reactions in viscera driven by anterior insular networks generate new ascending information through splanchnic and vagus nerves [55], thus providing new input to cortical and subcortical nociceptive targets. Hypnotic suggestions can influence the nociceptive, the second-order, or both matrices, depending on the instructions given to the subject (e.g., reexperiencing pleasant autobiographical memories [15], *versus* up and down modulation of the unpleasantness [48]). A dissociation between preserved activity in sensory cortices (posterior insula) but abated response in second-order parietal and temporal networks has been described under hypnosis (see Chapter 7).

The regions constituent of this second-order matrix can be activated in many contexts other than physical pain. For instance, the AI and ACC pertain to a "salience network" responding to behaviorally relevant stimuli, which they integrate into perceptual decision-making. These two regions are jointly activated not only in response to painful stimuli, but also when subjects are confronted to unpleasant situations such as observing expressions of disgust [61], feeling guilt [51], experiencing social and moral suffering [14, 28], or seeing/imagining other people in pain [25, 52]. This has led to considerable controversy as to whether subjects confronted to such unpleasant situations do *physically* feel pain [14, 28] and further, how similar the experiences of vicarious pain are to actual experiences of pain (see discussion in Chapter 14). Obviously, feeling pain and representing someone else's suffering is different, at least in physiological conditions†: neither the mid-AI nor the rostral ACC are nociceptive sensory areas, and therefore they cannot support by themselves the *corporal*

---

†Transformation of visual or auditory sensations into somatic experiences has been described as rare conditions such as vision–touch synesthesia (Blakemore et al., 2005;128:1571–83), which may be seen as an abnormal form of empathy (Fitzgibbon et al., 2010;34:500–12).

specificity that characterizes somatic pain, as shown in both stimulation and lesion studies [21, 38]. Their activation in response to unpleasant stimuli appears to reflect their belonging to a *broad system for salience detection* which may also include the ventral striatum, and which (a) generates internal state modifications, (b) alters the individual responsiveness to specific stimuli, and (c) may contribute *in fine* to modulate the subjective value of rewards. In this vein, responses in both AI and ACC can be triggered by *pleasant* stimuli to the same degree as unpleasant ones [50], and direct stimulation of the mid and AI in monkeys was able to elicit not only disgusting, but also socially *affiliative* behaviors [9].

The conscious perception of the noxious stimulus needs also the contribution of regions in this second-order matrix. Sensory inputs become conscious only if they create distributed brain activation: activity constrained to sensory areas does not produce reportable (i.e., declarative) conscious perceptions, which emerge only when sensory responses are associated to distributed fronto–parieto–temporal activation [11, 12], that is, areas integrating the second-order PM. Functional connectivity within the frontoparietal network appears crucial for declarative consciousness [29], and abundant evidence shows that the contribution of dorsolateral frontal and posterior parietal networks separates undetected versus detected stimulus changes, masked versus unmasked words, extinguished versus seen visual objects, and missed versus reported stimuli during attentional blinks (e.g., [7, 11, 49], and see Chapter 2). The functional coupling between stimulus-specific areas and such higher-order networks is currently considered an essential signature of the access of sensory information to consciousness, making it available to high-level processes, including perceptual categorization, long-term memorization, evaluation, and intentional action.[‡]

To sum up, while the *nociceptive matrix* provides the sensory specificity of the pain experience, the joint activity of the nociceptive and second-order matrices is essential to ensure (a) the modulation of vegetative reactions and internal feelings via anterior insular networks, (b) the attentional modulation of sensory gain by bottom–up/top–down transaction between dorsolateral frontal networks and sensory areas, and (c) the access of nociceptive information to declarative consciousness by activation of a distributed fronto–parieto–temporal network and top–down reentrance in sensory areas.

[‡]The literature in this matter being extensive and complex, the reader is strongly advised to refer to Chapters 2 and 6, which deal in more detail with this issue.

FROM IMMEDIATE PERCEPTION TO PAIN MEMORIES: THIRD-ORDER NETWORKS

While nociceptive and attentional/perceptual networks may suffice to achieve an immediate conscious perception of noxious stimuli, impressive changes of the pain experience can occur without changes in the matrices described above. For instance, the enhancement of subjective pain during the observation of other people's suffering [10, 20, 36] can develop in the absence of significant changes in thalamus, insula, operculum, or anterior cingulate, and has been associated instead with activity in high-level polymodal regions outside the "classical" PM, falling mostly within limbic/paralimbic systems, and including the perigenual cingulate, orbitofrontal cortex, temporal pole, and anterolateral prefrontal areas [19, 20]. Similarly, the pain-relieving effects derived from expectations and beliefs, including placebo effects, self-control over the stimulus, or strong religious values [42, 62, 63] have been associated with activity changes in the orbitofrontal, perigenual cingulate, and anterolateral prefrontal cortices, rather than in the classical PM. Orbitofrontal, perigenual, and anterolateral prefrontal activities were also described when the subjective perception of identical noxious stimuli changed from highly unpleasant to moderately pleasant by hedonic context manipulation [31]. A full dissociation between "core PM" activity and subjective pain reports was recently described during meditation-related analgesia, which was associated with *enhanced* activity in basic PM areas, but *decreased* activity in high-order prefrontal regions (see Chapter 8).

Although presented distinctly for clarity, it is apparent that the prefrontal cortex (PFC) participates in both the second and third-order matrices. The PFC, constitutes more than 12% of the total brain volume in humans, and is not a homogenous area. Growing evidence supports a control hierarchy within the PFC, whereby posterior-to-anterior development mediates progressively abstract control of perceptions and actions [4]. Thus, activities most clearly involved in attentional drive and access to immediate declarative percepts appear to converge in more posterior prefrontal subsections (BA 45-46-47, BA 24-32 dorsal ACC sections), while more rostral and ventromedial areas of the PFC are crucial for identification of the emotional significance of stimuli, production of affective states, and regulation of emotional responses [26]. In particular, the ventromedial PFC (orbitofrontal, perigenual) is considered as a region involved in the voluntary control of unpleasant emotions [34, 45]. While these areas are absent from the classically reported PM [2, 47], their activity appears able to sustain changes in subjective pain without involving sensory or low-level perceptive processes. At variance with pain modulations derived from selective attention or arousal, most emotional manipulations do not appear to change pain experiences by increasing the sensory gain (which would be reflected in enhanced sensory responses), but rather by a "reappraisal" of immediate pain perceptions, in the sense of a *reinterpretation* of the meaning of a stimulus. Such high-level processes require working memory resources, involve medial and lateral prefrontal cortices [19, 20, 26, 42], and appear to follow in time the activation of the basic PM, since the associated physiological changes only occur *after* the operculoinsular and cingulate activations have been elicited [20]. Activity in such third-order networks can therefore modify the immediate percepts driven by the nociceptive and second-order PMs.

Of importance, areas involved in the "reappraisal" matrix such as the perigenual cingulate and orbitofrontal cortices are themselves strongly interconnected with subcortical regions crucial for descending pain control (notably the periaqueductal gray matter). Tonic activation of these areas may therefore not only support modifications in the subjective value of the nociceptive stimulus, but also contribute to a feedback loop that changes the activity of ascending nociceptive systems, thus influence (i.e., bias) the ascending input to cortical targets (see reference [31]). This point is central to the discussion of PM activity changes during chronic pain, but clearly exceeds the scope of this chapter.

CONCLUSION: THE FULL PAIN EXPERIENCE AS AN INTERSECTION OF NEURAL MATRICES

The great merit of the PM concept was to underscore that pain experiences result from coordinated activity in a number of brain regions—that is, the absence of any single "pain center." While some investigators consider the PM as a genuine biomarker of the pain experience—a direct measure of the actual pain—others claim that the PM simply reflects a nonspecific system of salience detection. The viewpoint proposed elaborates and expands existing notions (see reference [35]): in essence, the final conscious experience of pain (the pain we shall remember) results from the interaction of several levels of processing with progressive complexity, in networks that we may tentatively label as "nociceptive," "perceptive-attentional," and "reappraisal-emotional" matrices. Cortical regions receiving spinothalamic afferents ensure the somatic-specific ("bodily") quality of the sensation; they trigger activity in parietal, frontal, and anterior insular circuits not receiving direct STT input but supporting conscious perception, vegetative reactions, and their modulation by attention and vigilance. The immediate perception issued from these activities can itself be modulated by higher-order networks driven by emotional contexts and internal states. This reappraisal determines a privately generated assessment of instant percepts, tuning them up or down as a function of affective states and previous memories, and building what will represent the "subjective experience" available to long-term memory buffers.

The dissociation of such different processing levels as described here, while useful for conceptualization purposes, should not occlude their interdependent and extremely fluid interactivity in real life. Also, this schema does not take into account rapid spinal-limbic routes such as the spino–parabrachio–amygdalar pathway, ensuring access of noxious input to limbic cortices with virtually identical timing as that needed to reach somatosensory areas. Although largely incomplete, existing data show that functional imaging is able to go beyond phenomenological descriptions, and propose testable hypotheses that will, or will not, come true in the following years. The perception of pain appears as an active, interpretative process of the brain, continuously reconstructing itself by integration of sensory inputs with ongoing memories and internal representations. Functional imaging has lent substance to the nociception–perception–suffering model. As stated by Loeser [35], "it is suffering, not pain, that brings patients into doctor's offices (...) Suffering is an emergent property of the human brain and is dependent upon consciousness." The internal experience of "affliction" underlies many distressing aspects shared by corporal and emotional suffering. Searching for this common ground will be with no doubt one of the strongest point of research and discussion in the following years.

ACKNOWLEDGMENTS

Work was supported by the Louise and Allan Edwards Foundation (Ronald Melzack Award 2012), the French Society for the Evaluation and Therapy of Pain, and the LABEX CORTEX (ANR-11-LABX-0042) of Université de Lyon, within the program "Investissements d'Avenir" (ANR-11-IDEX-0007) operated by the French National Research Agency (ANR). The Neurodis Foundation supported PLJ as a visiting scientist to the NeuroPain laboratory.

REFERENCES

1. Apkarian AV. A neural signature for pain. Trends Cogn Sci 2013;17:309–10.
2. Apkarian AV, Bushnell MC, Treede RD, Zubieta JK. Human brain mechanisms of pain perception and regulation in health and disease. Eur J Pain 2005;9:463–84.
3. Apkarian AV, Hodge CJ. Primate spinothalamic pathways: III. Thalamic terminations of the dorsolateral and ventral spinothalamic pathways. J Comp Neurol 1989;288:493–511.
4. Badre D. Cognitive control, hierarchy, and the rostro-caudal organization of the frontal lobes. Trends Cogn Sci 2008;12(5):193–200.

5. Bantick SJ, Wise RG, Ploghaus A, Clare S, Smith SM, Tracey I. Imaging how attention modulates pain in humans using functional MRI. Brain 2002;125:310–9.
6. Bastuji H, Mazza S, Perchet C, Frot M, Mauguière F, Magnin M, Garcia-Larrea L. Filtering the reality: functional dissociation of lateral and medial pain systems during sleep in humans. Hum Brain Mapp 2012;33:2638–49.
7. Beck DM, Rees G, Frith CD, Lavie N. Neural correlates of change detection and change blindness. Nat Neurosci 2001;4:645–50.
8. Biemond A. The conduction of pain above the level of the thalamus opticus. AMA Arch Neurol Psychiatry 1956;75:231–44.
9. Caruana F, Jezzini A, Sbriscia-Fioretti B, Rizzolatti G, Gallese V. Emotional and social behaviors elicited by electrical stimulation of the insula in the macaque monkey. Curr Biol 2011;21(3):195–9.
10. de Wied M, Verbaten MN. Affective pictures processing, attention, and pain tolerance. Pain 2001;90:163–72.
11. Dehaene S, Changeux JP, Naccache L, Sackur J, Sergent C. Conscious, preconscious, and subliminal processing: a testable taxonomy. Trends Cogn Sci 2006;10:204–11.
12. Del Cul A, Baillet S, Dehaene S. Brain dynamics underlying the nonlinear threshold for access to consciousness. PLoS Biol 2007;5(10):e260.
13. Dum RP, Levinthal DJ, Strick PL. The spinothalamic system targets motor and sensory areas in the cerebral cortex of monkeys. J Neurosci 2009;29:14223–35.
14. Eisenberger NI, Lieberman MD. Why rejection hurts: a common neural alarm system for physical and social pain. Trends Cogn Sci 2004;8:294–300.
15. Faymonville ME, Roediger L, Del Fiore G, Delgueldre C, Phillips C, Lamy M, Luxen A, Maquet P, Laureys S. Increased cerebral functional connectivity underlying the antinociceptive effects of hypnosis. Brain Res Cogn Brain Res 2003;17:255–62.
16. Frot M, Faillenot I, Mauguière F. Spatio-temporal gradient of pain evoked responses in the human insula. Hum Brain Mapp 2014;35:5486–99.
17. Frot M, Magnin M, Mauguière F, Garcia-Larrea L. Cortical representation of pain in primary sensory-motor areas (S1/M1)-a study using intracortical recordings in humans. Hum Brain Mapp 2013;34:2655–68.
18. Garcia-Larrea L. The posterior insular-opercular region and the search of a primary cortex for pain. Neurophysiol Clin 2012;42:299–313.
19. Godinho F, Faillenot I, Perchet C, Magnin M, Garcia-Larrea L. How the pain of others enhances our pain: searching the cerebral correlates of "compassional hyperalgesia." Eur J Pain 2012;16:748–59.
20. Godinho F, Magnin M, Frot M, Perchet C, Garcia-Larrea L. Emotional modulation of pain: is it the sensation or what we recall? J Neurosci 2006;26:11454–61.

21. Greenspan JD, Lee RR, Lenz FA. Pain sensitivity alterations as a function of lesion location in the parasylvian cortex. Pain 1999;81:273–82.
22. Head H, Holmes G. Sensory disturbances from cerebral lesions. Brain 1911;34:102–254.
23. Hutchison WD, Davis K, Lozano AM, Tasker RR, Dostrovsky JO. Pain-related neurons in the human cingulate cortex. Nat Neurosci 1999;2:403–405.
24. Iannetti GD, Mouraux A. From the neuromatrix to the pain matrix (and back). Exp Brain Res 2010;205:1–12.
25. Jackson PL, Meltzoff AN, Decety J. How do we perceive the pain of others? A window into the neural processes involved in empathy. Neuroimage 2005;24:771–9.
26. Kalisch R, Wiech K, Critchley HD, Dolan RJ. Levels of appraisal: a medial prefrontal role in high-level appraisal of emotional material. Neuroimage 2006;30:1458–66.
27. Kassubek J, Juengling FD, Els T, Spreer J, Herpers M, Krause T, Moser E, Lücking CH. Activation of a residual cortical network during painful stimulation in long-term postanoxic vegetative state: a $^{15}O\text{-}H_2O$ PET study. J Neurol Sci 2003;212:85–91.
28. Kross E, Berman MG, Mischel W, Smith EE, Wager TD. Social rejection shares somatosensory representations with physical pain. Proc Natl Acad Sci U S A 2011;108:6270–5.
29. Långsjö JW, Alkire MT, Kaskinoro K, Hayama H, Maksimow A, Kaisti KK, Aalto S, Aantaa R, Jääskeläinen SK, Revonsuo A, et al. Returning from oblivion: imaging the neural core of consciousness. J Neurosci 2012;32:4935–43.
30. Legrain V, Iannetti GD, Plaghki L, Mouraux A. The pain matrix reloaded: a salience detection system for the body. Prog Neurobiol 2010;93:111–24.
31. Leknes S, Berna C, Lee MC, Snyder GD, Biele G, Tracey I. The importance of context: when relative relief renders pain pleasant. Pain 2013;154:402–10.
32. Lenz FA, Gracely RH, Romanoski AJ, Hope EJ, Rowaland LH, Dougherty PM. Stimulation in the human somatosensory thalamus can reproduce both the affective and sensory dimensions of previously experienced pain. Nat Med 1995;1:910–3.
33. Lenz FA, Rios M, Chau D, Krauss GL, Zirh TA, Lesser RP. Painful stimuli evoke potentials recorded from the parasylvian cortex in humans. J Neurophysiol 1998;80:2077–88.
34. Levesque J, Eugene F, Joanette Y, Paquette V, Mensour B, Beaudoin G, Leroux JM, Bourgouin P, Beauregard M. Neural circuitry underlying voluntary suppression of sadness. Biol Psychiatry 2003;53:502–10.
35. Loeser JD. Pain and suffering. Clin J Pain 2000;16:S2–S6.
36. Loggia ML, Mogil JS, Bushnell MC. Empathy hurts: compassion for another increases both sensory and affective components of pain perception. Pain 2008;136:168–76.
37. Macdonald G, Leary MR. Why does social exclusion hurt? The relationship between social and physical pain. Psychol Bull 2005;131:202–23.

38. Mazzola L, Isnard J, Peyron R, Mauguière F. Stimulation of the human cortex and the experience of pain: Wilder Penfield's observations revisited. Brain 2012;135:631–40.

39. Mehler WR. The anatomy of the so-called "pain tract" in man: an analysis of the course and distribution of the ascending fingers of the fasciculus anterolateralis. In: French JD, Porter RW, editors. Basic research in paraplegia. Springfield, IL: Charles C. Thomas; 1962. pp. 26–55.

40. Melzack R. Phantom limb and the concept of a neuromatrix. Trends Neurosci 1990;13:88–92.

41. Melzack R, Casey KL. Sensory, motivational, and central control determinants of pain. In: Kenshalo DR, editor. The skin senses. Springfield, IL: Charles C. Thomas; 1968. pp. 423–35.

42. Mohr C, Leyendecker S, Petersen D, Helmchen C. Effects of perceived and exerted pain control on neural activity during pain relief in experimental heat hyperalgesia: a fMRI study. Eur J Pain 2012;16:496–508.

43. Montavont A, Mauguière F, Mazzola L, Garcia-Larrea L, Catenoix H, Ryvlin PH, Isnard J. On the origin of painful somatosensory seizures. Neurology 2015;84:594–601.

44. Ohara S, Anderson WS, Lawson HC, Lee HT, Lenz FA. Endogenous and exogenous modulators of potentials evoked by a painful cutaneous laser (LEPs). Acta Neurochir Suppl 2006;99:77–9.

45. Ohira H, Nomura, M, Ichikawa N, Isowa, T, Iidaka T, Sato, A, Fukuyama S, Nakajima T, Yamada J. Association of neural and physiological responses during voluntary emotion suppression. Neuroimage 2006;29:721–33.

46. Peyron R, Garcia-Larrea L, Gregoire MC, Costes N, Convers P, Lavenne F, Mauguiere F, Michel D, Laurent B. Haemodynamic brain responses to acute pain in humans: sensory and attentional networks. Brain 1999;122:1765–80.

47. Peyron R, Laurent B, Garcia-Larrea L. Functional imaging of brain responses to pain: a review and meta-analysis. Neurophysiol Clin 2000;30:263–88.

48. Rainville P, Duncan GH, Price DD, Carrier B, Bushnell MC. Pain affect encoded in human anterior cingulate but not somatosensory cortex. Science 1997;15;277:968–71.

49. Sergent C, Baillet S, Dehaene S. Timing of the brain events underlying access to consciousness during the attentional blink. Nat Neurosci 2005;8:1391–400.

50. Sescousse G, Redouté J, Dreher JC. The architecture of reward value coding in the human orbitofrontal cortex. J Neurosci 2010;30:13095–104.

51. Shin LM, Dougherty DD, Orr SP, Pitman RK, Lasko M, Macklin ML, Alpert NM, Fischman AJ, Rauch SL. Activation of anterior paralimbic structures during guilt-related script-driven imagery. Biol Psychiatry 2000;48(1):43–50.

52. Singer T, Seymour B, O'Doherty J, Kaube H, Dolan RJ, Frith CD. Empathy for pain involves the affective but not sensory components of pain. Science 2004;303:1157–62.

53. Sprenger C, Eippert F, Finsterbusch J, Bingel U, Rose M, Büchel C. Attention modulates spinal cord responses to pain. Curr Biol 2012;22:1019–22.

54. Talbot JD, Marrett S, Evans AC, Meyer E, Bushnell MC, Duncan GH. Multiple representations of pain in human cerebral cortex. Science 1991;251:1355–8.

55. Tattersall JE, Cervero F, Lumb BM. Viscerosomatic neurons in the lower thoracic spinal cord of the cat: excitations and inhibitions evoked by splanchnic and somatic nerve volleys and by stimulation of brain stem nuclei. J Neurophysiol 1986;56:1411–23.

56. Tracey I, Mantyh PW. The cerebral signature for pain perception and its modulation. Neuron 2007;55:377–91.

57. Tracey I, Ploghaus A, Gati JS, Clare S, Smith S, Menon RS, Matthews PM. Imaging attentional modulation of pain in the periaqueductal gray in humans. J Neurosci 2002;22:2748–52.

58. Valet M, Sprenger T, Boecker H, Willoch F, Rummeny E, Conrad B, Erhard P, Tolle TR. Distraction modulates connectivity of the cingulo-frontal cortex and the midbrain during pain—an fMRI analysis. Pain 2004;109:399–408.

59. Vogt BA. Pain and emotion interactions in subregions of the cingulate gyrus. Nat Rev Neurosci 2005;6:533–44.

60. Wager TD, Atlas LY, Lindquist MA, Roy M, Woo CW, Kross E. An fMRI-based neurologic signature of physical pain. N Engl J Med 2013;368:1388–97.

61. Wicker B, Keysers C, Plailly J, Royet JP, Gallese V, Rizzolatti G. Both of us disgusted in My insula: the common neural basis of seeing and feeling disgust. Neuron 2003;40:655–64.

62. Wiech K, Farias M, Kahane G, Shackel N, Tiede W, Tracey I. An fMRI study measuring analgesia enhanced by religion as a belief system. Pain 2008;139:467–76.

63. Wiech K, Ploner M, Tracey I. Neurocognitive aspects of pain perception. Trends Cogn Sci 2008;12:306–13.

64. Willer JC, Boureau F, Albe-Fessard D. Supraspinal influences on nociceptive flexion reflex and pain sensation in man. Brain Res 1979;179:61–8.

SECTION 2

Modulating Pain by Modulating Consciousness

Neurobiological Aspects of the Pain Experience during Psychophysiological Changes of the Conscious State

CHAPTER 5

Pain Perception during Sleep

Hélène Bastuji and Gilles Lavigne

Sleep is a state of altered consciousness associated with a decrease, not a total absence, of reactivity to most exogenous and endogenous somatic stimuli, distinct from hypnosis, anesthesia, and coma. A sleeping individual is thus able to filter all types of sensory inputs depending on sleep depth and on his or her relevance for body integrity, that is, threatening or not. What happens when a sleeper receives nociceptive information, with a potential to be painful, is not yet fully understood, but new knowledge has emerged in the last two decades.

PAIN

Pain experience reflects interacting sensory, affective, and cognitive dimensions. Garcia-Larrea and Peyron [15] recently proposed a conceptualization of the pain matrix as a system composed of several interacting networks. In their model, a nociceptive matrix receiving spinothalamic projections, and mainly composed of the posterior operculoinsular and midcingulate areas, ensures the bodily specificity of pain. Transition from cortical nociception to conscious pain relies on a second-order network, including posterior parietal, prefrontal, and anterior insular areas. Second-order regions are not nociceptive-specific but allow the modulation of vegetative reactions and internal feelings, the attentional modulation of sensory gain, and the access of nociceptive information to an organized declarative consciousness. The pain experience can still be modified as a function of beliefs, emotions, and expectations through activity of third-order areas, including the orbitofrontal and perigenual/limbic networks. During wakefulness, the interplay of these networks and sensory inputs are the principal components of the individualized and context-dependent pain experience. Environmental factors (i.e., past experience, mood influences, diet), neuroinflammatory mediators, and genes expression are contributing to the sensory and emotional/affection reaction to nociception and pain [29, 48].

SLEEP

Over the 24-hour circadian cycle, sleep lasts 7–9 hours, including a diurnal nap in some subjects, depending on the interplay of polymorphism of sleep and clock genes, and the environment [13]. Sleep is further divided into non-REM (NREM) and REM (for **R**apid **E**ye **M**ovements) sleep, the latter also named "Paradoxical sleep", which are repeated three to five times during the ultradian sleep cycle. The transition from waking to NREM sleep is accompanied by changes in the electroencephalographic (EEG) activity: from low-amplitude high-frequency to high-amplitude low-frequency activity (<4 Hz) and onset of sleep spindles [43]. Slow-waves EEG activity during NREM sleep reflect a slow oscillation (<1 Hz) of cortical neurons with up and down states, associated with neuronal depolarization and hyperpolarization respectively [43], reflecting the dynamic interaction between thalamic and cortical network activity [8]. During REM sleep, EEG shows low-amplitude high-frequency activity resembling that of wakefulness with a paradoxical state of nearly complete muscle atonia. Sleep is accompanied by global changes in neuromodulation, with decrease in norepinephrine, histamine, and orexin activity during NREM and REM sleep, and a decrease in acetylcholine neurotransmission during NREM sleep only [16]. Sleep is also important for synaptic plasticity and renormalization of synaptic strength in many functions including memory [45]. The regulation of cyclic alternations of NREM and REM sleep episodes also depends on circadian and homeostatic processes, which are under the control of brain stem and diencephalon structures, with "sleep promoting" and "wake promoting" areas mutually inhibiting each other [40].

While sleep was usually regarded as a global brain phenomenon, we now know that sleep is associated with localized changes in brain activity. At sleep onset the thalamic deactivation most often precedes that of numerous cortical areas by several minutes [26]. During NREM sleep, spindles are mostly local phenomena and slow waves propagate along major anatomical pathways [31]. Furthermore, slow-wave activity, prevalent over frontal cortex, can be locally regulated as a function of prior use and plastic processes [35, 45]. During REM sleep, while the cortex shows a low-amplitude, high-frequency activity, the activity of the posterior thalamus is characterized by low-frequency waves of high amplitude [25]. These local aspects of the sleeping brain may be involved in the fluctuations that occur in the processing of sensory information during sleep.

The lack of responsiveness toward external stimulation delivered during sleep led to hypothesize a functional disconnection between the cerebral cortex and the external world, due to a thalamic "gate" [44]. Despite the existence of these gating mechanisms controlling and attenuating the effect of external stimulations [9, 44], the hypothesis postulating a sensorial isolation of the sleeper has been now reconsidered. While such hypothesis was based on animal cellular studies, recent evidence suggests that during sleep the brain stem and the brain can react to significant or threatening situations including nociception. Indeed, fading of consciousness during sleep is not caused by a suspension of neural activity, since neural firing rates can be maintained and even increased during sleep [34, 46]. Evoked responses in primary sensory cortices are largely preserved during sleep [1, 33]. Furthermore, despite the absence of awareness and behavioral responsiveness, sleepers can still extract task-relevant information from external stimuli and covertly prepare for appropriate motor responses [1, 18]. Sleep is not anesthesia or coma (see Chapters 1 and 6): in physiological sleep, a gating system remains active to trigger a response that can preserve sleep continuity and allow the return of consciousness to external stimuli only for survival dimensions that will then awaken an individual.

PROCESSING AND REACTING TO NOCICEPTIVE STIMULI DURING SLEEP

During sleep, the reactivity to nociceptive stimuli expresses itself in different ways, including cortical and autonomic activation, simple motor reflex, periodic limb or jaw movement (bruxism), sleep stage shifts, and unconscious or conscious disruption of sleep continuity. While some of these expressions are systematically present, others occur inconsistently.

Obligatory Responses to Nociceptive Stimuli during Sleep

While phasic nociceptive stimuli delivered during sleep are followed by brief arousals or longer unconscious awakenings in only 30% of the cases [3, 22], they most frequently trigger a cardiac activation and a response of the somatosensory cortex, suggesting that the processing of nociceptive information is partly preserved during all sleep stages.

Nociceptive stimulations delivered during sleep give rise to a transient increase in heart rate, which exceeds that evoked by non-nociceptive stimuli [24]. Even when nociceptive stimuli did not produce cortical arousals, cardiac reactivity, sympathetically driven, was preserved, but of smaller magnitude than that observed in the absence of subsequent arousals [7]. Conversely, cardiac reactivity was not modulated by the sleep stage in which the stimulus occurred. Thus, the level of autonomic response to phasic nociceptive inputs seems to depend more on cortical activation rather than on a given state of vigilance. This autonomic reactivity might be considered as the first mechanism that allows a potential behavioral response and could partly modulate the occurrence of cortical arousals.

Even in the absence of behavioral arousal/awakening, the cortical processing of nociceptive stimuli is partly preserved during sleep. Nociceptive-specific brain responses can be produced using cutaneous infrared laser stimuli, which specifically activate thin myelinated (A-δ) and unmyelinated (C) fibers and yield cerebral potentials reflecting cortical pain processing [14]. Although early studies performed during short naps suggested a loss of cortical potentials to stimulation of A-δ or C-fibers during drowsiness and light sleep [17], it was later shown [3] that cortical responses to nociceptive laser stimuli remained present during all sleep stages (Fig. 5-1). Nevertheless, compared to wakefulness, sleep induced a decrease in the amplitude of the responses, as well as morphologic and topographic changes. In stage 2, this response was often followed by a high-amplitude negative wave with typical features of a K-complex. During REM, the morphology was similar to that of waking, but frontal components showed strong attenuation, consistent with the reported frontal metabolic deactivation in this stage (see [35]).

In an intracerebral study performed in epileptic patients receiving nociceptive stimuli, one of the three crucial areas of the pain matrix, the mid-anterior cingulate cortex (mid-ACC) had a markedly depressed activity [2] (Fig. 5-1), which was explicitly restored in case of behavioral response reactivation [28]. Since mid-ACC responses are mostly responsible for the scalp frontal distribution of laser-evoked responses [36], the absence of activation of the mid-ACC during REM could explain the topographic changes observed on scalp recordings. Furthermore, since this area is supposed to activate the attentional and motor components induced by pain [47], the suppression of its activation might also explain why oriented behavior to external sensory input is particularly depressed during this sleep stage [30]. Such differential attenuation appeared specific to REM, since during sleep stage 2 evoked potential amplitudes were similarly attenuated in both sensory and cingulate areas [2].

Interestingly, when the noxious stimulation was followed by an arousal, the cortical response included a late positive component [3]. During wakefulness, this component has been considered as an equivalent of the cognitive "P300" (or P3b) wave [41]. The strong association between the presence of this late positive wave and subsequent arousal reactions to nociceptive stimuli suggests that these stimulations have to undergo a certain level of cognitive processing to give rise to a behavioral response without declarative consciousness.

Inconsistent Responses to Nociceptive Stimuli during Sleep

Fig. 5-2 summarizes the sequence of events that can be observed from the application of nociceptive stimuli to a sleeping subject. The first level corresponds to a simple sensory cortical and heart rate activation, the second to a brief arousal with an increased cardiac activation and a possible body movement, the third to an unconscious awakening, and finally the conscious awakening during which the subject can express the sensory experience as "pain" with a sensory and/or emotional appreciation.

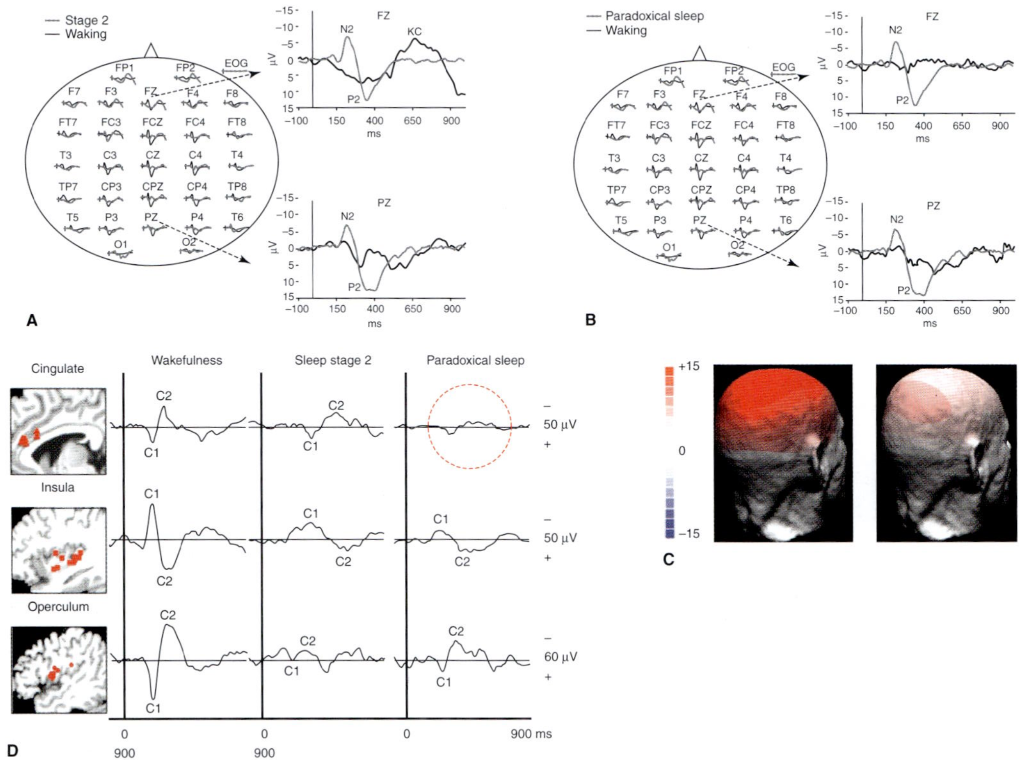

FIGURE 5-1 Superimposition of grand-averages of LEPs during waking and stage 2 **(A)** and REM sleep **(B)**. For both, Left: scalp distribution of LEPs. Right: traces obtained at Fz **(top)** and Pz **(bottom)** during waking **(gray)** and stage 2 or REM sleep **(black)**. Note that during stage 2 the response contains a negative late wave of K-complex on Fz and that on Pz N2/P2 is present with decreased amplitude. During REM sleep the response is virtually absent on Fz while it persists with reduced amplitude on Pz. **C:** 3D activity maps at the latency of the P2 component during waking **(left)** and REM sleep **(right)**. **D:** Grand average LEPs in referential recording mode during waking, sleep stage 2, and REM sleep in the operculum **(bottom)**, the insula **(middle)**, and the mid-anterior cingulate **(top)**. On the left part of the figure, for each structure, the contacts where the maximal amplitudes of the C1–C2 components were recorded are indicated. Note the depressed response in the cingulate during REM sleep. LEP, laser-evoked potential; REM, rapid eye movement. (Adapted from Bastuji et al. [2, 3].)

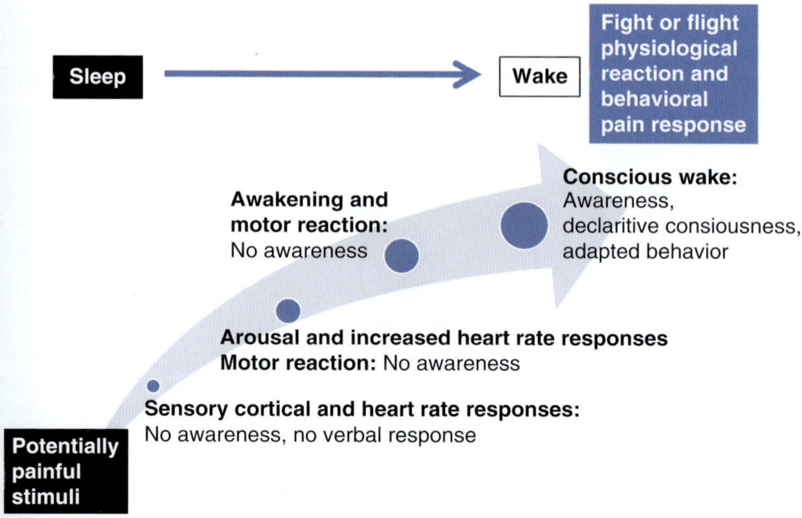

FIGURE 5-2 Crescendo of physiological response from unconscious nociception to consciousness of pain.

Nociceptive Reflex

The pain withdrawal reflex, classically used to behaviorally assess pain sensitivity, is an involuntary action aiming at taking away the part of the body receiving the nociceptive stimulus. This reflex can be mainly mediated at the spinal level (as the tail flick) or involve an upper brain motor response (hind paw withdrawal to paw lick).

Studies performed during sleep in animals provide contradictory results. In cats, the nociceptive tail flick reflex latency to radiant heat was increased (analgesic response) in non-REM to REM sleep as compared to wakefulness [19]. In rats, the hind paw withdrawal latency was found unchanged with laser heat across sleep/wake states but, surprisingly, was shorter (algesic response) during slow-wave sleep than during waking when light radiant heat was applied [27]. Despite the fact that rats remove their hind limb from noxious heat during sleep, and then quickly return to sleep afterward, these findings support that during sleep nociception remains an active protective process to preserve body integrity. In humans, the polysynaptic nociceptive flexion reflex threshold (R3 reflex) has also been used to assess nociception during sleep. The R3 reflex is induced by an electrical stimulation of a nerve and its threshold, amplitude, and duration are outcome measures. In comparison to wakefulness, the threshold to evoke a R3 reflex was increased during stage 2 and also in deep NREM sleep; it was even higher during REM sleep [39]. The amplitude and duration of the R3 reflex were higher during REM sleep than during wakefulness, suggesting a facilitating effect of REM sleep on spinal polysynaptic nociceptive reflexes. Thus, a paradoxical mechanism on one side preserves sleep continuity, and on the other side keeps a protective mechanism to prepare a reactive behavior, a "flight or fight" response.

Quantitative sensory testing (QST) protocols using thermal, mechanical, and chemical models of experimental pain have been also used to observe motor reactivity during sleep in humans. With a painful heat thermode [23] or laser [3] stimuli, a nocifensive behavioral–sensory–motor response was reported to occur during all sleep stages, and is more likely to occur in association with a sleep arousal (brief heart, brain, and muscle activation); these nocifensive responses were observed in the absence of cortical or behavioral arousals, following 2.5–11% of the stimulations. Therefore, sleep-reflex behaviors in response to nociceptive stimuli can be observed without triggering a discontinuation of sleep and, interestingly, without inducing any hyperalgesia in the morning following the experimental sleep session [4, 10, 23].

Sleep Disruption by Nociceptive Stimuli

In case of painful stimulation, sleep disruption is frequently observed both in clinical and experimental conditions [3, 4, 12, 22, 23]. As described above, the responsiveness to sleep disruption can be considered as an important protective mechanism that prepares the individual to react to homeostatic-threatening stimuli by enhancing his or her level of consciousness. Thereby and as expected, somatosensory nociceptive stimuli tend to induce more arousals than non-nociceptive somatic stimuli [3, 23] or repetitive auditory stimuli [1, 22] (Table 5-1). Awakening thresholds may differ according to sleep depth, suggesting that nociceptive inputs are submitted to a state-dependent gating [44]. As previously reported with other sensory stimuli [5], the intensity needed to trigger an arousal response in deep NREM and REM sleep was also reported to be higher than that needed to do so during light NREM sleep [4, 10, 11, 23]. Nevertheless, such sleep stage dependence was observed with thermal and mechanical stimulations, but was lost with longer stimulus durations (hypertonic muscular saline injections) [22], or brief cutaneous laser stimuli [3]. These latter stimuli induced an equipotent frequency of awakening responses across all NREM and REM sleep stages (see Table 5-1). Reactions to muscle or joint stimuli have also been described to be of higher magnitude than those to cutaneous stimuli [11], and as expected the duration of sleep disruption is longer with sustained [22] than with brief painful stimuli [3]. This suggests that the relevance of these stimulations might activate a top-down mechanism to override the brain stem neurons responsible for sleep maintenance and, consequently, activate the ascending arousal system to drive an awakening. Nevertheless, as mentioned above, it is of interest to note that brief pain-related stimuli, all perceived as painful during wakefulness, were not reported to be perceived by healthy volunteer subjects during sleep [2, 3, 22, 23]. The incorporation of nociceptive stimuli into dream contents is also unusual [32] and

TABLE 5-1 **Arousal Responsiveness in Approximate Percentage across Sleep Stages with Experimental External or Internal Stimulus Applied during Sleep in Humans**

Type of Stimulus	Duration	Light NREM (%)	Deep NREM (%)	REM Sleep
Sound (42 dB) [22]	1 s	6	0	0%
Vibration (70 Hz, 3 Giga) [22]	1 s	38	0	15%
Warm heat (37°C) No pain [23]	6–12 s	8	1	5%
Cold (24°C) No pain [23]	6–12 s	33	20	11%
Heat pain (47°C) [23]	6–12 s	48	28	31%
Laser pain [3]	5 ms	45	23	42% ns
Saline hypertonic infusion [22]	26 s	40	28	46% ns

Abbreviation: ns, no statistical difference between sleep stages.

might be more associated with stimulus-related unpleasantness and duration, rather than with intensity [22, 38].

INTERACTIONS BETWEEN PAIN, REM SLEEP, AND PLACEBO-INDUCED EXPECTATIONS OF PAIN RELIEF

As described above, external stimuli are processed differently during NREM and REM sleep. We showed that reactivity to combined auditory and vibrotactile stimuli is lower during deep NREM in comparison to light NREM and REM sleep, and were much more variable during REM [22]. Indeed, even if REM sleep is seen as a state isolated from the external milieu, it is not a homogenous state as it is made of tonic (i.e., muscle hypotonia and absence of REMs) and phasic periods (i.e., muscle hypotonia and REMs). These two REM patterns have different levels of reactivity since the incidence of behavioral reactions to external stimuli was found higher in tonic than in phasic REM periods with auditory [5] and with nociceptive ones [3], while nociceptive information remains similarly processed up to the cortex in both periods [3].

Furthermore, using an experimental protocol in which a healthy non–chronic pain subject is awaken during different sleep stages and in which sensory heat pain perception is assessed using visual analog scale (VAS), a reduction of 90% in pain intensity was observed if awakening is done from REM sleep [10]. This suggested that during REM sleep either sleep inertia, that is, longer time to get back to functional wake state, is more powerful or REM sleep may contribute to some form of analgesia. The relevance of such finding is further discussed below in relation to placebo analgesia conditioning (PAC) and role of REM sleep.

Before describing such experimental findings in more detail, we have to clarify that such effects are not specific to pain. In fact, sleep, and more specifically REM sleep, plays important roles in both memory consolidation and processing of emotion; this is of relevance to this chapter since pain perception and responsiveness are interrelated [35, 37]. In addition, the observation that prefrontal cortex activity during waking related to an experimental fear condition and the generic dimension of memory seem to be both REM sleep dependent [42], opens further considerations when assessing pain and sleep interaction.

Placebo Analgesia Conditioning (PAC) and Pain Relief Expectation

A commonly believed dogma establishes that the PAC requires full consciousness and vigilance to develop. We recently challenged such dogma by applying pain stimuli during wake and/or during or following sleep, after instructing participants that a medication will be analgesic in comparison to the application of an inert/control substance [20, 21]. The substance used in both PAC conditions was in fact an inert cream applied to the skin, and stimulus temperature was dropped to mimic analgesia. The experimental conditions to assess the subject's thermal pain threshold during waking were based on applying thermal stimuli from nonpainful ranges (32°–40°C) up to heat pain (around 45°–47°C) to the shoulder skin. Then the "active" cream was applied with instructions given that such *medical* cream had been shown in the scientific literature to be analgesic. In another session the cream was applied to the other side (crossover sequence between individuals), with the instruction that the cream was inert and was used as the "control substance." We then repeated the thermal stimulation at the pain threshold and, on the medication side only, the temperature was reduced by 2° to mimic an analgesic effect. More than half of the subjects are usually placebo analgesia responders to such procedure [37].

Three studies were done with such paradigm. In the first one, we observed that reinforcement (e.g., repeating the procedure) of the placebo conditioning before sleep onset, in comparison to basic instruction, was associated to longer REM sleep duration and less PAC effect on next morning tests, while leaving the subjects sleeping with initial conditioning reduced REM and potentiate PAC on pain relief expectation [20]. Hence, less REM during sleep of PAC subjects was associated with higher expectation of analgesia and pain relief.

In a second study, we used clonidine, an alpha autonomic blocker that suppresses most of the REM sleep, to assess if the absence of REM sleep modulated PAC across the sleep period. REM sleep suppression induced (1) stronger PAC, (2) unchanged expectations of pain relief, and (3) a positive and string correlation between placebo analgesia and pain relief expectations. This result suggests that REM sleep contributes to (inhibits) placebo analgesia independently of pain relief expectations [6].

Finally, a third study assessed whether full consciousness is required for placebo analgesia to take place. Pain stimuli were applied during sleep to subjects being instructed that an analgesic cream will prevent pain perception. We used the same PAC paradigm in a two consecutive crossover study nights design with full polysomnographic recordings in a sleep laboratory. Compared to a control night (inert cream), the night with the fake active analgesic cream condition (the PAC) was associated to (1) a lower response rate of arousal evoked by the noxious stimuli during REM sleep, (2) a reduction in the number of stimuli recalled the next morning, and (3) an increased activity of theta EEG activity in prefrontal cortex during the pain stimulus that was correlated with the level of the expected pain relief anticipated by the subject prior to sleep (Laverdure Dupont, IASP abstract [21]). These results further support some interaction of REM sleep with PAC pain relief expectation; less REM helps to consolidate expectations for pain relief, and pain during REM is partially blunted, attenuating its processing to a conscious experience reportable after sleep.

CONCLUSION

Overall, recent evidence supports that: (1) the access of nociceptive information to declarative consciousness is deficient during sleep; (2) the level of networking activity in the nociceptive matrix is attenuated during sleep in comparison to the higher-sensory specificity of the pain experience observed during wake state; (3) although some nociceptive network reactivity remains present during sleep, it is modulated according to sleep stage and the type of experimental sensory-nociceptive stimuli used; (4) brief and high-intensity painful stimuli seem to disrupt sleep in only 30% of the patients, suggesting fluctuations in the brain's ability to integrate and differentiate nociceptive information. The factors responsible for this, possibly related to fluctuations of the balance between local and global sleep phenomena, remain to be identified.

During sleep, any sensory inputs to the brain trigger the processing of dichotomic choice, either preserving the continuity of sleep or maintaining the survival protective reflex. Ultimately, many cognitive processes linked to pain perception and reaction are modulated or enhanced during sleep, such as memory, emotion, or placebo analgesia conditioning.

REFERENCES

1. Bastuji H, Garcia-Larrea L. Human auditory information processing during sleep assessed with evoked potentials. In: Parmeggiani PL, Velluti R, editors. The physiological nature of sleep. London: Imperial College Press; 2006. pp. 509–35.
2. Bastuji H, Mazza S, Perchet C, Frot M, Mauguière F, Magnin M, Garcia-Larrea L. Filtering the reality: functional dissociation of lateral and medial pain systems during sleep in humans. Hum Brain Mapp 2012;33:2638–49.
3. Bastuji H, Perchet C, Legrain V, Montes C, Garcia-Larrea L. Laser evoked responses to painful stimulation persist during sleep and predict subsequent arousals. Pain 2008;137:589–99.
4. Bentley AJ, Newton S, Zio CD. Sensitivity of sleep stages to painful thermal stimuli. J Sleep Res 2003;12:143–7.
5. Bonnet MH. Performance during sleep. In: Webb W, editor. Biological rhythms, sleep and performance. Chichester: John Wiley; 1982. pp. 205–37.
6. Chouchou F, Chauny JM, Rainville P, Lavigne G. Selective REM deprivation improves placebo analgesia. Plos One 2015 Dec 17;10(12):e0144992. doi: 10.1371/journal.pone.0144992.
7. Chouchou F, Pichot V, Perchet C, Legrain V, Garcia-Larrea L, Roche F, Bastuji H. Autonomic pain responses during sleep: a study of heart rate variability. Eur J Pain 2011;15:554–60.
8. Crunelli V, Hughes SW. The slow (<1 Hz) rhythm of non-REM sleep: a dialogue between three cardinal oscillators. Nat Neurosci 2010;13:9–17.
9. Czisch M, Wetter TC, Kaufmann C, Pollmächer T, Holsboer F, Auer DP. Altered processing of acoustic stimuli during sleep: reduced auditory activation and visual deactivation detected by a combined fMRI/EEG study. Neuroimage 2002;16:251–8.
10. Daya VG, Bentley AJ. Perception of experimental pain is reduced after provoked waking from rapid eye movement sleep. J Sleep Res 2010;19:317–22.
11. Drewes AM, Nielsen KD, Arendt-Nielsen L, Birket-Smith L, Hansen LM. The effect of cutaneous and deep pain on the electroencephalogram during sleep: an experimental study. Sleep 1997;20:632–40.
12. Finan PH, Goodin BR, Smith MT. The association of sleep and pain: an update and a path forward. J Pain 2013;14:1539–52.
13. Gaggioni G, Maquet P, Schmidt C, Dijk DJ, Vandewalle G. Neuroimaging, cognition, light and circadian rhythms. Front Syst Neurosci 2014;8:126. doi:10.3389/fnsys.2014.00126

14. Garcia-Larrea L, Frot M, Valeriani M. Brain generators of laser evoked potentials: from dipoles to functional significance. Neurophysiol Clin 2003;33:279–92.

15. Garcia-Larrea L, Peyron R. Pain matrices and neuropathic pain matrices: a review. Pain 2013;154(suppl 1):S29–S43.

16. Jones BE. From waking to sleeping: neuronal and chemical substrates. Trends Pharmacol Sci 2005;26:578–86.

17. Kakigi R, Wang X, Inui K, Qiu Y. Modulation of pain-related cortical activity by sleep and attention. In: Lavigne G, Sessle BJ, Choinière M, Soja PJ, editors. Sleep and pain. Seattle: IASP Press; 2007. pp. 175–87.

18. Kouider S, Andrillon T, Barbosa LS, Goupil L, Bekinschtein TA. Inducing task-relevant responses to speech in the sleeping brain. Curr Biol 2014;24:2208–14.

19. Kshatri AM, Baghdoyan HA, Lydic R. Cholinomimetics, but not morphine, increase antinociceptive behavior from pontine reticular regions regulating rapid-eye-movement sleep. Sleep 1998;21:677–85.

20. Laverdure-Dupont D, Rainville P, Montplaisir J, Lavigne G. Changes in rapid eye movement sleep associated with placebo-induced expectations and analgesia. J Neurosci 2009;29:11745–52.

21. Laverdure-Dupont D, Rainville P, Montplaisir J, Lavigne G. Relief expectation and sleep. Rev Neurosci 2010;21:381–95.

22. Lavigne G, Brousseau M, Kato T, Mayer P, Manzini C, Guitard F, Monplaisir J. Experimental pain perception remains equally active over all sleep stages. Pain 2004;110:646–55.

23. Lavigne G, Zucconi M, Castronova C, Manzini C, Marchettini P, Smirne S. Sleep arousal response to experimental thermal stimulation during sleep in human subjects free of pain and sleep problems. Pain 2000;84:283–290.

24. Lavigne GJ, Zucconi M, Castronovo V, Manzini C, Veglia F, Smirne S, Ferini-Strambi L. Heart rate changes during sleep in response to experimental thermal (nociceptive) stimulations in healthy subjects. Clin Neurophysiol 2001;112:532–5.

25. Magnin M, Bastuji H, Garcia-Larrea L, Mauguière F. Human thalamic medial pulvinar nucleus is not activated during paradoxical sleep. Cereb Cortex 2004;14:858–62.

26. Magnin M, Rey M, Bastuji H, Guillemant P, Mauguière F, Garcia-Larrea L. Thalamic deactivation at sleep onset precedes that of the cerebral cortex in humans. Proc Natl Acad Sci U S A 2010;107:3829–33.

27. Mason P, Escobedo I, Burgin C, Bergan J, Lee JH, Last EJ, Holub AL. Nociceptive responsiveness during slow-wave sleep and waking in the rat. Sleep 2001;24:32–8.

28. Mazza S, Perchet C, Frot M, Michael GA, Magnin M, Garcia-Larrea L, Bastuji H. Asleep but aware? Brain Cogn 2014;87:7–15.

29. Mogil JS. Pain genetics: past, present and future. Trends Genet 2012;28:258–66.

30. Morrison AR, Sanford LD, Ball WA, Mann G, Ross RJ. Stimulus-elicited behavior in rapid eye movement sleep without atonia. Behav Neurosci 1995;109:972–9.

31. Murphy M, Riedner BA, Huber R, Massimini M, Ferrarelli F, Tononi G. Source modeling sleep slow waves. Proc Natl Acad Sci U S A 2009;106:1608–13.

32. Nielsen TA, McGregor DL, Zadra A, Ilnicki D, Ouellet L. Pain in dreams. Sleep 1993;16:490–8.

33. Nir Y, Vyazovskiy VV, Cirelli C, Banks MI, Tononi G. Auditory responses and stimulus-specific adaptation in rat auditory cortex are preserved across NREM and REM sleep. Cereb Cortex 2015;25:1362–78.

34. Pedemonte M, Velluti RA. What individual neurons tell us about encoding and sensory processing in sleep. In: Parmeggiani PL, Velluti R, editors. The physiological nature of sleep. London: Imperial College Press; 2006. pp. 489–508.

35. Peigneux P. Neuroimaging studies of sleep and memory in humans. Curr Top Behav Neurosci 2015;25:239–68.

36. Perchet C, Godinho F, Mazza S, Frot M, Legrain V, Magnin M, Garcia-Larrea L. Evoked potentials to nociceptive stimuli delivered by CO_2 or Nd:YAP lasers. Clin Neurophysiol 2008;119:2615–22.

37. Price TJ, Inyang KE. Commonalities between pain and memory mechanisms and their meaning for understanding chronic pain. Prog Mol Biol Transl Sci 2015;131:409–34.

38. Raymond I, Nielsen TA, Lavigne G, Choinière M. Incorporation of pain in dreams of hospitalized burn victims. Sleep 2002;25:765–70.

39. Sandrini G, Milanov I, Rossi B, Murri L, Alfonsi E, Moglia A, Nappi G. Effects of sleep on spinal nociceptive reflexes in humans. Sleep 2001;24:13–7.

40. Saper CB, Fuller PM, Pederson NP, Lu J, Scammell TE. Sleep state switching. Neuron 2010;68:1023–42.

41. Siedenberg R, Treede RD. Laser-evoked potentials: exogenous and endogenous components. Electroencephalogr Clin Neurophysiol 1996;100:240–9.

42. Spoormaker VI, Gvozdanovic GA, Sämann PG, Czisch M. Ventromedial prefrontal cortex activity and rapid eye movement sleep are associated with subsequent fear expression in human subjects. Exp Brain Res 2014;232:1547–54.

43. Steriade M. Grouping of brain rhythms in corticothalamic systems. Neuroscience 2006;137:1087–106.

44. Steriade M, Jones EG, McCormick DA. The thalamus during brain disconnection. In: Steriade M, Jones EG, McCormick DA, editors. Thalamus. Amsterdam: Elsevier; 1997. pp. 536–49.

45. Tononi G, Cirelli C. Sleep and the price of plasticity: from synaptic and cellular homeostasis to memory consolidation and integration. Neuron 2014;81:12–34.

46. Tononi G, Massimini M. Why does consciousness fade in early sleep? Ann N Y Acad Sci 2008;1129:330–4.

47. Vogt BA. Pain and emotion interactions in subregions of the cingulate gyrus. Nat Rev Neurosci 2005;6:533–45.

48. Wiech K, Edwards R, Moseley GL, Berna C, Ploner M, Tracey I. Dissociable neural mechanisms underlying the modulation of pain and anxiety? An FMRI pilot study. PLoS One 2014;9:e110654.

CHAPTER 6

Pharmacological Approaches to Pain and Consciousness Using Functional Neuroimaging

Irene Tracey and Katie Warnaby

BACKGROUND

Powerful ways for better understanding pain, analgesia, relief, and altered states of consciousness are offered via pharmacological neuroimaging paradigms. This is where a drug is administered to volunteers alongside neuroimaging data acquisition. Most experiments to date have used functional magnetic resonance imaging (oftentimes called phFMRI), though there exists a strong early and periodic literature deploying positron-emission tomography (PET). Two modes of application are commonly used: (1) imaging the brain's response after acute or chronic administration of the drug and without any concurrent stimulation (i.e., no pain or sensory/cognitive task), and (2) imaging how the brain's response to a sensory stimulus or cognitive task is altered due to the concurrent presence of a drug (acutely or chronically administered). Relatedly, you can degrade the state of consciousness during anesthesia to determine how this impacts perception and awareness. The second mode of application is more commonly employed these days. The first mode is generally limited to PET studies where questions are focused on where and to what extent the drug binds within the human brain.

The popularity of phFMRI is growing as researchers recognize what a powerful tool it is for manipulating and probing the "state" of pain or consciousness to reveal underpinning mechanisms. Similarly, industry has long recognized the value of phFMRI and PET for the analgesic drug discovery process and has been pivotal in driving forward this field with their academic collaborations. We should note that although FMRI has been the predominant tool in such studies, there are many other physiological measures from the human brain that the MR modality can obtain which lend themselves to pharmacological studies—that is, neurochemical (magnetic resonance spectroscopy), structural, resting state networks (connectivity patterns and changes), arterial spin labeling, and diffusion imaging (white matter integrity/tracts). These measurements are now starting to be combined in "traditional" pharmacological imaging studies, and so the field generally refers to phMRI studies. Also, the reader should be aware that phMRI is used in preclinical studies, though to a lesser extent than human studies.

NEUROIMAGING ANESTHESIA–INDUCED ALTERED STATES OF CONSCIOUSNESS

Here, we will limit the discussion to studies exploring how anesthetic agents influence brain processing to produce altered states of consciousness. As the triad of anesthesia (analgesia, muscle relaxation, and hypnosis/awareness) has pain and awareness at its core, we will explore how such changes impact nociceptive processing and an awareness of pain alongside other sensory stimuli. This field is relatively young and very few laboratories work in this challenging arena. Conducting neuroimaging while subjects are under general anesthesia is one of the most difficult types of experiment to perform—both from a safety and practical perspective. This explains why the literature is relatively sparse compared to pain neuroimaging and phMRI. Understandably, there are far more electrophysiological-based studies, but we will discuss only a few of those briefly here. The interested reader is referred to the following reviews that summarize key aspects of this literature and relate it more broadly to issues surrounding consciousness, anesthesia, coma, and vegetative states [7, 29, 32, 37].

Fig. 6-1 nicely illustrates the complex relationship between behavior and increasing dose of anesthetic agent. Key features of this journey that neuroimaging/electrophysiological approaches might help identify and are relevant to the anesthetist, neuroscientist, and patient include the following:

1. What neural event(s) underpin loss of behavioral responsiveness (LOBR) and what does this mean in terms of interoceptive awareness?
2. What brain changes occur during further increases in dose of anesthetic agent that might indicate loss of perception to sensory events (e.g., nociceptive inputs and pain)? An efficacious *individualized brain-based biomarker* is much needed as most anesthetics are administered based upon population responses ("average") using nonbrain and indirect (e.g., heart and respiration rate) changes to indicate when it might be safe to start the surgical procedure without fear of pain, awareness, or movement.

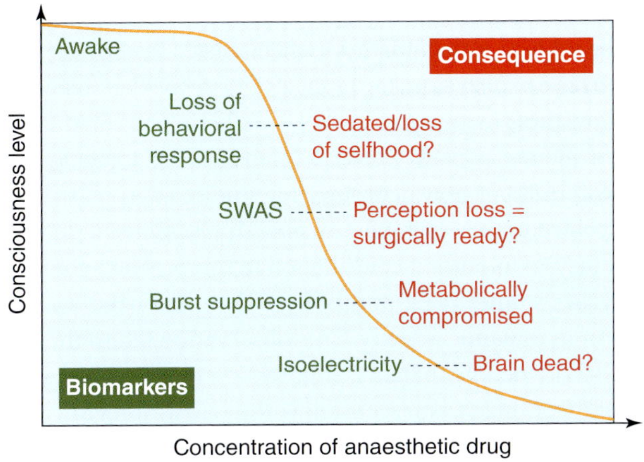

FIGURE 6-1 Schematic illustrating the relationship between state of consciousness, loss of behavioral response, and concentration of general anesthetic (GA) agent.

3. How robust are these measures across different anesthetic agents?
4. How variable are these measures based upon other subject parameters (e.g., age, sex, presence of other drugs, brain damage)?

Early Data—Is There a Thalamocortical "Switch" in Anesthesia?

Many models have been proposed to explain "consciousness," as discussed in the reviews recommended and this book. The "information integration" theory of consciousness states that when a percept, such as pain, is constructed then synchronous activity in distinct distributed nodes, each processing the discrete components of that percept, is necessary [10, 41]. Any breakdown of communication or connectivity between the nodes of these networks is thought to underlie loss of consciousness and will by definition impact that percept. Various studies have shown that changes in connectivity between discrete nodes occur during an anesthetic state [26, 27, 33]. An FMRI study performed by ourselves that examined the awake state and two propofol-induced sedated states (mild and moderate) in healthy subjects during concurrent auditory and nociceptive stimulation illustrates nicely how the connectivity of the thalamus and putamen to subcortical and cortical regions variably and independently changes at each of these transitional states.

When we group averaged the subjects' brain's responses to sensory stimulation at each of these states (awake, mild, and moderate sedation), we showed that this loss of connectivity decreased brain activity the deeper the subjects were sedated. As such, this data lends support to this theory, but the key to all these studies is our inability to know what the subjects *actually perceive* when sedated (as we have no behavioral measure or report). We have to *infer* from the brain activity map what subjects are likely perceiving based upon how these maps relate to the awake brain or a subject experiencing analgesia (if stimulus of interest is pain). Reverse inferences are fraught with assumptions—but right now it is commonly how neuroimaging studies interpret such data. Machine learning tools, discussed in the Machine-Learning Applications in phMRI section below, will undoubtedly play an important contribution to this problem going forward.

Several earlier studies (PET and FMRI) identified what was assumed to be a specific reduction in thalamic activity. This observation led to the concept of a "thalamocortical switch," whereby thalamic suppression blocks information flow and further processing of incoming sensory stimuli within cortical regions [2, 23, 48]. While this is an attractive and intuitive construct, it is starting to be questioned within the remit of anesthesia-induced unconsciousness [3, 31]. It should be remembered that there is an order of magnitude more connections from the cortex to the thalamus than vice versa. Therefore, the reduction observed during impaired consciousness in thalamic metabolism and blood flow may be secondary to the reduced inputs from cortex or brain stem to the thalamus producing a "functional thalamic deafferentation"-like state. Alternatively, failure of information integration may be due to disruption of corticocortical communication, as recently shown using advanced analysis methods [16, 22, 34] and reduction in thalamic connectivity [1, 17, 33]. Either way, based upon current literature the verdict is that thalamic deactivation is more likely to be a consequence of impaired consciousness rather than the cause.

We should stress this seems to be the case only for pharmacologically induced or "provoked" loss of consciousness, while in physiological unconsciousness (e.g., natural sleep) the thalamus deactivates earlier than the cortex [28]. This potential dissociation between "natural" and "provoked" unconsciousness, as discussed in Chapter 5, is extremely interesting and warrants further investigation and confirmation. Certainly, anesthesia-induced altered states of consciousness appear to share some brain processes with sleep-induced unconscious states, as discussed below. Interestingly, the mechanisms underlying induction of and emergence from anesthesia-induced states of altered consciousness might be different. They might have quite separate relationships to sleep-like states, and this is the focus of current research in some laboratories such as ours.

Current Data—Multimodal Imaging and Slow Waves

Previous work using pharmacological sedation, as a model for the study of consciousness, has been largely constrained by the assumptions underlying the application of population-based pharmacokinetic models to individuals. Therefore, it is unsurprising that no *individualized* neurophysiological marker of perceptual loss (e.g., to pain) has been identified. The approach used in many published neuroimaging studies of consciousness or anesthesia is to deliver the anesthetic agent at specific effector-site concentrations and collect data in response to sensory stimulation for all subjects at that dose. While this has been a valuable starting point for many studies and has provided valuable data showing how the brain's responsivity to sensory stimulation alters with increasing dose of anesthetic agent (see examples for ketamine [39] and propofol [33]), the subjects are at varying states of consciousness at each dose. The problem being that the averaged brain activation map at each dose cannot inform us about the specific link between a certain state of consciousness and the nociceptive processing relevant to pain perception. In order to achieve that understanding, we must examine each individual slowly as they transit in a continuous fashion down the curve described in Fig. 6-1. In short, we need a fundamentally different paradigm.

Due to the large and robust literature using electrophysiological measures (EEG) to explore how neural oscillations (e.g., α, δ, γ waves) alter during sleep and anesthesia [11, 35, 38], it is important to integrate these changes into any paradigm as they can inform the neuroimaging analysis. Further, we have known for a long time that under hyperpolarizing influences, including endogenous sleep drive and anesthetic drugs, cortical neurons oscillate at ~1 Hz, measurable as slow waves in the EEG. Also, it has been recently shown that in later stages of non-REM sleep, which are defined by the presence of slow waves, thalamic, and cortical responses to stimulation become less consistent [13]. Therefore, we hypothesized that the amplitude of slow-wave activity (SWA) upon reaching its maximum *for an individual* is the electrophysiological signature of an unresponsive yet active brain during anesthesia.

We used an ultraslow induction of propofol anesthesia (over 40 minutes induction rather than a few seconds—that is, allowing for a slow motion "video" of the brain as it transits through altered states of consciousness) and simultaneous EEG and FMRI during nociceptive and auditory stimulation—asking subjects to respond to the stimulus [36]. We showed that after LOBR each individual's EEG SWA rises to saturation (SWAS), and remains constant despite increasing drug levels. Impressively, the magnitude of SWAS response correlated positively with their prefrontal gray matter volume. Simultaneously collected FMRI and EEG during nociceptive/painful and auditory stimulation allowed us to interrogate the FMRI responses to auditory and nociceptive stimulation during time windows guided by behavior and the EEG slow-wave patterns. Pre-LOBR there is normal activity within the brain, and this is largely sustained post-LOBR but pre-SWAS (i.e., when SWA is still low). However, during the behavioral unresponsive transition to SWAS we see a dramatic change in brain activity in response to auditory and nociceptive stimulation—in effect, perception loss and thalamocortical isolation occur. Interestingly, based upon spindle patterns, we found that an internal thalamocortical exchange persists at this stage (possibly contradicting the "thalamocortical" switch hypothesis), and an alternative more fundamental cortical network occurs that includes precuneus activation to sensory stimulation. We have established for the first time the relationship between changes in SWA and functional imaging of the brain's response to sensory stimulation during anesthesia. From these results, we conclude that SWAS is a potential *individualized* biomarker for perception loss with profound implications for anesthesia and the study of altered states of consciousness [36].

This study nicely illustrates the potential for multimodal neuroimaging to reveal novel and important mechanisms related to states of consciousness and how they impact pain perception. We hope such studies provide a catalyst for other groups to work in this exciting arena.

phMRI STUDIES OF PAIN AND ANALGESIA

Stratification and Personalized Medicine

To date, most phMRI pharmacological studies have averaged the drug-induced neural response changes to a range of painful stimuli/experimental models (e.g., capsaicin model of secondary hyperalgesia and ongoing pain) within a group of approximately 20 healthy subjects to ascertain the "analgesic mechanism" [21, 25, 49, 53], or have combined FMRI with a pharmacokinetic model of the analgesic to explore the time course of its effect on pain processing [51]. As a whole, such studies show a good correlation between analgesia and reduced activity in response to these painful challenges within regions commonly found active in many pain studies (e.g., thalamus, S1, S2, anterior, mid, and posterior insula, anterior cingulate, brainstem nuclei, and prefrontal cortices). More complex mechanisms of analgesia can be identified—such as the amygdala-sensory uncoupling of connectivity during cannabinoid analgesia that correlated with the discrepancy between the change in pain intensity and unpleasantness ratings [25]. While such phMRI studies provide some validity for the neuroimaging measure relating to pain they do not confirm the specificity of these regions for pain (see below). Further, important individualized variances in network responses across these and other regions are commonly averaged out from the response, unless specific analyses are done as for the cannabinoid study. More recently, studies are being published that highlight how neuroimaging measures (functional, network, and neurochemical) at baseline, pretreatment, and posttreatment can contribute toward predicting and measuring behavioral and neuroimaging treatment responses at an *individualized* level. One example from our group showed that individual baseline reward system regional brain responsivity to painful stimulation predicted subsequent opioid analgesia [47]. Another study showed that posterior insula glutamate and glutamine levels and insula connectivity to other brain regions at baseline predicted subsequent pregabalin but not placebo analgesia [19]. Importantly, such studies can disambiguate drug from placebo mechanisms plus what might explain variances in the placebo response. As such, the personalized medicine and stratification goals that are much needed might be aided with the inclusion of neuroimaging. Further, they inform us about what role these brain regions contribute to pain perception and pain relief. This is important fundamental neuroscience.

The more we identify the neural systems involved in drug action and validate such markers as the ones affected by treatments in patients, the better we can generate novel hypotheses about combined treatments based on targeting complementary brain systems. Also, the better can we match individuals to appropriate treatments based on their brain systems that show abnormal responses and those targeted by a candidate treatment.

Verifying Pain Mechanisms Using phMRI—Drugs As "Probes"

This brings us to an important aspect of phMRI. Neuroimaging has powerfully contributed to our understanding of the mechanisms involved in developing, sustaining, and exacerbating a chronic pain state (e.g., central sensitization, alterations in descending pain modulation [DPMS], anxiety, catastrophizing, and depression). Further, neuroimaging has highlighted how the chronic pain condition itself directly and indirectly changes the brain and spinal cord. One way to test the clinical significance of any of these neuroimaging-based measures is to treat the patient pharmacologically and see how the specific measure changes relative to gold-standard clinical or behavioral measures. Such an approach is increasingly being used psychophysically without neuroimaging (e.g., aberrant conditioned pain modulation as indication of poor DPMS relating to increased duloxetine analgesia) [55]. However, given the differences in sensitivity between behavioral and neuroimaging measures, the issue discussed below regarding effect sizes alongside the complex relationship between brain processing of nociceptive inputs and subjective pain ratings, it is possible that a treatment can change structure, function, or neurochemistry in the absence of a significantly altered pain rating or behavior. If a patient's brain is "normalized" post pharmacological treatment to that of an age-matched healthy control subject, but there is no pain relief, is that meaningful and does it make the measure/mechanism any more or less relevant? This is discussed in a recent editorial [42]. Correcting identified mechanisms with or without concomitant pain relief is now measurable because of brain imaging, but it raises interesting questions for the community. What has certainly been shown, thankfully, is that even patients with years of chronic pain and measurable changes in chemistry and structure when treated (pharmacologically or surgically) for their pain successfully reverse these changes and have "normal"-looking brains from a structural and functional perspective [18, 19, 40].

Are the phMRI Changes "Clinically Significant"?

The potential "disconnect" between what phMRI might show up as a significant effect on neural networks in the absence of any analgesia—sometimes explained away as imaging having an improved SNR—should be considered in the light of the fact that MRI and FMRI images have measures anywhere between 50,000 and 200,000 voxels approximately. This means there is activity in coherent, but spatially distributed systems across the brain—akin to other measures distributed across many variables, such as genome-wide scans. As such, MRI analyses may show many statistically significant differences that are not large enough to be clinically significant. This can lead to an overestimation of effect sizes for brain correlations. Some machine-learning approaches (discussed further below) integrate brain information across regions to make a *single* prediction about a patient's level of pain (whether on drug or not), and as such can robustly track acute pain magnitude [46], and even provide diagnostic information [43]. Such approaches powerfully contribute to our basic understanding of what brain regions are important for conscious pain perception.

Machine-Learning Applications in phMRI

There is a many-to-one mapping between psychological or physiological processes and activity in each voxel, which it should be remembered integrates activity across hundreds of thousands to millions of neurons with distinct functional properties [54]. fMRI correlates of pain have been identified in the anterior cingulate and insula (among other regions)—these regions are important for pain, but they are often activated in many other tasks (e.g., emotion, decision-making). As such, when reported as single brain regions they are not *specific* to pain or any other function for that matter, questioning their utility as a single diagnostic marker. However, whereas any one voxel in a region such as the anterior cingulate may not be highly diagnostic of pain, a particular local pattern across voxels within the anterior cingulate may be highly diagnostic and biologically relevant to pain [46].

To circumnavigate this problem, "machine-learning" algorithms that identify distributed patterns of fMRI activity within and across regions are being increasingly used in neuroimaging. Such "multivoxel pattern analysis" has been applied to pain and identified patterns maximally predictive of a pain state [9, 30, 43, 46]. As such, these patterns are potentially better suited to diagnostic development and testing because they are designed to optimize the prediction of outcomes such as pain (e.g., be sensitive to pain) and differentiate pain from related conditions (e.g., be specific to pain). Similarly, they can be applied in phMRI studies to better inform us about what constitutes a pharmacological-related "analgesic network" versus a "placebo or no treatment network," as highlighted in a recent study from our group [15]. Here, we pooled many phMRI studies across a range of drug classes tested in either experimental pain

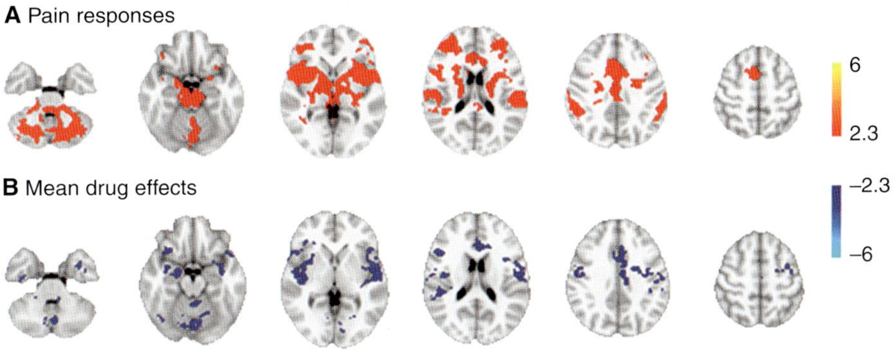

FIGURE 6-2 Multistudy activation maps. **A:** *Z*-statistic maps of a mixed-effects analysis of the average pain response across eight phMRI studies. Red corresponds to brain regions showing significant response to the painful stimuli. **B:** Mixed-effects analysis of modulation of pain responses by analgesics across all eight analgesic studies. Blue corresponds to regions showing a significantly reduced response to the painful stimuli in the analgesic sessions = "analgesic network." (Adapted from Duff et al. [15].)

models, healthy controls, or patients and developed a novel machine-learning paradigm ideally suited for analgesic drug development. It allows single subject and single cohort prediction of drug or placebo treatment. Further, the study design also enabled us to examine across drugs and types of painful experiences the "averaged" brain network subservient to pain and drug-induced analgesia. This is illustrated in Fig. 6-2.

In summary, many examples now exist of brain markers based on distributed patterns of activity within and across brain regions that can be used to predict forms of acute pain [9, 30, 43, 46], identify brain targets of analgesic drugs (e.g., remifentanil; [46]), identify placebo responders [20, 45], and predict whether a subject is on drug or placebo arm [15].

Specificity versus Sensitivity in phMRI

Currently, there is growing interest on the diagnostic value of brain patterns for clinical pain conditions [4] and treatment responses using the accepted criteria of *specificity and sensitivity*. For acute nociception-driven pain, a distributed pattern of regions that matches well with prototypical "pain-processing" regions in humans accurately tracks the magnitude of pain [46]. If two conditions are moderately different in pain (e.g., two points on a 10-point VAS), activity in the "neurologic pain signature" (NPS), as coined by Wager, can correctly predict which is more painful for an individual person with 90–100% accuracy. It has been successfully tested across different sites, and in addition, it was shown to have 90% or greater sensitivity and specificity to somatic pain in comparison with nonpainful warmth, pain anticipation, pain recall, and emotionally evocative images. This "NPS" responded to remifentanil administration; however, it was not affected by a placebo treatment suggesting it is sensitive to certain aspects of pain. Again, such approaches in phMRI are contributing in fundamental ways to our understanding of what brain networks are core to the complex and subjective experiences that are pain and analgesia.

Analgesic Drug Discovery

Industry has suffered from a lack of tools that provide objective in vivo information on whether their drugs have, first, target engagement and, second, efficacy toward the mechanism being targeted. Over-reliance on subjective ratings that are influenced or biased by several extraneous factors means that novel compounds with genuine antinociceptive, antihyperalgesic, and so forth activity are discarded in early phase studies. The attrition rate for analgesics is larger than for any other disease area. Many factors contribute, but one relates to the problem that pain is a multifactorial experience subject to many influences. Therefore, irrespective of the nociceptive input or even the presence of strong analgesics divergences and complex relationships occur between what a subject reports and what is measured using regional brain activity [14].

The fact that subjects might not show a statistical improvement in subjective rating when using any of our developed pain scales is not a binary reason to discard the drug at very early stages of drug development, and yet this happens. Recent studies highlighting how negative expectation can mask true analgesic efficacy [6, 24], and how correction of aberrant neurochemistry and network connectivity can occur in patients without necessarily good analgesia [19], illustrate these points well.

The sad truth is that few drugs make it to Phase IV testing in humans; therefore, it is important that an appropriate range of tools are used to assess potential efficacy at this stage. From what has been previously discussed in this chapter, it should be apparent that imaging can provide the following novel insights into a new compound:

1. CNS penetration and drug dosing
2. Identification of neural circuits targeted
3. Assessment of potential efficacy, based on neural circuitry of activation and its connectivity
4. Potential side effects based on changes in brain regions involved with sleepiness, addiction, and nausea/vomiting

The use of imaging in early clinical trials (and drug evaluation for analgesia) is increasing: of the 70 drugs reported on clinicaltrials.gov that included imaging, 10 involved analgesics. Currently, there are few phase 3 imaging analgesia studies; however, this situation is likely to change [8, 44].

Additionally, the ability of phMRI to measure the responsivity of neural circuits with respect to pharmacological manipulation means these circuits provide "a language of translation" between preclinical species and humans, and as such phMRI studies allow for extrapolation of efficacy from preclinical models to humans more objectively [5, 8] and identification of potential side effect profiles based upon circuitry affected (e.g., nausea and vomiting) [12].

For the interested reader, several excellent reviews provide a comprehensive overview of phMRI's potential application and benefit for analgesic drug development [8, 50, 52]. Neuroimaging is being slowly adopted into analgesic drug development in both translational and clinical trials. Many large companies have realized the benefit of phMRI to provide objective readouts and, as such, help with their "go/no-go" decision-making processes. En route, we are learning more about how our drugs work and fundamental aspects regarding pain and analgesic mechanisms.

CONCLUSION

From the literature discussed, phMRI is a significant and growing component of neuroimaging-based studies, exploring pain and altered states of consciousness. Such paradigms provide insight into the neural bases of analgesia and pain relief, in the context of pain-related drugs, as well as enable a translational agenda by aiding analgesic drug development within industry. phMRI will play an increasing role in both clinical decision-making and drug discovery in the years to come. Further, as we improve our neurobiological understanding of the neural networks core to consciousness, pain perception and analgesia through phMRI studies alongside new analysis approaches, such as machine learning, so we can better interpret brain patterns generated during anesthesia-induced altered states of consciousness during surgical procedures. The link between pain and the conscious brain is an old but complex one. Our hope is that phMRI can continue to unravel and simplify this relationship.

REFERENCES

1. Akeju O, Loggia ML, Catana C, Pavone KJ, Vazquez R, Rhee J, Ramirez VC, Chonde DB, Izquierdo-Garcia D, Arabasz G, et al. Disruption of thalamic functional connectivity is a neural correlate of dexmedetomidine-induced unconsciousness. eLife 2014;3:e04499.

2. Alkire MT, Haier RJ, Fallon JH. Toward a unified theory of narcosis: brain imaging evidence for a thalamocortical switch as the neurophysiologic basis of anesthetic-induced unconsciousness. Conscious Cogn 2000;9:370–86.
3. Alkire MT, Hudetz AG, Tononi G. Consciousness and anesthesia. Science 2008;322:876–80.
4. Baliki MN, Petre B, Torbey S, Herrmann KM, Huang L, Schnitzer TJ, Fields HL, Apkarian AV. Corticostriatal functional connectivity predicts transition to chronic back pain. Nat Neurosci 2012;15:1117–9.
5. Becerra L, Navratilova E, Porreca F, Borsook D. Analogous responses in the nucleus accumbens and cingulate cortex to pain onset (aversion) and offset (relief) in rats and humans. J Neurophysiol 2013;110:1221–6.
6. Bingel U, Wanigasekera V, Wiech K, Ni Mhuircheartaigh R, Lee MC, Ploner M, Tracey I. The effect of treatment expectation on drug efficacy: imaging the analgesic benefit of the opioid remifentanil. Sci Transl Med 2011;3:70ra14.
7. Boly M, Sanders RD, Mashour GA, Laureys S. Consciousness and responsiveness: lessons from anaesthesia and the vegetative state. Curr Opin Anaesthesiol 2013;26: 444–9.
8. Borsook D, Becerra L, Fava M. Use of functional imaging across clinical phases in CNS drug development. Transl Psychiatry 2013;3:e282.
9. Brodersen KH, Wiech K, Lomakina EI, Lin C, Buhmann JM, Bingel U, Ploner M, Stephan KE, Tracey I. Decoding the perception of pain from fMRI using multivariate pattern analysis. Neuroimage 2012;63:1162–70.
10. Buzsaki G. Neuronal oscillations in cortical networks. Science 2004;304:1926–9.
11. Casali AG, Gosseries O, Rosanova M, Boly M, Sarasso S, Casali KR, Casarotto S, Bruno M-A, Laureys S, Tononi G, Massimini M. A theoretically based index of consciousness independent of sensory processing and behavior. Sci Transl Med 2013;5:198ra105.
12. Chin C-L, Fox GB, Hradil VP, Osinski MA, McGaraughty SP, Skoubis PD, Cox BF, Luo Y. Pharmacological MRI in awake rats reveals neural activity in area postrema and nucleus tractus solitarius: relevance as a potential biomarker for detecting drug-induced emesis. Neuroimage 2006;33:1152–60.
13. Dang-Vu TT, Bonjean M, Schabus M, Boly M, Darsaud A, Desseilles M, Degueldre C, Balteau E, Phillips C, Luxen A, et al. Interplay between spontaneous and induced brain activity during human non-rapid eye movement sleep. Proc Natl Acad Sci U S A 2011;108:15438–43.
14. Denk F, McMahon SB, Tracey I. Pain vulnerability: a neurobiological perspective. Nat Neurosci 2014;17:192–200.

15. Duff EP, Vennart W, Wise RG, Howard MA, Harris RE, Lee M, Wartolowska K, Wanigasekera V, Wilson FJ, Whitlock M, et al. Learning to identify CNS drug action and efficacy using multistudy fMRI data. Sci Transl Med 2015;7:274ra16.

16. Ferrarelli F, Massimini M, Sarasso S, Casali A, Riedner BA, Angelini G, Tononi G, Pearce RA. Breakdown in cortical effective connectivity during midazolam-induced loss of consciousness. Proc Natl Acad Sci U S A 2010;107:2681–6.

17. Gili T, Saxena N, Diukova A, Murphy K, Hall JE, Wise RG. The thalamus and brainstem act as key hubs in alterations of human brain network connectivity induced by mild propofol sedation. J Neurosci 2013;33:4024–31.

18. Gwilym SE, Filippini N, Douaud G, Carr AJ, Tracey I. Thalamic atrophy associated with painful osteoarthritis of the hip is reversible after arthroplasty: a longitudinal voxel-based morphometric study. Arthritis Rheum 2010;62:2930–40.

19. Harris RE, Napadow V, Huggins JP, Pauer L, Kim J, Hampson J, Sundgren PC, Foerster B, Petrou M, Schmidt-Wilcke T, Clauw DJ. Pregabalin rectifies aberrant brain chemistry, connectivity, and functional response in chronic pain patients. Anesthesiology 2013;119:1453–64.

20. Hashmi JA, Baria AT, Baliki MN, Huang L, Schnitzer TJ, Apkarian AV. Brain networks predicting placebo analgesia in a clinical trial for chronic back pain. Pain 2012;153:2393–402.

21. Iannetti GD, Zambreanu L, Wise RG, Buchanan TJ, Huggins JP, Smart TS, Vennart W, Tracey I. Pharmacological modulation of pain-related brain activity during normal and central sensitization states in humans. Proc Natl Acad Sci U S A 2005;102:18195–200.

22. Jordan D, Ilg R, Riedl V, Schorer A, Grimberg S, Neufang S, Omerovic A, Berger S, Untergehrer G, Preibisch C, et al. Simultaneous electroencephalographic and functional magnetic resonance imaging indicate impaired cortical top-down processing in association with anesthetic-induced unconsciousness. Anesthesiology 2013;119:1031–42.

23. Kaisti KK, Metsahonkala L, Teras M, Oikonen V, Aalto S, Jaaskelainen S, Hinkka S, Scheinin H. Effects of surgical levels of propofol and sevoflurane anesthesia on cerebral blood flow in healthy subjects studied with positron emission tomography. Anesthesiology 2002;96:1358–70.

24. Kessner S, Wiech K, Forkmann K, Ploner M, Bingel U. The effect of treatment history on therapeutic outcome: an experimental approach. JAMA Intern Med 2013;173:1468–9.

25. Lee MC, Ploner M, Wiech K, Bingel U, Wanigasekera V, Brooks J, Menon DK, Tracey I. Amygdala activity contributes to the dissociative effect of cannabis on pain perception. Pain 2013;154:124–34.

26. Lee U, Mashour GA, Kim S, Noh G-J, Choi B-M. Propofol induction reduces the capacity for neural information integration: implications for the mechanism of consciousness and general anesthesia. Conscious Cogn 2009;18:56–64.

27. Liu X, Lauer KK, Ward BD, Li S-J, Hudetz AG. Differential effects of deep sedation with propofol on the specific and nonspecific thalamocortical systems: a functional magnetic resonance imaging study. Anesthesiology 2013;118:59–69.

28. Magnin M, Rey M, Bastuji H, Guillemant P, Mauguière F, Garcia-Larrea L. Thalamic deactivation at sleep onset precedes that of the cerebral cortex in humans. Proc Natl Acad Sci U S A 2010;107:3829–33.

29. Marchant N, Sanders R, Sleigh J, Vanhaudenhuyse A, Bruno M-A, Brichant JF, Laureys S, Bonhomme V. How electroencephalography serves the anesthesiologist. Clin EEG Neurosci 2014;45:22–32. doi:10.1177/1550059413509801.

30. Marquand A, Howard M, Brammer M, Chu C, Coen S, Mourão-Miranda J. Quantitative prediction of subjective pain intensity from whole-brain fMRI data using Gaussian processes. Neuroimage 2010;49:2178–89.

31. Mashour GA, Alkire MT. Consciousness, anesthesia, and the thalamocortical system. Anesthesiology 2013;118:13–5.

32. Mashour GA, Alkire MT. Evolution of consciousness: phylogeny, ontogeny, and emergence from general anesthesia. Proc Natl Acad Sci U S A 2013;110:10357–64.

33. Mhuircheartaigh RN, Rosenorn-Lanng D, Wise R, Jbabdi S, Rogers R, Tracey I. Cortical and subcortical connectivity changes during decreasing levels of consciousness in humans: a functional magnetic resonance imaging study using propofol. J Neurosci 2010;30:9095–102.

34. Monti MM, Lutkenhoff ES, Rubinov M, Boveroux P, Vanhaudenhuyse A, Gosseries O, Bruno M-A, Noirhomme Q, Boly M, Laureys S. Dynamic change of global and local information processing in propofol-induced loss and recovery of consciousness. PLoS Comput Biol 2013;9:e1003271.

35. Mukamel EA, Pirondini E, Babadi B, Wong KFK, Pierce ET, Harrell PG, Walsh JL, Salazar-Gomez AF, Cash SS, Eskandar EN, et al. A transition in brain state during propofol-induced unconsciousness. J Neurosci 2014;34:839–45.

36. Ni Mhuircheartaigh R, Warnaby C, Rogers R, Jbabdi S, Tracey I. Slow-wave activity saturation and thalamocortical isolation during propofol anesthesia in humans. Sci Transl Med 2013;5:208ra148.

37. Owen AM. Detecting consciousness: a unique role for neuroimaging. Annu Rev Psychol 2013;64:109–33.

38. Purdon PL, Pierce ET, Bonmassar G, Walsh J, Harrell PG, Kwo J, Deschler D, Barlow M, Merhar RC, Lamus C, et al. Simultaneous electroencephalography and functional magnetic resonance imaging of general anesthesia. Ann N Y Acad Sci 2009;1157:61–70.

39. Rogers R, Wise RG, Painter DJ, Longe SE, Tracey I. An investigation to dissociate the analgesic and anesthetic properties of ketamine using functional magnetic resonance imaging. Anesthesiology 2004;100:292–301.

40. Seminowicz DA, Wideman TH, Naso L, Hatami-Khoroushahi Z, Fallatah S, Ware MA, Jarzem P, Bushnell MC, Shir Y, Ouellet JA, Stone LS. Effective treatment of chronic low back pain in humans reverses abnormal brain anatomy and function. J Neurosci 2011;31:7540–50.

41. Tononi G. An information integration theory of consciousness. BMC Neurosci 2004;5:42.

42. Tracey I. "Seeing" how our drugs work brings translational added value. Anesthesiology 2013;119:1247–8.

43. Ung H, Brown JE, Johnson KA, Younger J, Hush J, Mackey S. Multivariate classification of structural MRI data detects chronic low back pain. Cereb Cortex 2014;24: 1037–44.

44. Upadhyay J, Anderson J, Baumgartner R, Coimbra A, Schwarz AJ, Pendse G, Wallin D, Nutile L, Bishop J, George E, et al. Modulation of CNS pain circuitry by intravenous and sublingual doses of buprenorphine. Neuroimage 2012;59:3762–73.

45. Wager TD, Atlas LY, Leotti LA, Rilling JK. Predicting individual differences in placebo analgesia: contributions of brain activity during anticipation and pain experience. J Neurosci 2011;31:439–52.

46. Wager TD, Atlas LY, Lindquist MA, Roy M, Woo C-W, Kross E. An fMRI-based neurologic signature of physical pain. N Engl J Med 2013;368:1388–97.

47. Wanigasekera V, Lee MC, Rogers R, Kong Y, Leknes S, Andersson J, Tracey I. Baseline reward circuitry activity and trait reward responsiveness predict expression of opioid analgesia in healthy subjects. Proc Natl Acad Sci U S A 2012;109:17705–10.

48. White NS, Alkire MT. Impaired thalamocortical connectivity in humans during general-anesthetic-induced unconsciousness. Neuroimage 2003;19:402–11.

49. Wise RG, Lujan BJ, Schweinhardt P, Peskett GD, Rogers R, Tracey I. The anxiolytic effects of midazolam during anticipation to pain revealed using fMRI. Magn Reson Imaging 2007;25:801–10.

50. Wise RG, Preston C. What is the value of human FMRI in CNS drug development? Drug Discov Today 2010;15:973–80.

51. Wise RG, Rogers R, Painter D, Bantick S, Ploghaus A, Williams P, Rapeport G, Tracey I. Combining fMRI with a pharmacokinetic model to determine which brain areas activated by painful stimulation are specifically modulated by remifentanil. Neuroimage 2002;16:999–1014.
52. Wise RG, Tracey I. The role of fMRI in drug discovery. J Magn Reson Imaging 2006;23:862–76.
53. Wise RG, Williams P, Tracey I. Using fMRI to quantify the time dependence of remifentanil analgesia in the human brain. Neuropsychopharmacol 2004;29:626–35.
54. Yarkoni T, Poldrack RA, Nichols TE, Van Essen DC, Wager TD. Large-scale automated synthesis of human functional neuroimaging data. Nat Methods 2011;8:665–70.
55. Yarnitsky D, Granot M, Nahman-Averbuch H, Khamaisi M, Granovsky Y. Conditioned pain modulation predicts duloxetine efficacy in painful diabetic neuropathy. Pain 2012;153:1193–8.

CHAPTER 7

Hypnosis and Pain Modulation

Audrey Vanhaudenhuyse, Aline Gillet, Anne-Sophie Nyssen, and Marie-Elisabeth Faymonville

BACKGROUND

The clinical use of hypnosis to manage pain has a long history, with surgeons and medical staff using hypnosis as a substitute for chemical anesthesia to alleviate the suffering of injured patients (for a review, see reference [17]). From the 18th century to the present day, scientific interest in hypnosis has steadily increased and significant contributions to the development of hypnosis as a theory have been made. First, hypnosis was defined as a state of consciousness characterized by enhanced and involuntary suggestibility. Currently, hypnosis is discussed in relation to three main schools of thought. The first focuses on the "state," elucidating the neurocognitive mechanisms underlying hypnosis. The second looks at the "trait," and is concerned with the qualities associated with an individual that might affect hypnotic responsiveness and considers why hypnosis produces greater effects on some people than others. A third interesting field is the experimental use of both "state" and "trait" considerations as starting points to elucidate particular neuropsychological processes of brain functions. In 2013, the Hypnosis Definition Committee of the American Psychological Association (Division 30) proposed a revised definition of hypnosis: "A state of consciousness involving focused attention and reduced peripheral awareness characterized by an enhanced capacity for response to suggestion" [6]. However, there is no unanimous definition and no common agreement on how the term "hypnosis" is to be regarded. One can consider hypnosis a "procedure" or a "product." The late 20th century saw increasing neuropsychological experiments designed to test theoretical assertions regarding the existence, or not, of a special trance or altered state of consciousness. The neodissociation theory characterizes hypnosis as a special condition that is fundamentally different from normal waking consciousness. In short, the theory proposes that during hypnosis dissociation takes place and a sense of involuntariness and direction of attention emerges without awareness. Suggestions made during hypnosis directly bring about responses or behaviors with little or no sense of effort or conscious control. Meanwhile, "nonstate" theories consider hypnosis to be a social and psychological phenomenon, which can be explained by referring to processes such as beliefs, expectations, and motivation. In our opinion, hypnosis can be seen as a particular waking state in which the subject can experience vivid, multimodal, and coherent mental imagery that invades and fills the subject's consciousness. Current neurophysiology studies tend to support the "state" view.

PAIN PERCEPTION AND BRAIN MODULATION UNDER HYPNOSIS

As hypnotic procedures have found application in various clinical situations it is important for us to understand the mechanisms underlying the reported changes in pain perception. The neurobiological correlates of hypnosis have been difficult to interpret given the multiple variables involved, such as the type of suggestions targeted (which include analgesia, visual or motor imagery, altered perception, and others). Studies have shown that hypnotic procedures and hypnotic instructions activate a process that modifies the functional organization of the brain, depending on the individual's level of susceptibility.

Early neuroimaging studies showed that the anterior cingulate cortex (ACC), a brain area known to be related to the internal monitoring of sensory information, was involved in the modulatory effect of hypnosis [22]. Modulation of the ACC combined with a large cortical and subcortical network (encompassing prefrontal, anterior insular, and pregenual cortices, pre-SMA, thalami, striatum, and brain stem) was shown to increase with hypnosis (for a review, see reference [34]). The usual brain activations observed when subjects received painful stimulation in a normal alert state (i.e., within the pain matrix—ACC, premotor, dorsolateral, prefrontal, primary somatosensory and bilateral insular cortices, thalamus, bilateral striatum, and brain stem) were significantly decreased with hypnosis [31]. In addition, hypnosis is characterized by a modulation of ACC activation as well as an increased functional connectivity between the ACC and the rest of the pain matrix (i.e., insula, pregenual cortex, superior frontal gyrus, thalamus, caudate nucleus, and brain stem) [10, 22]. Pain modulation through hypnosis has also been investigated using electroencephalography (EEG) combined with other imaging techniques. For example, a study conducted in EEG and positron-emission tomography (PET) reported a reduction of the hypnosis-related increases in occipital activity (measured with PET) and delta power (measured with EEG) when subjects received painful stimulation [24], reflecting, according the authors, an alteration of consciousness associated with decreased arousal. Studies note that by modulating ACC and pain matrix brain activity, hypnosis decreases both pain sensation and the unpleasantness of painful stimulation (for a review, see reference [17]). Derbyshire et al. [5] have used hypnosis to induce pain in the absence of noxious stimulation and showed that pain-related brain areas activity was increased by hypnotic suggestions of pain (i.e., activity in thalamus, cerebellum, insula, ACC, primary and secondary somatosensory cortices, and prefrontal cortex). These activations were more significant during hypnosis than while simply imagining pain [5]. These results are not limited to healthy volunteers but are also observed in patients in pathological states. For example, some studies associate hypnosis with a modulation of brain areas involved in pain perception, as well as modulation of the brain activity at rest, in patients suffering from fibromyalgia and other chronic pain pathologies (for a review, see reference [34]). Neuroimaging studies have reported that patients with fibromyalgia show increased connectivity between the insular cortex (i.e., left, middle, and posterior insula), left secondary somatosensory cortex, and default mode network (encompassing midline brain structures such as precuneus and mesiofrontal) at rest. Some authors proposed that this "hyperconnectivity" may be a marker for chronic pain intensity [26]. Indeed, several studies have shown that decreases in connectivity between the default mode network and insular cortex following treatment were associated with reductions in clinical pain [20, 26].

According to theories (for a review, see reference [34]), hypnosis is characterized by the inhibition of afferent nociceptive transmission, which is explained by the extremely decreased activity in the thalamus observed. In addition, the sensory component of pain (pain perception threshold) related to the intensity of the stimulation involves activation in the lateral thalamic nuclei and its projections to the primary and secondary somatosensory cortices, while medial thalamic nuclei and its projections to the anterior cingulate and prefrontal cortices are related to the unpleasantness of the stimulation (i.e., affective component) (for more information, see reference [31]). Some authors proposed that the increased functional connectivity between midcingulate cortex, thalamus, and brain stem might be related to pain-relevant arousal or attention mechanisms. The ACC increased functional relationships with premotor areas and striatum during hypnosis, reported in a neuroimaging study [10], is proposed to allow the midcingulate cortex to organize the most appropriate behavioral response taking into account the affective component of perceived pain stimuli. Furthermore, basal ganglia are known to encode and initiate basic movement patterns expressed through premotor pathways and have also been proposed to support basic attentional mechanisms facilitating the calling up of motor programs and thoughts [10]. The modulated activations in brain regions involved in sensory as well as in affective component of stimulation perception, combined with the modification of connectivity observed between cortical (encompassing premotor regions) and subcortical areas (encompassing ACC, basal ganglia), support the hypothesis that hypnosis may diminish anxiety-related, defensive and emotional reactions to pain by reducing the activation of both cortical and subcortical areas [31]. The increased modulation of insular activity is in line with the role of this structure in pain affect and pain intensity coding. Moreover, the perception of environmental stimulation during hypnosis is modified. These changes can be explained by the disruption in cognitive attentional, appraisal, and memory systems during the hypnotic procedure. Finally, the ACC is involved in executive attention, error detection, and the monitoring of conflict between competing cognitive processes (for more information, see reference [23]). It's activity correlated with the relaxation state among subjects, and was implicated in the "suffering" component of pain and affective reactions associated with pain unpleasantness [23]. According to current literature on the ACC and its function in modulation of the affective component of pain, its decreased activity during hypnosis can be interpreted as reflecting the decreased unpleasantness of the stimulation reported by subjects under hypnosis (for a review, see reference [35]). Some theories suggest that engagement of the cognitive and neurophysiologic processes involved in each of these accounts may be accompanied by a subjective experience of increased mental absorption as reported by subjects under hypnosis [23].

Awareness can be subdivided in two major components [13]. External awareness or awareness of the environment can be defined as the conscious perception of one's environment through the sensory modalities, while internal awareness or awareness of self can be defined as encompassing mental processes that do not require the mediation of external stimuli or sensory input (e.g., mind wandering, daydreaming, inner speech, mental imagery) [32]. We previously showed that external/environmental awareness was mediated by the lateral frontoparietal cortices, whereas internal/self-awareness was associated with activation in precuneus/posterior cingulate, anterior cingulate/mesiofrontal cortices, and parahippocampal areas. Studies have shown that hypnotic processes modify brain networks involved in internal/self-awareness as well as brain network involved in external/environmental awareness (for a review, see reference [34]) (Fig. 7-1). These brain activity modifications were correlated with the subjects' self-reports: in hypnosis, subjects reported an increased internal/self-awareness and a decreased external/environmental awareness as compared to normal wakefulness state [4]. The observed changes in the internal/self-awareness network can be understood as a modification of the degree of continuous information being retrieved from the external world in terms of its relation to oneself, while the decreased connectivity in the external/environmental awareness system might reflect a blockage of the sensory systems that receive stimuli, as a result of hypnotic suggestion [3]. Alterations observed in the internal/self- and external/environmental awareness networks can thus explain the modifications of pain perceptions reported by subjects and patients suffering from acute or chronic pain.

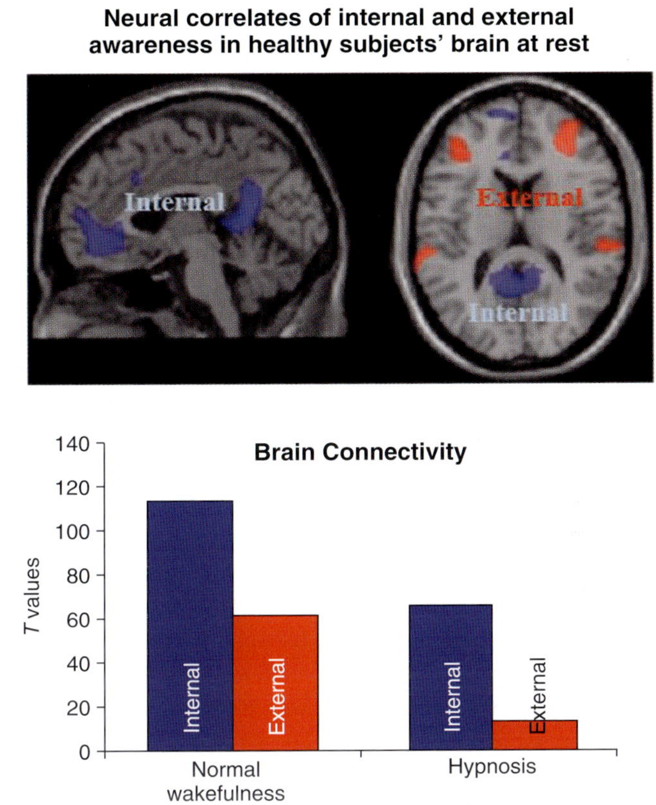

FIGURE 7-1 Brain areas showing a correlation between blood oxygen level dependent (BOLD) signal and the intensity of internal/self- *(blue)* and external/environmental awareness *(red)* in healthy volunteers. Graphical representation shows the hypnosis brain connectivity modulation of the internal/self-awareness *(blue)* and external/environmental *(red)* networks, as compared to normal wakefulness state. (Adapted from references [3, 32].)

HYPNOSIS AND CLINICAL MANAGEMENT OF PAIN

Hypnosis and Chronic Pain

Chronic pain is a complex phenomenon characterized by prolonged and persistent pain (lasting at least 3 months), involving biological, psychosocial, and socioprofessional factors that affect the patient, their loved ones, and society in many ways. Currently, no single medication or treatment addresses all aspects of this condition, which can obey to multiples etiologies. Available treatments provide modest improvements in managing pain and daily functioning. There is a real need for an assessment of combinations of treatments. In recent years, studies have shown interest in nonpharmacological approaches to manage chronic pain (for a review, see reference [33]). Physical rehabilitation and psychological treatments are often incorporated as part of multimodal treatment approaches. In addition, studies on pain management should concentrate on functional and psychological disabilities as well as on quality of life, since we have observed that these variables were usually reported as influenced by pain in chronic pain patients. Recently, self-hypnosis combined with self-care activities have demonstrated benefits in a wider variety of biological, psychological, and social dimensions associated with chronic pain when compared with other treatments such as physiotherapy or psychoeducation, in both neuropathic and nonneuropathic pain patients [33]. Indeed, pain intensity, pain interference, anxiety, and depression were shown to decrease after self-hypnosis and self-care treatment in a group of 158 patients suffering from chronic pain (25 male, mean duration of pain 125 ± 89 months; 133 female 98 ± 13 months of pain) with different etiologies (including both neuropathic and nonneuropathic etiologies), while these patients reported an improved quality of life. A meta-analysis on 12 clinical trials shows that for chronic pain patients (both neuropathic and nonneuropathic etiologies) hypnosis is more efficacious than other psychological interventions such as biofeedback, cognitive–behavior therapy, and muscle relaxation [1].

Pain management for chronic pain patients is largely focused upon pain relief or control. The pursuit of pain control is associated with high costs and few positive results. However, some patients seem to be fixated on this strategy despite the negative consequences. As shown in the literature, an exclusive focus on pain control may lead to greater suffering and disability [2] and may hinder adaptation to pain and paradoxically increase frustrations and limitations due to pain. In our opinion, interventions aiming at improving the patient's capacity for dealing with daily life, and developing strategies to promote positivism and live well in the presence of pain, may indirectly help these patients to gain more control over their pain. In a recent work, we concentrated on patient attitudes and beliefs about pain in a clinical nonrandomized prospective study [33]. Our aim was to assess the effectiveness of different treatments based on psychological and/or physiological approaches, such as physiotherapy, psychoeducation, physiotherapy combined with psychoeducation, and self-hypnosis/self-care learning.

In our clinical and research work, we focus on treatment routines delivered in multidisciplinary pain programs. Indeed, in 2005, the National Institute for Health and Disability Insurance of Belgium (NIHDI) concluded an agreement with multidisciplinary pain centers, permitting a predetermined number of chronic pain patients to receive a multidisciplinary pain diagnosis and an adapted treatment program (for details, see reference [33]). Therapeutic interventions were proposed to patients with chronic pain in our Algology and Palliative Care Department. In our last study, we include both neuropathic and nonneuropathic etiologies patients with a long history of chronic pain from January 2007 to December 2012. The method used was the same as that previously published [33]. In summary, the study included four phases: (1) an initial screening phase during which the algologist elaborated an appropriate pain diagnosis and proposed the patient as suitable for a multidisciplinary approach, (2) a baseline pretreatment assessment of patient health using questionnaires, (3) a treatment delivery phase, and (4) a posttreatment assessment of patient health using the same questionnaires. The multidisciplinary team allocated patients to a treatment group based on patients' physical and psychological conditions, individual pain history, daily functioning, and the treatments they had already tried. In this study, we compared two treatment plans, namely (a) physiotherapy combined with psychoeducation and (b) self-hypnosis/self-care learning, with a control group. A detailed description of the treatment groups can be read in [33]. In this study, three measures were used in pre- and postintervention assessment. First, the Visual Analog Scale (VAS) was used in order to assess pain. Second, the Survey of Pain Attitudes-35 (SOPA-35) [15] was used in order to identify and monitor pain-related beliefs. Finally, the Patients' Global Impression of Change (PGIC) scale [12] assessed overall quality of life by considering pain intensity and disability during daily living activities, and anxiety, depression, fear avoidance, and locus of control behavior during social activities. In this study, the multidisciplinary team allocated 415 patients with chronic pain to the treatment program. Of these, 89 patients were assigned to the control group, 169 to the physiotherapy/psychoeducation group, and 157 to the self-hypnosis/self-care group. Different chronic pain etiologies were equally represented across groups (i.e., fibromyalgia, lower back pain, chronic pain syndrome, polyalgia, neuropathic, osteoarticular, psychiatric, and visceral pain) [8]. The results showed improvement in the patients' global condition reflected by an increase in all scores of each subscales of the SOPA (i.e., pain disability, harm, need of medication, solicitude, belief in medical cure, pain control, and emotion) for both treatment groups. Specifically, an increase in the pain control subscale, which assesses perceived control over pain, was observed for all patients. Pain control is proposed to be positively associated with coping responses thought to reflect a self-management orientation [15]. We can hypothesize that all patients who decided to come in an algology center have initiated an automanagement process in order to improve their quality of life and/or to diminish the disability associated with daily pain. Pain control was shown to be negatively correlated with pain perception, that is, improved pain control was linked to a lower VAS score reported by patients. In addition, we found correlation between the pain control score and PGIC, showing that improved pain control was linked to an improved perception of quality of life, activity limitations, symptoms, and emotions. These results are in line with studies highlighting that pain control is associated with positive psychological functioning [27]. Patients included in the self-hypnosis/self-care treatment group showed a decrease in the medical cure subscale score similar to patients of the physiotherapy/psychoeducation group. The medical cure subscale assesses maladaptive beliefs and includes habits such as placing responsibility for pain management onto the medical profession. Patients involved in the treatment groups seem to have less belief in an eventual cure for pain. These results can be explained by the indirect objective of self-hypnosis/self-care learning tasks, as well as psychoeducation. Both forms of treatment aimed to correct patients' negative beliefs about pain and reinforce their positive beliefs about pain management, while patients in the control group did not receive any teaching about attitudes toward pain. Patients of the two treatment groups were involved in discussions that aimed to empower them to become active participants in their own treatment. In addition, we provided patients with a comprehensible model of pain mechanisms, an understanding of the rationales for pharmacological, physical, and psychological therapy, and guidance for making lifestyle changes. The effects of self-hypnosis/self-care treatment were also observed on pain disability subscales (belief in oneself as disabled by pain) and pain medication subscales (belief in the appropriateness of medications to manage pain). Self-hypnosis/self-care learning assisted the process of encouraging patients to reject their passive role, in order to expand their awareness and amplify positive experiences [33]. The aim was to induce modifications in their attitudes toward pain. Belief that pain indicates disability reflects the belief that pain is damaging and uncontrollable. We can hypothesize that self-hypnosis/self-care may have an effect on this erroneous belief by increasing patients' sense of control over their pain. In addition, we believe that patients who practiced self-hypnosis have learned a new tool to help manage their pain. Hypnosis offers patients an alternative form of pain management, helping them to avoid reliance on painkiller medications. Finally, we found that patients reported an impression of improvement when they received self-hypnosis/self-care treatment, as compared to patients included in the psychoeducation group and control group (Table 7-1). Indeed, 84% of patients included in the self-hypnosis/self-care treatment group considered their overall quality of life to be better than before the treatment, while 54% reported improvement in the psychoeducation treatment group and 45% in the control group. Some authors proposed that, in chronic pain, low quality of life may originate from a high level of pain

TABLE 7-1 **Patient's Global Impression of Change [12] Frequencies (%) of Responses according to Treatment Group**

Patient's Global Impression of Changes	Control (%)	Psychoeducation & Physiotherapy (%)	Self-hypnosis & Self-care (%)
Improvement	45	54	84
No change	25	19	9
Aggravation	25	18	4
Missing data	5	9	3

Note: Total number of patients: 415.

catastrophizing (defined as an exaggerated negative orientation toward pain stimuli and pain experience [28]), often observed in chronic pain patients [16]. We can hypothesize that self-hypnosis/self-care interventions, with the aim of changing the usual focus on pain observed in chronic pain patients, are increasing the patients' sense of control over their pain, and thus has a positive influence on their quality of life.

Nowadays, few studies have directly compared outcomes of different treatment interventions in chronic pain patients. Studies showed that patients who have beneficiated from hypnosis as treatments reported greater decreases in pain and pain interference, anxiety, depression, and quality of life as compared to patients involved in other treatments [14, 33]. Other reported small benefits in patients included in physiotherapy interventions group as compared with education interventions [19, 30].

Hypnosis allows the health specialist to modify the patient's perceived pain disability in daily life by using suggestions that encourage them to take a new perspective, enhancing their own resources. Indeed, with the appearance of pain and chronic pain, patients seem to let pain take a central place in their life. With the hypnosis/self-care learning tasks, we directly worked on the abilities of patients to feel in control of their pain sensation and perception rather than feeling controlled by their pain [21]. With these exercises, we enable patients to get back their sense of control over pain, as well as to (re)discover the power they are able to have over their pain. Internal locus of control refers to the patient's belief that they can control their life. We previously discussed the effect of hypnosis on consciousness brain networks and showed that it modifies the internal/self-awareness network. By changing the functional activity of the internal/self-awareness network (i.e., increased connectivity between the middle frontal and bilateral angular gyri, and decreased connectivity between the restrosplenial/posterior cingulate and bilateral parahippocampal [3]), we can hypothesize that hypnosis involves modification to the patients' sense of self. We can assume that these changes in self-awareness have consequences on patients' sense of control by increasing the internal locus of control, allowing patients to recover the feeling of being an actor/controller over their own pain rather than a passive observer.

Hypnosis As an Anesthesia Tool

Hypnosis can also be used as an anesthetic technique. Hypnosedation combines hypnosis with local anesthesia and conscious intravenous sedation in patients undergoing surgery. This technique can be used in various minor surgical situations such as, plastic surgery (e.g., corrections of scars, correction of prominent ears, liposuction), extraction of wisdom teeth, turbinoplasty, nose fracture, burn dressing changes, as well as in major surgical indications like surgery of thyroid, major plastic surgery (e.g., head and neck lifting, breast prosthesis), and gynecological interventions [34]. Hypnosedation is associated with improved intraoperative comfort, reduced anxiety and pain, diminished intraoperative requirements for anxiolytic and analgesic drugs, optimal surgical conditions, and faster patient recovery [9], independently of the type of surgery. Retrospective and prospective studies on large cohorts of patients showed that hypnosis as an adjunct procedure to conscious intravenous sedation provides better peri- and postoperative pain and anxiety relief, decreased signs of discomfort, and better surgical conditions as compared to control groups of patients undergoing a simple intravenous sedation or relaxation procedure (for a review, see reference [34]). For example, studies on hypnosis and breast reduction surgery indicate that use of a hypnotic intervention can accelerate postoperative wound healing [11], decreases postoperative nausea, vomiting, and need of analgesics [7]. A meta-analysis comprising a total of 2597 patients undergoing surgical or medical procedures reported positive effects of hypnosis on various pre- and postoperative factors such as emotional distress, pain, medication consumption, physiological parameters, recovery, and surgical procedure time as compared to standard care alone or an attention control [29]. Studies showed that patients who beneficiated from hypnosis showed a decrease of 56% in their anxiety on entrance to the operating rooms and were less anxious after surgery, as compared to other patients on postintervention [25]. In addition, hypnosis had a larger effect when delivered face to face than via tape, and was more effective when implemented preoperatively [29]. Some authors explained the observed benefits of hypnosis in acute pain management and surgery as an opportunity for patients to escape the vicious circle of anxiety and pain. Indeed, anticipatory anxiety related to treatment leads to increased pain, while higher pain generates more anxiety [18]. In addition, affective or unpleasantness as well as the sensory or perceived intensity components of pain perception were shown to be reduced when hypnosis was used in acute pain (for a review, see reference [34]).

INTEREST IN HYPNOSIS, IN BRIEF

Currently, clinical research has shown benefits of hypnosis in both acute and chronic pain management. Hypnosis combined with local anesthesia allows patients to avoid general anesthesia in several surgical indications (e.g., surgery of thyroid, plastic surgery), improves pre- and postoperative comfort of patients, and demands less medication. In addition, hypnosis combined with self-care learning enables patients suffering from chronic pain to improve their quality of life by increasing their ability to take advantage of their own resources. Neuroimaging studies showed the hypnotic modulation of the brain mechanisms involved in pain perception, lending support to the positive impact of this technique on acute and chronic pain observed in clinical research. Indeed, activation and functional connectivity of brain areas involved in attentional and emotional processing, as well as in internal/self- and external/environmental awareness, were modified when subjects used hypnosis as compared to normal alert state. Finally, self-awareness brain network modifications induced by self-hypnosis could be proposed as leading to a modification of patients' sense of control. It can enable patients to recover and/or to increase their internal locus of control and thus to become an actor over their pain rather than a mere observer.

Despite of the scientific evidence regarding the interest of hypnosis in acute pain management, more studies are needed to reinforce the idea that not only pharmacological but also psychological treatment can relieve pain by modulating brain activation involved in pain perception. Currently, financial support for this type of study is still missing and should be promoted. Indeed, in the literature, we can observe an increased number of studies reporting efficiency of biopsychological approaches in the management of different pathologies. Leading changes in the medical practices need scientific evidence-based results on large cohort of patients. Future studies are needed with large samples of patients as well as a randomized double-blind methodology. These studies are essential to highlight the robust effect of hypnosis as treatment approaches and to enhance its use in medicine.

ACKNOWLEDGMENTS

We thank V. Bonhivers, M-C. Charles, R. Fontaine, L. Galloy, N. Jamoulle, M-P. Lecart, C. Lequarre, D. Libbrecht, N. Malaise, I. Salamun, S. Smitz, S. Teuwis, and M. Tomasella for their significant help in our daily clinical work.

REFERENCES

1. Adachi T, Fujino H, Nakae A, Mashimo T, Sasaki J. A meta-analysis of hypnosis for chronic pain problems: a comparison between hypnosis, standard care, and other psychological interventions. Int J Clin Exp Hypn 2014;62(1):1–28.
2. Crombez G, Eccleston C, De Vlieger P, Van Damme S, De Clercq A. Is it better to have controlled and lost than never to have controlled at all? An experimental investigation of control over pain. Pain 2008;137(3):631–9.
3. Demertzi A, Soddu A, Faymonville M, Bahri M, Gosseries O, Vanhaudenhuyse A, Phillips C, Maquet P, Noirhomme Q, Luxen A, Laureys S. Hypnotic modulation of resting state fMRI default mode and extrinsic network connectivity. Prog Brain Res 2011;193:309–22.
4. Demertzi A, Vanhaudenhuyse A, Noirhomme Q, Faymonville ME, Laureys S. Hypnosis modulates behavioural measures and subjective ratings about external and internal awareness. J Physiol Paris 2015; Epub Nov 10.

5. Derbyshire SW, Whalley MG, Stenger VA, Oakley DA. Cerebral activation during hypnotically induced and imagined pain. Neuroimage 2004;23(1):392–401.

6. Elkins GR, Barabasz AF, Council JR, Spiegel D. Advancing research and practice: the revised APA Division 30 definition of hypnosis. Int J Clin Exp Hypn 2015;63(1):1–9.

7. Enqvist B, Bjorklund C, Engman M, Jakobsson J. Preoperative hypnosis reduces postoperative vomiting after surgery of the breasts: a prospective, randomized and blinded study. Acta Anaesthesiol Scand 1997;41(8):1028–32.

8. Faymonville M, Blavier A, Palmaricciotti V, Malaise N, Salamun I, Fontaine R, Libbrecht D, Tomasella M, Smitz S, Malengreaux C, et al. The analysis of biopsychosocial characteristics of 1832 chronic pain patients consulting a tertiary pain center. Douleur et Analgésie 2014;27:181–91.

9. Faymonville ME, Meurisse M, Fissette J. Hypnosedation: a valuable alternative to traditional anaesthetic techniques. Acta Chir Belg 1999;99(4):141–6.

10. Faymonville ME, Roediger L, Del Fiore G, Delgueldre C, Phillips C, Lamy M, Luxen A, Maquet P, Laureys S. Increased cerebral functional connectivity underlying the antinociceptive effects of hypnosis. Brain Res Cogn Brain Res 2003;17(2):255–62.

11. Ginandes C, Brooks P, Sando W, Jones C, Aker J. Can medical hypnosis accelerate post-surgical wound healing? Results of a clinical trial. Am J Clin Hypn 2003;45(4):333–51.

12. Hurst H, Bolton J. Assessing the clinical significance of change scores recorded on subjective outcome measures. J Manipulative Physiol Ther 2004;27(1):26–35.

13. James W. The principles of psychology. New York, NY: Dover Press; 1890.

14. Jensen MP, Barber J, Romano JM, Molton IR, Raichle KA, Osborne TL, Engel JM, Stoelb BL, Kraft GH, Patterson DR. A comparison of self-hypnosis versus progressive muscle relaxation in patients with multiple sclerosis and chronic pain. Int J Clin Exp Hypn 2009;57(2):198–221.

15. Jensen MP, Turner J, Romano J. Pain belief assessment: a comparison of the short and long versions of the surgery of pain attitudes. J Pain 2000;1(2):138–50.

16. Lame IE, Peters ML, Vlaeyen JW, Kleef M, Patijn J. Quality of life in chronic pain is more associated with beliefs about pain, than with pain intensity. Eur J Pain 2005;9(1):15–24.

17. Lanfranco RC, Canales-Johnson A, Huepe D. Hypnoanalgesia and the study of pain experience: from Cajal to modern neuroscience. Front Psychol 2014;5:1126.

18. Marvin J, Muller M, Blakeney P, Meyer W. Pain response and pain control. In: Herndon DN, editor. Total burn care. London: Saunders; 1996. pp. 529–43.

19. Miyamoto GC, Costa LO, Galvanin T, Cabral CM. Efficacy of the addition of modified Pilates exercises to a minimal intervention in patients with chronic low back pain: a randomized controlled trial. Phys Ther 2013;93(3):310–20.

20. Napadow V, Kim J, Clauw DJ, Harris RE. Decreased intrinsic brain connectivity is associated with reduced clinical pain in fibromyalgia. Arthritis Rheum 2012;64(7):2398–403.

21. Nyssen AS. The paradox of hypnosis and pain: from the power of the hypnotherapist to the patient's sense of control. Douleur et Analgésie 2008;21:44–7.

22. Rainville P, Duncan GH, Price DD, Carrier B, Bushnell MC. Pain affect encoded in human anterior cingulate but not somatosensory cortex. Science 1997;277(5328):968–71.

23. Rainville P, Hofbauer RK, Bushnell MC, Duncan GH, Price DD. Hypnosis modulates activity in brain structures involved in the regulation of consciousness. J Cogn Neurosci 2002;14(6):887–901.

24. Rainville P, Hofbauer RK, Paus T, Duncan GH, Bushnell MC, Price DD. Cerebral mechanisms of hypnotic induction and suggestion. J Cogn Neurosci 1999;11(1):110–25.

25. Saadat H, Drummond-Lewis J, Maranets I, Kaplan D, Saadat A, Wang SM, Kain ZN. Hypnosis reduces preoperative anxiety in adult patients. Anesth Analg 2006;102(5):1394–6.

26. Schmidt-Wilcke T, Ichesco E, Hampson JP, Kairys A, Peltier S, Harte S, Clauw DJ, Harris RE. Resting state connectivity correlates with drug and placebo response in fibromyalgia patients. Neuroimage Clin 2014;6:252–61.

27. Shen MJ, Redd WH, Winkel G, Badr H. Associations among pain, pain attitudes, and pain behaviors in patients with metastatic breast cancer. J Behav Med 2014;37(4):595–606.

28. Sullivan M, Bishop S, Pivik J. The pain catastrophizing scale: development and validation. Psychol Assess 1995;7(4):524–32.

29. Tefikow S, Barth J, Maichrowitz S, Beelmann A, Strauss B, Rosendahl J. Efficacy of hypnosis in adults undergoing surgery or medical procedures: a meta-analysis of randomized controlled trials. Clin Psychol Rev 2013;33(5):623–36.

30. Toth C, Brady S, Gagnon F, Wigglesworth K. A randomized, single-blind, controlled, parallel assignment study of exercise versus education as adjuvant in the treatment of peripheral neuropathic pain. Clin J Pain 2014;30:111–8.

31. Vanhaudenhuyse A, Boly M, Balteau E, Schnakers C, Moonen G, Luxen A, Lamy M, Degueldre C, Brichant JF, Maquet P, et al. Pain and non-pain processing during hypnosis: a thulium-YAG event-related fMRI study. Neuroimage 2009;47(3):1047–54.

32. Vanhaudenhuyse A, Demertzi A, Schabus M, Noirhomme Q, Bredart S, Boly M, Phillips C, Soddu A, Luxen A, Moonen G, Laureys S. Two distinct neuronal networks mediate the awareness of environment and of self. J Cogn Neurosci 2011;23(3):570–8.
33. Vanhaudenhuyse A, Gillet A, Malaise N, Salamun I, Barsics C, Grosdent S, Maquet D, Nyssen AS, Faymonville ME. Efficacy and cost-effectiveness: a study of different treatment approaches in a tertiary pain center. Eur J Pain 2015;19:1437–46.
34. Vanhaudenhuyse A, Laureys S, Faymonville ME. Neurophysiology of hypnosis. Neurophysiol Clin 2014;44(4):343–53.
35. Vogt BA, Sikes RW. The medial pain system, cingulate cortex, and parallel processing of nociceptive information. Prog Brain Res 2000;122:223–35.

CHAPTER 8

Mindfulness Meditation Modulates the Conscious Experience of Pain: A Neuroscientific Account

Joshua A. Grant and Fadel Zeidan

Pain is a subjectively available experience, sensitive to change arising from interactions with a great many factors, often in parallel with the underlying nociceptive activity, but not necessarily so. As defined by the International Association for the Study of Pain (IASP), "pain is an unpleasant sensory or emotional experience associated with actual or potential damage" and "is always subjective" in nature. Thus, to be considered pain at least some degree of conscious awareness is necessary.

Known modulators of pain could be said to exert their influence directly (i.e., altering the pain and/or nociceptive activity itself), or indirectly (i.e., by modifying the state in which the experience is embedded). This could be viewed as having a primarily influence on either the content or background of consciousness. Meditative states are one example of the latter, in which practices are said to alter the context of our conscious environment. During mindfulness meditation one attempts to adopt a more accepting attitude toward their experience. The practice is said to have profound implications for fundamental schemas in which experience is embedded, such as the concept of self. It is then fitting that mindfulness meditation has been shown to attenuate the subjective experience of pain. Interestingly, it appears to do so through quite unique neuronal mechanisms.

The goal of this chapter is to explore the experience of pain in relation to mindfulness-based meditation practices. The chapter builds on our previous work [22, 63] by shifting the focus to examining how changes to our consciousness or awareness, arising from these techniques, might help explain their influence on pain. We begin with a description of mindfulness meditation, providing an overview of several popular techniques, as well as their putative neural correlates. This is followed by a short summary describing the conscious experience of pain and how mindfulness meditation may relate. We then move to the scientific literature examining the effects of mindfulness on pain from a state perspective and then from a trait perspective. Finally, we discuss how other meditation-related work supports our interpretation of the influence of mindfulness on the experience of pain.

WHAT IS MINDFULNESS MEDITATION?

Mindfulness meditation is a fairly loose term to which many meditation practices apply. These practices have been found to improve a wide spectrum of clinically relevant cognitive and health outcomes [25]. In patients, training in mindfulness improves to different extents the self-reports of anxiety [21, 34, 66], depression [3, 57], stress [1, 6, 7, 35], and cognition [29, 41–43, 64]. Mindfulness-related health benefits are associated with enhancements in cognitive control, emotion regulation, positive mood, and acceptance [25], and interestingly, each of these phenomena have also been associated with pain modulation.

Generally, mindfulness has been described as a "nonelaborative, nonjudgmental awareness" of the present moment experience [32]. However, one does not need to be meditating, or even trained in meditation, to be mindful. Varying degrees of "trait mindfulness" exist in the general population, outside of any formal training [11, 13]. However, mindfulness can also be developed with mental training routines such as meditation. A variety of different practices are subsumed under the general rubric of "mindfulness meditation." Thus, it is critical that the specifics of the practice being taught or employed be recognized [13, 41, 53]. In the present chapter, we will focus on two rather coarse categories of mindfulness practice, namely, focused attention (*samatha* in the Pali language) and open monitoring (*vipassana* in the Pali language) [41]. In general, these two groups of practices are centered on developing a number of distinct cognitive skills.

During focused attention, or *samatha* [59], the practitioner is taught to develop cognitive control and attentional stability by training the mind to sustain focus on the moment-to-moment quality and characteristics of sensory, emotional, and cognitive events [41]. In brief, *samatha* involves directing one's attention to the dynamic nature of the chosen object of meditation, most often the sensations of breath or body. When attention drifts from the object of focus, to a distracting sensory event, for example, the practitioner is taught to acknowledge the event and to disengage by returning their attention back to the meditative object (e.g., the breath). Often *samatha* is taught as a series of distinct practices increasing in complexity (e.g., mindfulness of breath, of emotions, of thoughts). While *samatha* practices aim primarily at gaining mental control and stabilization of attention, they naturally lead, and in a somewhat ambiguous way, to the traits associated with open monitoring meditation, or *vipassana*. Indeed, it is difficult to see where *samatha* ends and *vipassana* begins.

As a developmental derivative of focused attention practice, the mindfulness practitioner finds himself or herself almost naturally transitioning into the open monitoring mental stance known as *vipassana*. Whereas *samatha* often entails focus on a single, dynamic, meditative object, open monitoring practices are more inclusive. When applied to the full extent, these practices are associated with a nondirected acknowledgment of any sensory, emotional, or cognitive event that arises in the mind. While practicing open monitoring, the practitioner is said to experience their current "event" without evaluation, interpretation, or preference. Fittingly, open monitoring meditation has been described as a state of nonappraisal and/or a nonelaborative mental stance [23, 63].

Traditionally, focused attention is taught before, or as a *prerequisite* to, open monitoring practice. The reason for this is likely that a greater capacity for attentional stability and mental control [28, 64] would allow more success in the daunting task of relaxing one's tendency to automatically engage with, and appraise, ongoing experience. As the practitioner becomes more adept in meditation, he or she will be able to employ a unique cognitive approach where consciously available sensory events can be simply "let go," presumably leading to significant reductions in affective or cognitive appraisals/reactions to the event. It should be noted, however, that the goal of mindfulness is not to simply train what might be termed a "Teflon mind," incapable of holding a sensory or cognitive percept. Rather, a balance between sustained attention on one hand and "letting go" on the other should provide the ability to adaptively and flexibly shift between mindful and more reactive or absorbed thought processes.

THE SHAPING OF PAINFUL EXPERIENCE

Pain is a complex, and subjective, conscious experience. Psychophysical evaluations of painful experiences demonstrate that dissociable differences exist between the sensory aspects (i.e., intensity) and the affective aspects (i.e., unpleasantness), although these two dimensions are usually highly correlated [45, 47, 50]. Further, the integration of a constellation of sensory, cognitive, and affective factors including the mood, psychological disposition, meaning-related cognitions (e.g., suffering), prepain cognitive state (e.g., expectations), etc. interact to provide a continually changing experience. In short, the experience of pain can be significantly influenced by the context in which it occurs. One example of this comes from studies assessing pain in cancer patients and in women giving birth [46]. The pain of labor was rated as significantly higher on sensory aspects compared to the affective dimension. In contrast, cancer pain was rated significantly higher on pain unpleasantness than pain intensity [48]. The suggestion here is that the contextual evaluation of welcoming a new baby into the world when compared to facing one's own death has profound implications for what might have been very similar experiences otherwise. In what follows we suggest that mindfulness, in a similar albeit less profound manner than giving birth or dying, also alters the meaning, interpretation, and appraisal of nociceptive information. First, we will give an overview of what these practices appear to be doing in the brain.

A CAVEAT AND THE NEURAL CORRELATES OF MINDFULNESS MEDITATION

Elucidating the brain networks underlying any experiential state is complicated by many factors, not least of which is often the lack of outward behavioral markers preventing even a coarse orientation with the mental landscape. Specifically concerning mindfulness, most studies apply the construct to something, such as pain, and cannot make statements about what the state of mindfulness, in itself, might reveal in the brain. What these studies can say is that "mindfulness of pain," or, "mindfulness of the breath during pain" activates a specific and distinct pattern of neural activation. Here we make the assumption, rightly or wrongly, that there is something to mindfulness, in terms of brain activity, beyond the object to which it is being applied. This postulation is supported by claims of the existence of mindful but nonreferential awareness [13, 30]. Nevertheless, repeated experimentation, literature reviews, and meta-analyses paint a slowly emerging picture of what *is happening* in the brain during mindfulness.

Contrasting Hindu and Buddhist meditative practices, Tomasino et al. [58] conducted a meta-analysis of functional imaging studies which (a) reported the style of meditation used, (b) asked participants to meditate, and (c) reported whole brain activation (i.e., not simply regions of interest). Consistent with the idea that Buddhist practices are associated more with the cognitively oriented concept of mindfulness, and Hindu practices more with absorptive attention, the authors reported primarily medial and lateral prefrontal loci for Buddhism versus parietal and cingulate cortices for Hindu practices. These results are largely consistent with another recent meta-analysis of 21 meditation studies, looking at structural brain correlates [16]. These authors found significantly greater gray matter of the anterior insula (aINS), dorsal anterior cingulate cortex (dACC), prefrontal cortex (PFC) (including lateral and orbitofrontal [OFC] regions), hippocampus, and several temporal lobe regions. Interestingly, when looking at only novices, gray matter differences were observed selectively in the cingulate (posterior cingulate cortex [PCC/ACC]) and insula. The structural changes to PFC were restricted to more advanced meditators. Together, these two meta-analyses support our previous suggestion that as skill and proficiency of mindfulness increase, there is a shift from active prefrontal regulation to more effortless regulation, which we suggest requires less prefrontal recruitment. That is, novice meditators show increased activation of PFC while attempting to be mindful whereas advanced practitioners show lower activity in comparison to both their own control conditions and control groups [22, 23, 63]. Of course, the context and meditative object being regulated in individual functional imaging studies will dictate which other brain regions and networks are activated.

NEURAL MECHANISMS SUPPORTING MINDFULNESS-BASED ANALGESIA

Several approaches have been taken to studying the influence of mindfulness on pain. The first approach we review is state induction. That is, the active practice of mindfulness meditation. While studies have looked at both advanced practitioners and beginners, the latter is particularly salient, as the transition from mindfully "naïve" to mindful seems to be profound, allowing observation of large effects. As one advances in skill and proficiency the baseline itself begins to change. One begins to have greater "trait" mindfulness, not necessarily needing to sit and meditate to produce a nonevaluative cognitive approach. One possible consequence of this, for research, is that state inductions in advanced practitioners may seem less remarkable than in beginners. Indeed, this may explain why certain effects appear to be much larger in novices. One solution to this is to take a trait approach, comparing practitioners and controls in nonmeditative states. This approach is also important as it provides an indication of whether meditative training has any long-term impact on daily life, which is ultimately the goal.

State-Induced Mindfulness Meditation during Pain

Practicing mindfulness involves focusing on a dynamic, and automatic, stimulus such as the breath and "letting go" of distracting mental events as they arise, typically in the form of cognitive evaluation, emotion, and/or narratives. Given the difference of this "mind set" with our often mindless, ruminative, full head of steam, thought trains, it then seems reasonable that mindfulness would alter the experience of pain. Zeidan and colleagues [65] examined state-related meditative pain relief with a brief mindfulness training protocol in naïve participants. Using a perfusion-based fMRI technique they examined the effects of 4 days (20 minutes/day) of mindfulness meditation training on pain-related brain processing. Training consisted of a combination of a focused attention and open monitoring techniques. After training, meditating in the presence of noxious heat significantly reduced pain intensity (40%) and pain unpleasantness (57%) compared to a posttraining rest condition. These training-related effects were associated with activity reductions in contralateral primary somatosensory cortex (S1), (i.e., corresponding to the stimulation site), consistent with a reduction of low-level sensory processing. Reductions in pain unpleasantness were correlated with deactivation of the thalamus, a region crucially involved in processing sensory and nociceptive information. Therefore, at one level, one could postulate that brief mindfulness training modulates the conscious experience of pain by gating the nociceptive signal prior to its distribution throughout the cortex. While this sounds similar to distraction, there appear to be clear differences. Zeidan et al. [65] directly compared mindfulness to an attention-to-breath (ATB) condition, a task characterized by divided attention. Mindfulness was associated with a distinct pattern of neural activation, including the ACC, OFC, and reduced activation of PCC, compared to ATB. This suggests the mechanisms underlying mindfulness are more than simple distraction.

In the same study [65], regression analyses of the posttraining session revealed that greater activity of the rostral (r) ACC and anterior (a) INS during meditation and pain predicted pain intensity reductions. The rACC is a brain region implicated in executive-level regulation of cognitive and affective processes. The insula links somatosensory processing areas with brain regions such as the PFC, amygdala, and ACC [18, 44]. Finally, the study also found that greater activity in areas involved in the contextual evaluation of pain and positive mood (OFC) was related to pain unpleasantness decreases, from the posttraining baseline, during meditation and noxious stimulation. In sum, brief mindfulness training seems to have a profound impact on pain, which manifests through multiple channels in the brain.

Concurrent work with more advanced practitioners, also actively generating mindful states, is quite consistent with the findings just described. Gard and colleagues [19] examined the influence of *vipassana* meditation on pain processing using BOLD fMRI. Experientially, long-term mindfulness practitioners reported significant reductions in pain unpleasantness during meditation (with electrically evoked pain), when compared to a well-matched control group. Interestingly, pain intensity did not differ between groups. In the brain, contrary to the novice meditators described above, meditators exhibited greater activation in sensory-related regions, including contralateral S2 and posterior insula [19] which, predicted pain relief during the mindful state. Further, lateral PFC, bilaterally, was found to be deactivated, that is, activated less during mindfulness than during a baseline condition. These effects were interpreted as evidence for increased sensory and decreased executive processing during mindfulness meditation. Nearly the same pattern has been observed for advanced Tibetan meditators performing open monitoring during pain [40] where again a selective reduction in pain unpleasantness was observed and both aINS and dACC were more active in meditators than in control subjects during pain.

The two studies just mentioned also looked at how actively meditating influences the anticipation of pain. Gard and colleagues [19] reported increased activation of rACC and ventromedial (vm) PFC for meditators anticipating electrical shocks, in contrast to their report of decreased PFC activity during the stimulus. Similarly, Lutz et al. [40] found that the increased activity of aINS and dACC for meditators during pain was predicted by lower activity of these regions in the anticipatory period, compared to controls. Finally, Brown and Jones [5] demonstrated reductions in expectations of impending noxious stimuli reduced behavioral and electrophysiological markers of pain. Thus, it appears that mindfulness can operate during the prestimulus phase of conscious processing and may predict the subsequent meditation-induced reductions in pain and pain-related activation increases.

As a whole the state-related studies of meditators, novice or advanced, suggest that mindfulness is likely "active," or being applied, prior to stimulus presentation and enhances the activity of pain related, but domain general, brain areas (aINS, ACC). However, rather than being associated with increased painful experience, as is typical of such activation change in pain research [9, 10, 12], pain was decreased, particularly unpleasantness. Multiple other mechanisms also seem to be involved, such as the regulation of affective appraisal and expectation. Interestingly, advanced meditators and novices seem to differ in terms of sensory-related activation. In novices, there appears to be attenuation of low-level sensory processing not observed in more advanced practitioners, who if anything, show activation increases. Next, we will review studies taking a trait approach to these same questions, which combined with the state-related studies present a clear pattern.

Trait Effects of Mindfulness Meditation on Pain Processing

Extensive training in mindfulness-based meditation is postulated to produce robust, long-term changes in conscious awareness. With a more stable mind, the repeated attempts to refrain from automatic appraisal and acceptingly attend to the present moment, becomes nearly reflexive. The result is said to be a loosening of the concept of an unchanging or static "self," which in turn frees the practitioner of attachments and the tendency to grasp or cling to them. In relation to pain, this may mean the ability to sit, calmly, in the face of a noxious stimulus, with full experiential awareness of the quality of the stimulus but with less fear or anxiety of its implications. Combined with the state effects described above, work with trait effects suggests this may actually be the case.

In their first study, rather than have participants meditate, Grant and Rainville [24] instructed advanced Zen practitioners and controls to try to sustain their attention on painful and nonpainful heat stimuli. In this "focused attention" condition, compared to their respective baselines, pain increased in meditation-naive controls, as would be expected when attending to pain, but did not differ in meditators. When instructed to engage the same stimuli without judgment (i.e., mindfully) pain intensity and unpleasantness were significantly reduced in meditators, with no change in controls. This was taken as evidence that the baseline of practitioners involves a high degree of attentiveness to one's experience, and, that they may be unable to refrain from exerting some degree of mindfulness automatically. This was supported by the fact that the meditators also required significantly higher stimulus intensities to report moderate pain, assessed prior to the attention conditions as well as less autonomic reactivity throughout the experiment [24].

In a follow-up study, Zen practitioners and matched controls were scanned while experiencing pain in a nonmeditative waking state [23]. Similar to the state-related studies of advanced practitioners, meditators exhibited greater activation of INS, thalamus, and midcingulate cortex. These areas are involved in pain experience but also modulation and importantly, salience [52]. Interestingly, widespread brain activity decreases were also observed for meditators in regions involved in emotion, memory, and appraisal (i.e., medial-PFC [mPFC], dorsolateral [DL] PFC, OFC, amygdala, caudate, and hippocampus among others). The most advanced practitioners had the largest activation decreases in many of these areas, paralleled by the lowest pain ratings. What was striking was that decreased connectivity between DLPFC (deactivated) and dACC (activated) predicted baseline pain sensitivity of the meditators (i.e., how hot they required stimuli to be to report moderate pain). These results were interpreted as reflecting a state wherein the meditators were fully engaged with the experiential nature (i.e., the qualia of pain) of the stimulus (reflected by higher activity in dACC, aINS, thalamus) but simultaneously "let go" of the typical appraisal, elaboration, and emotional reactivity (deactivated DLPFC, OFC, mPFC, amygdala, hippocampus). Grant [22] argued that truly being "in the moment" theoretically precludes engagement of a host of mental processes, which directly or indirectly require reference to the past or future for assessment of the present situation. This in turn led to the suggestion that the multifaceted construct of mindfulness may be a cascade that is initiated by remaining focused on the present moment. As discussed in the following section, there is evidence, outside of pain research, that attending to the present moment can alter conscious experience.

MINDFULNESS MEDITATION AND PRESENT-MOMENT EXPERIENCE

The temporal dynamics of the human mind are influenced, or perhaps even dictated, by fluctuations of various neural networks. Networks involved in task-related activities, involving pretty much anything, can be distinguished from task-unrelated networks, such as the "default mode network" (DMN) which is associated with self-referential thought, mind wandering [8, 37] and lapses in attentional stability [61]. The DMN, active during rest and deactivated during other tasks, involves the mPFC, PCC, precuneus, and medial parietal cortices [17, 49, 51], all regions implicated in self-related processing. While mind wandering is likely an extremely important and adaptive mental process [54, 55], in the absence of control, it may run wild and perpetuate mental disorders such as anxiety [21, 66] or depression [15]. Concerning the experience of pain, several studies have shown that self-referential thought has an influence on experimentally induced and chronic pain [2, 14, 36, 39, 60]. Importantly, it has been suggested that over time, persistent pain-related thought may become intertwined with self-referential thought and be an exacerbating factor in chronic pain [62]. In other words, the concept of pain may become indistinguishable from the concept of "self." The antithesis of this effect would seemingly be mindfulness and indeed evidence suggests these practices modulate, and provide control over, self-referential thought or mind wandering.

Adept meditators exhibit alterations between DMN nodes [56] and significantly greater decreases in DMN activation [4, 20, 26, 27] paralleling significant reductions in mind wandering [26, 27]. Interestingly, the functional connections between the PCC and the ACC and DLPFC (involved in executive-level cognitive and affective control) were stronger in adept meditators than controls, even at baseline [4]. This suggests meditation practitioners have less "anticorrelation" between brain networks, potentially allowing control-related regions to influence resting-related networks like the DMN. Impressively, even brief meditation training (4–5 days) leads to state anxiety reductions coupled to deactivation of the PCC [66]. Taken together, it seems that mindfulness practice, rather quickly, can bestow a level of control on the practitioner, which influences the contents of their consciousness. We suggest that this paring down of narrative elaboration would have a major impact on one's sense of self by reducing the associations (e.g., pain-related thought) that may become embedded through rumination. Ultimately, the meditation practitioner can develop to the extent that he or she can *interpret or realize* even the sense of self as a "distractor" or an affective obscuration of *being,* leading to what psychologists call "ego death" [38] or *samadhi* [59]. The chance to study this level of proficiency on pain may indeed be enlightening.

CONCLUSIONS

We have offered a view of how mindfulness-related meditative practices and states can influence the conscious experience of pain, starting with beginners and experts actively generating mindfulness, and moving to long-term mindfulness-related traits in advanced practitioners. The literature suggests that many neural mechanisms are involved but also suggest the pain-modulatory effects of mindfulness are quite distinct from other known modulators. We postulate that applying mindfulness to pain, with varying degrees of self- or ego retraction, associated with different skill levels, leads to an interpretation of the event more in line with "a sensation" than "a painful sensation involving suffering." Some behavioral evidence for this hypothesis comes from the very first works with mindfulness and pain by Jon Kabat-Zinn.

Chronic pain patients who successfully completed the mindfulness meditation intervention reported that their pain-related symptoms did not diminish significantly, but that their *interpretations* or affective *reactions* to pain were markedly reduced. Patients reported that they were more *accepting* of their pain, which was related to a "decoupling" of pain intensity and emotional aspects of pain [31, 33].

What may be unique about mindfulness, in terms of a modulatory strategy, is that the goal is not to blunt sensations typically interpreted as pain. Rather, it involves an attempt to alter the context, through changes in appraisal, which seems to subsequently influence the associated suffering. These effects seem to be largely dependent on experience level of the meditator. Novices appear to reduce low-level, presumably sensory, pain-related activity (thalamus, S1) and show greater activation of higher-order evaluative regions such as aINS and OFC. In contrast, advanced practitioners significantly attenuate multiple prefrontal regions, including the OFC and DLPFC. Concurrently, activity is maintained or increased in sensory and pain-related regions such as INS, S2, thalamus, and ACC. We have suggested previously that these discrepant effects may reflect two approaches to mindfulness. Novices may require more cognitive effort and ultimately be implementing an active reappraisal-like form of mindfulness. The literature, particularly the trait-related studies [23, 24], suggest that more advanced practitioners apply the mental stance more reflexively in what might be termed a "no-appraisal" form of mindfulness. Nevertheless, both novices and expert meditators seem to alter the contextual evaluation of arising nociceptive and sensory events in a fashion that is largely consistent with the concept of mindfulness. This raises the intriguing question of whether a fully mindful experience of noxious stimulation still fits the definition of pain.

REFERENCES

1. Astin JA. Stress reduction through mindfulness meditation: effects on psychological symptomatology, sense of control, and spiritual experiences. Psychother Psychosom 1997;66(2):97–106.
2. Baliki MN, Chialvo DR, Geha PY, Levy RM, Harden RN, Parrish TB, Apkarian AV. Chronic pain and the emotional brain: specific brain activity associated with spontaneous fluctuations of intensity of chronic back pain. J Neurosci 2006;26(47):12165–73.
3. Barnhofer T, Crane C, Hargus E, Amarasinghe M, Winder R, Williams JM. Mindfulness-based cognitive therapy as a treatment for chronic depression: a preliminary study. Behav Res Ther 2009;47(5):366–73.
4. Brewer JA, Worhunsky PD, Gray JR, Tang YY, Weber J, Kober H. Meditation experience is associated with differences in default mode network activity and connectivity. Proc Natl Acad Sci U S A 2011;108(50):20254–9.

5. Brown CA, Jones AK. Meditation experience predicts less negative appraisal of pain: electrophysiological evidence for the involvement of anticipatory neural responses. Pain 2010;150(3):428–38.
6. Carlson LE, Speca M, Patel KD, Goodey E. Mindfulness-based stress reduction in relation to quality of life, mood, symptoms of stress, and immune parameters in breast and prostate cancer outpatients. Psychosom Med 2003;65(4):571–81.
7. Carlson LE, Ursuliak Z, Goodey E, Angen M, Speca M. The effects of a mindfulness meditation-based stress reduction program on mood and symptoms of stress in cancer outpatients: 6-month follow-up. Support Care Cancer 2001;9(2):112–23.
8. Christoff K, Gordon AM, Smallwood J, Smith R, Schooler JW. Experience sampling during fMRI reveals default network and executive system contributions to mind wandering. Proc Natl Acad Sci U S A 2009;106(21):8719–24.
9. Coghill RC, McHaffie JG, Yen YF. Neural correlates of interindividual differences in the subjective experience of pain. Proc Natl Acad Sci U S A 2003;100(14):8538–42.
10. Coghill RC, Sang CN, Maisog JM, Iadarola MJ. Pain intensity processing within the human brain: a bilateral, distributed mechanism. J Neurophysiol 1999;82(4):1934–43.
11. Creswell JD, Way BM, Eisenberger NI, Lieberman MD. Neural correlates of dispositional mindfulness during affect labeling. Psychosom Med 2007;69(6):560–5.
12. Derbyshire SW, Jones AK, Gyulai F, Clark S, Townsend D, Firestone LL. Pain processing during three levels of noxious stimulation produces differential patterns of central activity. Pain 1997;73(3):431–45.
13. Dunne J. Toward an understanding of non-dual mindfulness. Contemporary Buddhism 2011;12(1):69–86.
14. Emerson NM, Zeidan F, Lobanov OV, Hadsel MS, Martucci KT, Quevedo AS, Starr CJ, Nahman-Averbuch H, Weissman-Fogel I, Granovsky Y, et al. Pain sensitivity is inversely related to regional grey matter density in the brain. Pain 2014;155(3):566–73.
15. Farb NA, Anderson AK, Mayberg H, Bean J, McKeon D, Segal ZV. Minding one's emotions: mindfulness training alters the neural expression of sadness. Emotion 2010;10(1):25–33.
16. Fox KC, Nijeboer S, Dixon ML, Floman JL, Ellamil M, Rumak SP, Sedlmeier P, Christoff K. Is meditation associated with altered brain structure? A systematic review and meta-analysis of morphometric neuroimaging in meditation practitioners. Neurosci Biobehav Rev 2014;43:48–73.
17. Fransson P, Marrelec G. The precuneus/posterior cingulate cortex plays a pivotal role in the default mode network: evidence from a partial correlation network analysis. Neuroimage 2008;42(3):1178–84.

18. Friedman DP, Murray EA, O'Neill JB, Mishkin M. Cortical connections of the somatosensory fields of the lateral sulcus of macaques: evidence for a corticolimbic pathway for touch. J Comp Neurol 1986;252(3):323–47.

19. Gard T, Holzel BK, Sack AT, Hempel H, Vaitl D, Ott U. Pain attenuation through mindfulness is associated with decreased cognitive control and increased sensory processing in the brain. Cerebral Cortex 2011;191(1):36–43.

20. Garrison KA, Santoyo JF, Davis JH, Thornhill TA, Kerr CE, Brewer JA. Effortless awareness: using real time neurofeedback to investigate correlates of posterior cingulate cortex activity in meditators' self-report. Front Hum Neurosci 2013;7:440.

21. Goldin PR, Gross JJ. Effects of mindfulness-based stress reduction (MBSR) on emotion regulation in social anxiety disorder. Emotion 2010;10(1):83–91.

22. Grant JA. Meditative analgesia: the current state of the field. Ann N Y Acad Sci 2014;1307:55–63.

23. Grant JA, Courtemanche J, Rainville P. A non-elaborative mental stance and decoupling of executive and pain-related cortices predicts low pain sensitivity in Zen meditators. Pain 2011;152(1):150–6.

24. Grant JA, Rainville P. Pain sensitivity and analgesic effects of mindful states in Zen meditators: a cross-sectional study. Psychosom Med 2009;71(1):106–14.

25. Grossman P, Niemann L, Schmidt S, Walach H. Mindfulness-based stress reduction and health benefits: a meta-analysis. J Psychosom Res 2004;57(1):35–43.

26. Hasenkamp W, Barsalou LW. Effects of meditation experience on functional connectivity of distributed brain networks. Front Hum Neurosci 2012;6:38.

27. Hasenkamp W, Wilson-Mendenhall CD, Duncan E, Barsalou LW. Mind wandering and attention during focused meditation: a fine-grained temporal analysis of fluctuating cognitive states. Neuroimage 2011;59(1):750–60.

28. Holzel BK, Lazar SW, Gard T, Schuman-Olivier Z, Vago DR, Ott U. How does mindfulness meditation work? Proposing mechanisms of action from a conceptual and neural perspective. Perspect Psychol Sci 2011;6:537–59.

29. Jha AP, Krompinger J, Baime MJ. Mindfulness training modifies subsystems of attention. Cogn Affect Behav Neurosci 2007;7(2):109–19.

30. Josipovic Z. Neural correlates of nondual awareness in meditation. Ann N Y Acad Sci 2014;1307:9–18.

31. Kabat-Zinn J. An outpatient program in behavioral medicine for chronic pain patients based on the practice of mindfulness meditation: theoretical considerations and preliminary results. Gen Hosp Psychiatry 1982;4(1):33–47.

32. Kabat-Zinn J. Full catastrophe living. New York, NY: Delta Publishing; 1990.

33. Kabat-Zinn J, Lipworth L, Burney R. The clinical use of mindfulness meditation for the self-regulation of chronic pain. J Behav Med 1985;8(2):163–90.

34. Kabat-Zinn J, Massion AO, Kristeller J, Peterson LG, Fletcher KE, Pbert L, Lenderking WR, Santorelli SF. Effectiveness of a meditation-based stress reduction program in the treatment of anxiety disorders. Am J Psychiatry 1992;149(7):936–43.

35. Kabat-Zinn J, Wheeler E, Light T, Skillings A, Scharf MJ, Cropley TG, Hosmer D, Bernhard JD. Influence of a mindfulness meditation-based stress reduction intervention on rates of skin clearing in patients with moderate to severe psoriasis undergoing phototherapy (UVB) and photochemotherapy (PUVA). Psychosom Med 1998;60(5):625–32.

36. Kucyi A, Moayedi M, Weissman-Fogel I, Goldberg MB, Freeman BV, Tenenbaum HC, Davis KD. Enhanced medial prefrontal-default mode network functional connectivity in chronic pain and its association with pain rumination. J Neurosci 2014;34(11):3969–75.

37. Kucyi A, Salomons TV, Davis KD. Mind wandering away from pain dynamically engages antinociceptive and default mode brain networks. Proc Natl Acad Sci U S A 2013;110(46):18692–7.

38. Leveton A. Time, death and the ego-chill. J Existent 1965;6(21):69–80.

39. Loggia ML, Kim J, Gollub RL, Vangel MG, Kirsch I, Kong J, Wasan AD, Napadow V. Default mode network connectivity encodes clinical pain: an arterial spin labeling study. Pain 2013;154(1):24–33.

40. Lutz A, McFarlin DR, Perlman DM, Salomons TV, Davidson RJ. Altered anterior insula activation during anticipation and experience of painful stimuli in expert meditators. Neuroimage 2013;64:538–546.

41. Lutz A, Slagter HA, Dunne JD, Davidson RJ. Attention regulation and monitoring in meditation. Trends Cogn Sci 2008;12(4):163–9.

42. Lutz A, Slagter HA, Rawlings NB, Francis AD, Greischar LL, Davidson RJ. Mental training enhances attentional stability: neural and behavioral evidence. J Neurosci 2009;29(42):13418–27.

43. Maclean KA, Ferrer E, Aichele SR, Bridwell DA, Zanesco AP, Jacobs TL, King BG, Rosenberg EL, Sahdra BK, Shaver PR, et al. Intensive meditation training improves perceptual discrimination and sustained attention. Psychol Sci 2010;21:829–39.

44. Mufson EJ, Mesulam MM. Insula of the old world monkey. II: afferent cortical input and comments on the claustrum. J Comp Neurol 1982;212(1):23–37.

45. Price DD. Psychological and neural mechanisms of the affective dimension of pain. Science 2000;288(5472):1769–72.

46. Price DD, Barell JJ. Inner experience and neuroscience. Cambridge, MA: MIT Press; 2012.
47. Price DD, Bush FM, Long S, Harkins SW. A comparison of pain measurement characteristics of mechanical visual analogue and simple numerical rating scales. Pain 1994;56(2):217–26.
48. Price DD, Harkins SW, Baker C. Sensory-affective relationships among different types of clinical and experimental pain. Pain 1987;28(3):297–307.
49. Raichle ME, MacLeod AM, Snyder AZ, Powers WJ, Gusnard DA, Shulman GL. A default mode of brain function. Proc Natl Acad Sci U S A 2001;98(2):676–82.
50. Rainville P, Carrier B, Hofbauer RK, Bushnell MC, Duncan GH. Dissociation of sensory and affective dimensions of pain using hypnotic modulation. Pain 1999;82(2):159–71.
51. Scheeringa R, Bastiaansen MC, Petersson KM, Oostenveld R, Norris DG, Hagoort P. Frontal theta EEG activity correlates negatively with the default mode network in resting state. Int J Psychophysiol 2008;67(3):242–51.
52. Seeley WW, Menon V, Schatzberg AF, Keller J, Glover GH, Kenna H, Reiss AL, Greicius MD. Dissociable intrinsic connectivity networks for salience processing and executive control. J Neurosci 2007;27(9):2349–56.
53. Shapiro SL, Carlson LE, Astin JA, Freedman B. Mechanisms of mindfulness. J Clin Psychol 2006;62(3):373–86.
54. Smallwood J, Fitzgerald A, Miles LK, Phillips LH. Shifting moods, wandering minds: negative moods lead the mind to wander. Emotion 2009;9(2):271–6.
55. Smallwood J, McSpadden M, Schooler JW. The lights are on but no one's home: meta-awareness and the decoupling of attention when the mind wanders. Psychon Bull Rev 2007;14(3):527–33.
56. Taylor VA, Daneault V, Grant J, Scavone G, Breton E, Roffe-Vidal S, Courtemanche J, Lavarenne AS, Marrelec G, Benali H, Beauregard M. Impact of meditation training on the default mode network during a restful state. Soc Cogn Affect Neurosci 2013;8(1):4–14.
57. Teasdale JD, Segal ZV, Williams JM, Ridgeway VA, Soulsby JM, Lau MA. Prevention of relapse/recurrence in major depression by mindfulness-based cognitive therapy. J Consult Clin Psychol 2000;68(4):615–23.
58. Tomasino B, Chiesa A, Fabbro F. Disentangling the neural mechanisms involved in Hinduism- and Buddhism-related meditations. Brain Cogn 2014;90:32–40.
59. Wallace BA. The attention revolution: unlocking the power of the focused mind. Somerville, MA: Wisdom Publications; 2006.

60. Wasan AD, Loggia ML, Chen LQ, Napadow V, Kong J, Gollub RL. Neural correlates of chronic low back pain measured by arterial spin labeling. Anesthesiology 2011;115(2):364–74.

61. Weissman DH, Roberts KC, Visscher KM, Woldorff MG. The neural bases of momentary lapses in attention. Nat Neurosci 2006;9(7):971–8.

62. Zeidan F, Coghill RC. Functional connections between self-referential thought and chronic pain: a dysfunctional relationship. Pain 2012;154(1):3–4.

63. Zeidan F, Grant JA, Brown CA, McHaffie JG, Coghill RC. Mindfulness meditation-related pain relief: evidence for unique brain mechanisms in the regulation of pain. Neurosci Lett 2012;520(2):165–73.

64. Zeidan F, Johnson SK, Diamond BJ, David Z, Goolkasian P. Mindfulness meditation improves cognition: evidence of brief mental training. Conscious Cogn 2010;19(2):597–605.

65. Zeidan F, Martucci KT, Kraft RA, Gordon NS, McHaffie JG, Coghill RC. Brain mechanisms supporting the modulation of pain by mindfulness meditation. J Neurosci 2011;31(14):5540–8.

66. Zeidan F, Martucci KT, Kraft RA, McHaffie JG, Coghill RC. Neural correlates of mindfulness meditation-related anxiety relief. Soc Cogn Affect Neurosci 2014;9(6):751–9.

CHAPTER 9

Consciousness, Placebo, and Nocebo Effects on Pain

Luana Colloca

There are moments of existence when time and space are more profound, and the awareness of existence is immensely heightened.
—Charles Baudelaire

During the last three decades, theories of placebo and nocebo effects have primarily relied on consciousness. Some argue that conscious components are pivotal to create desires, beliefs, and hence placebo and nocebo effects, and awareness in placebo and nocebo effects per se has been poorly investigated. Despite these beliefs, there is compelling evidence of placebo and nocebo effects present under different states of consciousness which includes effects with and without awareness, effects observed during sleep and hypnosis, as well as placebo effects in infants and animals.

AWARENESS, VERBALLY INDUCED PLACEBO AND NOCEBO EFFECTS

Not surprisingly, awareness and language play a pivotal role when we explore placebo and nocebo effects in humans. In particular, "language turns the self into a thing and gives it attributes and powers" [10]. Being informed about the effects of a treatment and becoming aware of being treated is extremely relevant for the formation of placebo and nocebo effects in daily clinical practice [18].

Interesting translational research has shown that patients undergoing treatment for pain respond better when they are aware of receiving pain medication. These observations are based on open/hidden paradigms in which identical doses of medication are given either overtly (open) or covertly (hidden). In the overt scenario, the patient receives treatment from a health practitioner and is fully aware of its administration, whereas in the covert scenario, medication is administered via a computer-programmed infusion pump. Patients in postoperative acute pain who underwent overt morphine treatment (10 mg) required 50% less drug intake as compared to those who were treated covertly [23]. Similar results have been observed across different painkillers such as buprenorphine, tramadol, ketorolac, and metamizol, indicating that the reinforcing awareness is a widespread phenomenon [2].

Awareness about the treatment results in an enhancement of therapeutic placebo effects and improvement of clinical outcomes. For example, semantic and verbal information such as those embedded in drug labeling has a powerful suggestive impact on clinical outcomes, as illustrated in a recent study. In this study, half of the participants were randomly administered 10 mg rizatriptan (Maxalt) and half were administered a placebo pill [39]. However, the labels for the pills were also randomly and equally assigned. One-third of the pills were labeled "Maxalt," corresponding to positive information, one-third were labeled "Maxalt or Placebo," representing neutral information, and the remaining third were labeled "Placebo," representing negative information. Pain relief was greatest when given positive information followed by neutral and then by negative information. Although Maxalt correctly labeled was more effective than placebo correctly labeled, Maxalt labeled as "placebo" was surprisingly just as effective as placebo labeled as "Maxalt." Moreover, actual placebo pills in each of the different information categories (positive, neutral, or negative) accounted for more than 50% of the drug effect [39]. This study represents another example of how awareness about treatments through patient–clinician communication leads to significant differences in the perception of efficacy and can influence decision-making processes.

The findings described above have been extended in studies with healthy subjects. For example, being aware of receiving remifentanil potentiated its pharmacological analgesic effect in healthy subjects receiving acute thermal painful stimulation. Importantly, knowledge about the discontinuation of the treatment when, in actuality, the treatment was continuously administered reversed the analgesic effect. Being aware of the administration of remifentanil doubled the analgesic effect, while believing that the treatment had been stopped blocked the remifentanil-induced analgesia. These effects produced significant changes in functional magnetic resonance imaging (fMRI)-assessed neural activity in specific brain areas related to coding of pain intensity and experience. The blocking of analgesia due to negative beliefs was reflected in the activation of the hippocampus [9], a region that has been linked to nocebo effects [41].

Remarkably, the degeneration and disconnection of the frontal lobes in Alzheimer disease (AD) are associated with a reduction or complete loss of the verbally induced placebo analgesic response. The impairment of language processing and cognitive functions can potentially alter the meaning of the psychosocial component of any treatments, therefore minimizing placebo effects. Benedetti et al. [7] applied a local anesthetic, either overtly or covertly, to the skin of patients with AD to reduce venipuncture-induced pain. Placebo responses were then correlated with both cognitive status and functional connectivity among different brain regions as assessed by EEG measurements. AD patients with reduced prefrontal executive control and decreased EEG connectivity of the prefrontal lobes with the rest of the brain presented a reduced placebo component of the analgesic treatment lidocaine. The loss of these placebo-related mechanisms is associated with a reduction of treatment efficacy.

PLACEBO AND NOCEBO EFFECTS ACQUIRED WITHOUT AWARENESS

Implicit learning refers to complex information acquired in an incidental manner, without awareness. Frensch and Rünger [29] pointed out that the general definition of implicit learning is still subject to some controversy, although the topic has had some significant developments since the 1960s. Certainly, implicit learning is fundamental for cognition and a determinant actor in the genesis of placebo and nocebo effects [17, 24, 25].

Implicit learning boosts the magnitude and persistence of placebo and nocebo effects. Subjects received painful stimulation while the intensity was manipulated to make subjects experience the mastery of analgesia. Subjects were randomized to a 40 or 10 conditioning trials. Placebo and nocebo effects were larger and lasted over the entire experimental session when the long conditioning session was used to acquire the information [26]. Recently, we studied the effects of long (4 days) versus short (1 day) conditioning in combination with an intentional disclosure about the sham nature of the treatment. Immediately following the conditioning phase, placebo analgesia was measured during the testing phase both before and after subjects were told the treatment was a placebo (placebo reveal). Being aware of the fact that they had never received an active drug did not abolish the effect of implicit learning. Placebo analgesia was indeed retested, and we observed that the effects persisted after the revelation in the long conditioning group but not in the short conditioning group (Fig. 9-1). These findings suggest that automatic processes may persist despite awareness of placebo treatments and that these effects are independent of conscious expectations for pain relief [50].

Jensen and colleagues [37] compared conscious versus unconscious conditions in a placebo and nocebo effect study using a behavioral conditioning paradigm. The paradigm consisted of a conditioning procedure in which clearly recognizable images of two male faces were consistently paired with a high- and low-heat painful stimulus delivered on the volar forearm. After an acquisition phase, high and low cues were paired with identical moderate heat stimuli to test for placebo and nocebo effects.

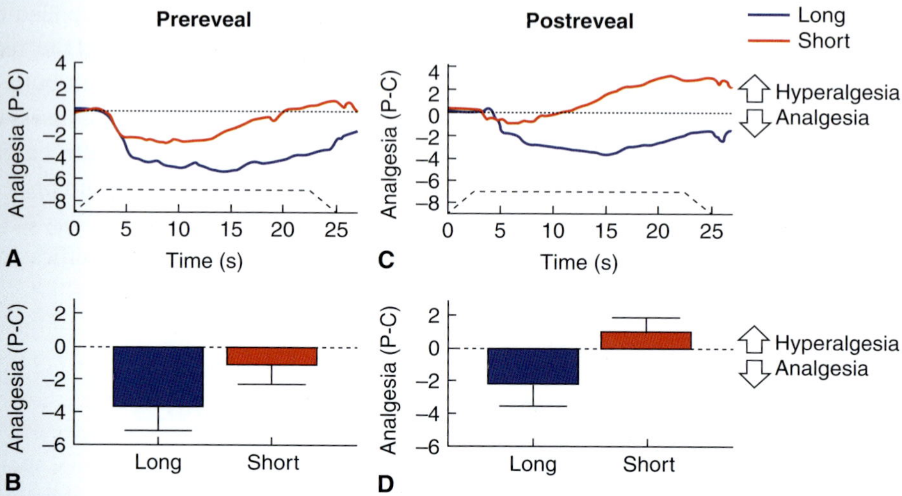

FIGURE 9-1 The solid blue and red lines represent the analgesic responses within the long and short conditioning groups, respectively. The dashed line shows the onset and offset of the painful stimulus, as well as the duration of peak temperature. **A:** Prereveal placebo analgesia during thermal painful stimulation. **B:** Average of prereveal placebo analgesia. Long conditioning group had significant placebo analgesia, but short conditioning did not. **C:** Postreveal placebo analgesia. Subjects in the long conditioning group continued to demonstrate placebo analgesia postreveal, and had significantly greater placebo analgesia than the short conditioning group. **D:** There was no significant postreveal placebo effect in the short group. Data are presented as mean ± sem. (Data from Schafer et al. [50].)

During this phase, 50% of the cues were presented long enough (100 ms) so that participants were able to recognize them. The remaining 50% of the cues were masked to prevent conscious recognition (backward masking) and cues were presented for 12 ms only (nonconscious masked exposures). Significant placebo and nocebo effects were found even when masked cues, not consciously perceptible, were used to test the behavioral responses [37], indicating that placebo and nocebo mechanisms can partially operate without conscious awareness.

More recently, Jensen and colleagues extended these findings by investigating the neural counterparts of nonconscious placebo and nocebo pain responses, using fMRI in healthy participants [36]. Nonconscious placebo analgesia showed increased activation of the orbitofrontal cortex as compared with conscious placebo analgesic effects. During the presentation of the masked cues, nocebo effects induced an increased activation of the thalamus, amygdala, and hippocampus as compared to the unmasked cues. Nocebo responses on pain induced an activation of the hippocampus along with the activation of the amygdala as previously reported [9, 41]. The activation of the amygdala during nonconscious nocebo responses was more highly correlated with the pain ratings indicating an unconscious motivation that may affect participants' rating. Thus, placebo and nocebo responses can occur independently of conscious awareness [36]. These results are in line with previous studies demonstrating that fear responses also occur without conscious perception of the fear cues [47], and that the amygdala and adjacent subcortical structures facilitate an immediate, likely unconscious, recognition of threat [13].

In humans, learning is cognitively mediated and can elicit analgesia when relationships between events are acquired [48, 49]. Instructions can amplify the effect of automatic processes. A recent study included two groups of healthy subjects each receiving a conditioning procedure with or without explicit information about the cues, which consisted in distinct-colored lights anticipating either analgesia or a control level of pain, as previously used [12]. An N2–P2 component of laser-evoked potentials (LEP) was used as an index of brain responses to nociceptive stimuli and pain modulation. The group who received verbal information along with the conditioning manipulation experienced a decrease in pain rating and LEP amplitude, indicating that conscious components can reinforce automatic visual-analgesic associations [12].

Furthermore, Au Yeung and colleagues [4] investigated how partial and full reinforcement learning paradigms influence placebo analgesia. Healthy volunteers were randomly assigned continuous reinforcement, partial reinforcement, or a control (no conditioning) group. For the continued reinforcement group, the placebo was always followed by a reduction in pain during the acquisition phase. For the partial reinforcement group, the placebo treatment was followed by a reduction in pain stimulation in 62% of trials only. In the testing phase, both full and partial conditioning induced placebo analgesia, with the magnitude of analgesia being larger after the continuous conditioning. However, responses elicited by partial conditioning were less sensitive to extinction. This result indicates that partial reinforcement schedules can potentially be exploited to prevent extinction of placebo effects [4].

Also to compare continuous and partial reinforcement procedures, we tested how partial reinforcement modulates nocebo hyperalgesia and whether the effects established under partial reinforcement were more resistant to extinction as compared to those induced by full conditioning. Three key findings emerged. First, nocebo hyperalgesia can be established under partial reinforcement, although it is weaker than that established under continuous reinforcement. Second, nocebo hyperalgesia is resistant to extinction independently of whether it is established via continuous or partial reinforcement. Third, there is strong concordance between the level of hyperalgesia expected and the level experienced. These findings have a number of important theoretical and practical implications [16]. Partial reinforcement affected nocebo hyperalgesia differently than its effects on placebo analgesia. These findings were in line with previous studies showing that nocebo effects are stronger than placebo effects even when participants were merely informed about the possibility to receive high level of painful electrical shocks. Although subjects were given either tactile or low-intensity painful electrical stimuli, they reported tactile stimuli as painful and low-intensity stimuli as highly painful, indicating the possibility to create verbally induced allodynic and hyperalgesic responses. The magnitudes of the nocebo hyperalgesic effect following either verbal suggestions alone or following the conditioning procedure were not significantly different [27]. From an evolutionary viewpoint, nocebo effects may represent a form of short-term innate responses, aimed at enhancing responses to negative outcomes to initiate defensive behaviors.

AWARENESS: HOW OBSERVATION SHAPES PAIN PERCEPTION

Self-awareness is a composite of the way we see ourselves and we see others. The awareness of our identity (therefore our perceptions) results from the integration of information acquired through first-hand experiences and observation of both others' experiences and environmental cues outside of our self. Both direct experience and observation influence the formation of placebo and nocebo effects. Healthy subjects who have witnessed a benefit in another person showed strong placebo analgesic effects comparable in magnitude to those induced through direct conditioned experiences [20]. When tested for pain following the observational phase, observers experienced as analgesic, stimuli that were actually set at a painful level. Interestingly, observation modulates behavioral nocebo effects: observing another person in pain induced hyperalgesic effects when control painful stimuli were delivered later [54]. Psychosocial cues and the entire set of interpersonal interactions also contribute to induce expectations and potentially consolidate analgesia.

Recently, a social contagion has been demonstrated, whereby informing a single subject of the possibility of headache produces a propagation of this negative information across several subjects, who will also experience headache. Interestingly, this social propagation may change the brain biochemistry of the socially infected individuals, as shown by the increase in cyclooxygenase activity and prostaglandins synthesis [8]. This phenomenon occurs in clinical encounters whereby patients interact with each other sharing experiences, feelings, and emotions. The relevance of these factors has not been investigated, but it is evident that placebo and nocebo effects have clinical implications [6, 23, 45].

MEMORY OF EFFICACIOUS OUTCOMES

Learning from prior positive experience can create strong memory analgesic responses, and likewise negative previous experiences can elicit nocebo effects. We designed a study in which one group received a treatment perceived as efficacious (actually, the intensity of painful stimulations was surreptitiously decreased) and a second group received a treatment perceived as ineffective (verbal suggestions with no manipulation of the intensity of painful stimulation). When tested for placebo analgesia the first group reported significant reduction of pain (49.3%), while the second group reported a smaller pain reduction (9.7%) [19]. After 4–7 days, both groups were retested for placebo analgesia, and we found that the placebo responses following the effective procedure were significantly higher than that observed after the ineffective treatment (29% vs. 18% pain reduction). Therefore, placebo and nocebo effects are shaped by learning (either positive or negative prior experience), and the effect of initial treatment exposure influences the response to subsequent placebo responses with obvious clinical implications [19].

Distinct neural correlates underpin the role of treatment history in placebo and nocebo effects. After randomizing healthy volunteers to two groups, either a positive or negative treatment experience, Kessner et al. [40] introduced a new analgesic to test for the effect of treatment history in an elegant fMRI study. The therapeutic effect of the tested treatment was lower in the negative compared to the positive treatment history group. The adverse effect of the negative treatment history was sustained in the brain by a higher activation of posterior insula bilaterally, a region implicated in the afferent nociceptive processing, and a lower activation of the right dorsolateral prefrontal cortex (dl-PFC), involved in pain modulatory system [40]. These findings showed how therapeutic experiences affect modulatory systems and responses to subsequent treatments and placebos.

Notably, similar effects have been documented in patients with chronic neuropathic pain [3]. André-Obadia and colleagues studied the effects of true and sham repetitive transcranial magnetic stimulation (rTMS) in a crossover design in neuropathic pain patients resistant to pharmacological treatment. Patients were assigned to one of two conditions: (1) sham rTMS delivered before the conventional stimulation of the motor cortex, and (2) sham rTMS delivered after the conventional stimulation of the motor cortex. Those patients who received the sham rTMS after a session of real rTMS perceived an analgesic effect (11% pain reduction), suggesting that the exposure to effective treatments induces the formation of significant hypoalgesic responses [3].

PLACEBO EFFECTS UNDER ALTERED STATES OF CONSCIOUSNESS: SLEEP AND HYPNOSIS

Sleep and specific related activity appear to be a potential actor in regulating placebo analgesia [15]. Laverdure-Dupont and colleagues [42] recently showed that sleep, and more specifically rapid eye movement (REM) sleep, a state that contributes to information processing, regulates placebo analgesia, conditioning effects as well as expectations of pain relief. Before sleep, healthy participants received a conditioning manipulation wherein the intensity of thermal pain stimulation was surreptitiously reduced after the application of a topical placebo cream. Expectations and placebo analgesic effects were measured the following morning and compared with those of a control daytime group without sleep. Placebo effects were observed in both groups. However, correlation analyses indicated that the mediating effect of expectations on placebo analgesia was strongest in the overnight group. The relative duration of REM sleep decreased in subjects showing higher analgesic expectations and placebo responses the next morning. Interestingly, REM sleep predicted placebo-induced expectations of pain relief. More recently, Chouchou and colleagues [14] studied placebo analgesia, following pharmacological REM deprivation to test the hypothesis that placebo analgesia would be improved by experimental REM deprivation in healthy participants. Following an adaptive night in a sleep laboratory, participants underwent classical experimental placebo analgesic conditioning in the evening and were randomized to either clonidine or inert control pills in a double-blind fashion. Placebo analgesia was tested in the morning. The authors found that placebo analgesia increased with REM sleep deprivation. Expectations of pain relief did not differ between REM sleep deprivation and control groups, but placebo analgesia correlated positively and strongly with pain relief expectations in REM sleep deprivation but not in control group. Overall these findings indicate a key role of REM sleep in modulating placebo analgesia.

Psychological traits such as dispositional optimism [30, 31], somatic focus [38], empathy [20, 35, 52], neuroticism [46], and altruism [46] have been linked to individual placebo effects (for a review, see reference [22]). Particularly interesting for this topical book is the hypnotic suggestibility trait. Responsiveness of an individual to suggestions has been also linked to behavioral placebo effects [28] and neural conditioned placebo responses [34]. De Pascalis and colleagues [28] tested individual differences in suggestibility, verbal expectancy for drug efficacy, and manipulation procedure for pain reduction as possible mediators of placebo analgesia. Dependent variables such as (1) subjective expectancy for drug efficacy in pain relief, (2) expected pain intensity and unpleasantness, (3) concurrent pain intensity and unpleasantness, and (4) remembered pain intensity and unpleasantness were measured. Verbal expectancy for drug efficacy and individual differences in suggestibility were found to contribute significantly to the magnitude of placebo analgesia. Interestingly, the highest suggestibility trait was associated with the highest placebo effect. Placebo effects established on remembered pain were at least twice as great as those obtained on concurrent placebo effects. Moreover, remembered placebo effects, like the concurrent placebo effects, were highly correlated with expected pain scores obtained just after manipulation trials. These results indicate that although multiple factors contribute to the placebo effect, suggestibility is a critical determinant of placebo-induced pain relief [28].

After studying fMRI conditioned placebo analgesia in subjects receiving brief laser-heat stimuli delivered to one foot (either right or left) that were preceded by different visual cues, signaling either painful stimuli alone, or painful stimuli accompanied by a (sham) analgesic procedure [44], Huber et al. [34] retrospectively contacted the same subjects to explore the connection between conditioning and hypnosis. High hypnotic susceptibility was associated with increased anticipatory activity in the right dl-PFC, and the ability to reduce functional connectivity of that focus with other brain regions such as the anterior midcingulate cortex and medial-PFC that are involved in emotional and evaluative pain processes. Subjects with low hypnotic susceptibility presented a reverse pattern of fMRI changes and functional connectivity [34].

PLACEBO EFFECTS IN INFANTS

Another important open question to be addressed is how and when conscious processes start to take place in the formation of neurobiological placebo analgesic responses. An interesting way to address this question is to look at learned placebo effects in infants. Indeed, it is well-known that a newborn lacks self-awareness. However, newborns process complex visual stimuli and attend to sounds and sights in the world, such as looking at faces. Actually, the capability to activate self-healing processes and create placebo effects seems to be present very early in the stage of development. Infants respond to noxious stimulation from birth (and likely before birth), and these responses produce reflex movements, autonomic and metabolic responses that are distinct from the complex pain experience, and ability to report pain reliefs. A few studies have described modulation of nociception in infants (for a review, see reference [51]). A case study reported that an infant with complex cardiopathy and agenesis of the trachea showed conditioned analgesic response after repeated, frequent bronchoscopies performed under the effects of midazolam and fentanyl [5]. After 61 bronchoscopies performed by the same clinician, medication was not needed because the patient indicated no signs of distress while watching the clinician performing the intervention. By contrast, the infant began demonstrating compliant behaviors by positioning her body to receive treatment, indicating a sort of conditioned antinociceptive response [5].

Similar acquired antinociception responses were observed in hospitalized full-term infants of diabetic mothers who underwent repeated venipuncture consisting in heel lancing without anesthesia for monitoring blood glucose concentration in the first 24–36 hours [53]. Infants exposed to frequent heel lancing showed more pronounced pain behaviors, or signs of increased distress, than normal infants following venipuncture for newborn screening only. Notably, cleaning the skin elicited pain behaviors in the infants of diabetic mothers, suggesting that likewise, the infants presented anticipatory hyperalgesic effects [53].

PLACEBO EFFECTS IN ANIMALS

The topic of placebo effects in animals as well as animal consciousness or animal awareness is besieged with a number of difficulties. Animals lack the ability to express human language and cannot tell us about their pain experiences but, like infants, show the ability to experience or to feel as well as initiate defensive behaviors [21].

Recently, a few studies of pain and placebo analgesia have been published using animal models. Guo et al. [32] created an animal model to evoke, in mice, opioid and non-opioid placebo responses that were either naloxone-reversible or naloxone-insensitive, depending on the drug used in conditioning procedure. With this animal model the opioid placebo analgesia was found to be mediated exclusively through μ-opioid receptor. Amanzio and Benedetti [1] showed that both expectation and conditioning are crucial for the activation of opioid or non-opioid systems: expectation triggers endogenous opioids, whereas conditioning activates specific subsystems [1]. If conditioning is performed with opioids, placebo analgesia is mediated via opioid receptors, but if conditioning is performed with non-opioid drugs, other non-opioid mechanisms tend to be involved. On the basis of these experiments and previous animal work on placebo responses, Guo et al. performed a 4-day drug conditioning experiment in female Imprinting Control Region (ICR) mice. A hot-plate test was used to measure response latencies according to the method described by Hargraves and Hentall [33]. The reason for using the hot-plate test was the likely involvement of supraspinal mechanisms in this pain model [43], in contrast with other nociceptive tests such as the tail-flick test, which are indicative of spinal reflexes, as it persists after section or cold block of upper parts of the spinal cord. After a conditioning with morphine, mice were treated with saline solution, exposed to the conditioned cue cage and then, tested for pain tolerance [32]. Saline solution induced enhanced pain tolerance compared with control levels, indicating that the previous morphine conditioning was sufficient to evoke a morphine-like analgesic effect. A pretreatment with naloxone blocked the placebo-induced analgesia. The same procedure described above was repeated after a pharmacological conditioning with aspirin. Interestingly, similar placebo responses were observed except that the pretreatment with naloxone did not block the conditioned analgesic response established by prior conditioning with the non-opioid aspirin. This research suggested that mice learn to associate contextual cues with elevated pain tolerance producing conditioned analgesia similar to the response previously observed in humans, namely, conditioning with morphine-produced placebo analgesia that was completely antagonized by naloxone in animals and humans. Similarly, conditioning with aspirin elicited a placebo effect that was not blocked by naloxone in mice and humans.

Zhang et al. [55] also investigated the role of μ-, δ-, and κ-opioid receptors in animal placebo analgesia. Rats were treated with intra-rACC injection of

D-Phe-Cys-Tyr-D-Trp-Orn-Thr-Pen-Thr-NH2 (CTOP), a selective μ-opioid receptor antagonist, naltrindole (NTI), a highly selective δ-opioid receptor antagonist, or nor-binaltorphimine (nor-BNI), a highly selective κ-opioid receptor antagonist, before the hot-plate tests. Rats underwent the 4-day placebo analgesic conditioning, and saline solution along with the exposure to the conditioned cue compartment was used to test for pain tolerance. CTOP inhibited placebo analgesia dose-dependently. Neither NBI nor NTI affected the placebo analgesia in rats. Not surprisingly, a conditioning with morphine elicited opioid-mediated placebo analgesia that was blocked by microinjection of CTOP into rACC, but not the NTI and nor-BNI, δ-, or κ-opioid receptor antagonists, respectively outlining the specificity of selective μ-opioid receptors in morphine-like effects [55].

Obviously, conditioned effects in animals are extensively studied and are not limited to placebo analgesia. For example, Bryant and colleagues [11] tested in male C57BL/6J mice the effect of a pharmacological conditioning with selective μ-opioid receptor agonist fentanyl (0.2 mg/kg, i.p.) on locomotor activity, straub tail, hot-plate sensitivity, and conditioned place preference. Mice exhibited multiple conditional opioid-like responses including conditional hyperlocomotion, a conditional pattern of opioid-like locomotion, straub tail, analgesia, and place preference. The authors also explored the potential modeling effect by administrating fentanyl to a "demonstrator" mice in the home cage, "the observer" mice was watching his cage mate. The observation did not affect the expression of conditioned place preference or the concomitant locomotor activity in the "observer" mice, suggesting that observationally induced analgesia may require distinct levels of awareness.

CONCLUSIVE REMARKS

Although enormous advances have been achieved in understanding the psychological and neurobiological mechanisms of placebo and nocebo effects, knowledge about the role of consciousness on modulatory pain systems and associated learning mechanisms is still in its infancy. It is worth exploring to what extent conscious mechanisms are necessary to trigger a placebo and nocebo effect. Answering this question may have profound clinical and neuroscientific implications ranging from evoking beneficial therapeutic placebo effects in patients with altered consciousness states to understanding the interplay between brain modulatory pain systems and altered states of consciousness.

ACKNOWLEDGMENTS

This research was supported by University of Maryland Baltimore (UMB).

REFERENCES

1. Amanzio M, Benedetti F. Neuropharmacological dissection of placebo analgesia: expectation-activated opioid systems versus conditioning-activated specific subsystems. J Neurosci 1999;19(1):484–94.
2. Amanzio M, Pollo A, Maggi G, Benedetti F. Response variability to analgesics: a role for non-specific activation of endogenous opioids. Pain 2001;90(3):205–15.
3. Andre-Obadia N, Magnin M, Garcia-Larrea L. On the importance of placebo timing in rTMS studies for pain relief. Pain 2011;152(6):1233–7.
4. Au Yeung ST, Colagiuri B, Lovibond PF, Colloca L. Partial reinforcement, extinction, and placebo analgesia. Pain 2014;155(6):1110–7.
5. Bachiocco V, Mondardini MC. Julia's placebo effect. Pain 2010;150(3):582–5.
6. Benedetti F. Placebo and the new physiology of the doctor–patient relationship. Physiol Rev 2013;93(3):1207–46.
7. Benedetti F, Arduino C, Costa S, Vighetti S, Tarenzi L, Rainero I, Asteggiano G. Loss of expectation-related mechanisms in Alzheimer's disease makes analgesic therapies less effective. Pain 2006;121(1–2):133–44.
8. Benedetti F, Durando J, Vighetti S. Nocebo and placebo modulation of hypobaric hypoxia headache involves the cyclooxygenase-prostaglandins pathway. Pain 2014;155(5):921–8.
9. Bingel U, Wanigasekera V, Wiech K, Ni Mhuircheartaigh R, Lee MC, Ploner M, Tracey I. The effect of treatment expectation on drug efficacy: imaging the analgesic benefit of the opioid remifentanil. Science Transl Med 2011;3(70):70ra14.
10. Blackmore S. Demolishing the self. J Conscious Stud 1994;1(2):280–2.
11. Bryant CD, Roberts KW, Culbertson CS, Le A, Evans CJ, Fanselow MS. Pavlovian conditioning of multiple opioid-like responses in mice. Drug Alcohol Depend 2009;103(1–2):74–83.
12. Carlino E, Torta DM, Piedimonte A, Frisaldi E, Vighetti S, Benedetti F. Role of explicit verbal information in conditioned analgesia. Eur J Pain 2015;19:546–53.
13. Carlsson K, Petersson KM, Lundqvist D, Karlsson A, Ingvar M, Ohman A. Fear and the amygdala: manipulation of awareness generates differential cerebral responses to phobic and fear-relevant (but nonfeared) stimuli. Emotion 2004;4(4):340–53.
14. Chouchou F, Chauny JM, Rainville P, Lavigne GJ. Selective REM sleep deprivation improves expectation-related placebo analgesia. PLoS One 2015;10(12):e0144992.
15. Chouchou F, Lavigne GJ. Placebo analgesia and sleep [in French]. Pathol Biol (Paris) 2014;62(5):270–5.

16. Colagiuri B, Quinn VF, Colloca L. Nocebo hyperalgesia, partial reinforcement, and extinction. J Pain 2015;16:995–1004.
17. Colloca L. Placebo, nocebo, and learning mechanisms. Handb Exp Pharmacol 2014;225:17–35.
18. Colloca L, Benedetti F. Placebos and painkillers: is mind as real as matter? Nat Rev Neurosci 2005;6(7):545–52.
19. Colloca L, Benedetti F. How prior experience shapes placebo analgesia. Pain 2006;124(1–2):126–33.
20. Colloca L, Benedetti F. Placebo analgesia induced by social observational learning. Pain 2009;144(1–2):28–34.
21. Colloca L, Flaten MA, Meissner K. Placebo and pain: from bench to bedside. Oxford: Elsevier; 2013.
22. Colloca L, Grillon C. Understanding placebo and nocebo responses for pain management. Curr Pain Headache Rep 2014;18(6):419.
23. Colloca L, Lopiano L, Lanotte M, Benedetti F. Overt versus covert treatment for pain, anxiety, and Parkinson's disease. Lancet Neurol 2004;3(11):679–84.
24. Colloca L, Miller FG. Harnessing the placebo effect: the need for translational research. Philos Trans R Soc Lond B Biol Sci 2011;366(1572):1922–30.
25. Colloca L, Miller FG. How placebo responses are formed: a learning perspective. Philos Trans R Soc Lond B Biol Sci 2011;366(1572):1859–69.
26. Colloca L, Petrovic P, Wager TD, Ingvar M, Benedetti F. How the number of learning trials affects placebo and nocebo responses. Pain 2010;151(2):430–9.
27. Colloca L, Sigaudo M, Benedetti F. The role of learning in nocebo and placebo effects. Pain 2008;136(1–2):211–8.
28. De Pascalis V, Chiaradia C, Carotenuto E. The contribution of suggestibility and expectation to placebo analgesia phenomenon in an experimental setting. Pain 2002;96(3):393–402.
29. Frensch PA, Rünger D. Implicit learning. Curr Dir Psychol Sci 2003;12:13.
30. Geers AL, Helfer SG, Kosbab K, Weiland PE, Landry SJ. Reconsidering the role of personality in placebo effects: dispositional optimism, situational expectations, and the placebo response. J Psychosom Res 2005;58(2):121–7.
31. Geers AL, Wellman JA, Fowler SL, Helfer SG, France CR. Dispositional optimism predicts placebo analgesia. J Pain 2010;11(11):1165–71.
32. Guo JY, Wang JY, Luo F. Dissection of placebo analgesia in mice: the conditions for activation of opioid and non-opioid systems. J Psychopharmacol 2010; 24(10):1561–7.

33. Hargraves WA, Hentall ID. Analgesic effects of dietary caloric restriction in adult mice. Pain 2005;114(3):455–61.

34. Huber A, Lui F, Porro CA. Hypnotic susceptibility modulates brain activity related to experimental placebo analgesia. Pain 2013;154(9):1509–18.

35. Hunter T, Siess F, Colloca L. Socially induced placebo analgesia: a comparison of a pre-recorded versus live face-to-face observation. Eur J Pain 2014;18:914–22.

36. Jensen KB, Kaptchuk TJ, Chen X, Kirsch I, Ingvar M, Gollub RL, Kong J. A neural mechanism for nonconscious activation of conditioned placebo and nocebo responses. Cereb Cortex 2015;25:3903–10.

37. Jensen KB, Kaptchuk TJ, Kirsch I, Raicek J, Lindstrom KM, Berna C, Gollub RL, Ingvar M, Kong J. Nonconscious activation of placebo and nocebo pain responses. Proc Natl Acad Sci U S A 2012;109(39):15959–64.

38. Johnston NE, Atlas LY, Wager TD. Opposing effects of expectancy and somatic focus on pain. PLoS One 2012;7(6):e38854.

39. Kam-Hansen S, Jakubowski M, Kelley JM, Kirsch I, Hoaglin DC, Kaptchuk TJ, Burstein R. Altered placebo and drug labeling changes the outcome of episodic migraine attacks. Sci Transl Med 2014;6(218):218ra215.

40. Kessner S, Wiech K, Forkmann K, Ploner M, Bingel U. The effect of treatment history on therapeutic outcome: an experimental approach. JAMA Intern Med 2013;173:1468–9.

41. Kong J, Gollub RL, Polich G, Kirsch I, Laviolette P, Vangel M, Rosen B, Kaptchuk TJ. A functional magnetic resonance imaging study on the neural mechanisms of hyperalgesic nocebo effect. J Neurosci 2008;28(49):13354–62.

42. Laverdure-Dupont D, Rainville P, Montplaisir J, Lavigne G. Changes in rapid eye movement sleep associated with placebo-induced expectations and analgesia. J Neurosci 2009;29(38):11745–52.

43. Le Bars D, Gozariu M, Cadden SW. Animal models of nociception. Pharmacol Rev 2001;53(4):597–652.

44. Lui F, Colloca L, Duzzi D, Anchisi D, Benedetti F, Porro CA. Neural bases of conditioned placebo analgesia. Pain 2010;151(3):816–24.

45. Miller FG, Colloca L, Kaptchuk TJ. The placebo effect: illness and interpersonal healing. Perspect Biol Med 2009;52(4):518–39.

46. Pecina M, Azhar H, Love TM, Lu T, Fredrickson BL, Stohler CS, Zubieta JK. Personality trait predictors of placebo analgesia and neurobiological correlates. Neuropsychopharmacology 2013;38(4):639–46.

47. Phelps EA, LeDoux JE. Contributions of the amygdala to emotion processing: from animal models to human behavior. Neuron 2005;48(2):175–87.

48. Reiss S. Pavlovian conditioning and human fear: an expectancy model. Behav Ther 1980;11:380–96.

49. Rescorla RA. Pavlovian conditioning: it's not what you think it is. Am Psychol 1988;43:151–60.

50. Schafer SM, Colloca L, Wager TD. Conditioned placebo analgesia persists when subjects know they are receiving a placebo. J Pain 2015;16:412–20. doi:10.1016/j.jpain.2014.12.008.

51. Simmons K, Ortiz R, Kossowsky J, Krummenacher P, Grillon C, Pine D, Colloca L. Pain and placebo in pediatrics: a comprehensive review of laboratory and clinical findings. Pain 2014;155(11):2229–35.

52. Swider K, Babel P. The effect of the sex of a model on nocebo hyperalgesia induced by social observational learning. Pain 2013;154(8):1312–7.

53. Taddio A, Shah V, Gilbert-MacLeod C, Katz J. Conditioning and hyperalgesia in newborns exposed to repeated heel lances. JAMA 2002;288(7):857–61.

54. Vogtle E, Barke A, Kroner-Herwig B. Nocebo hyperalgesia induced by social observational learning. Pain 2013;154(8):1427–33.

55. Zhang RR, Zhang WC, Wang JY, Guo JY. The opioid placebo analgesia is mediated exclusively through μ-opioid receptor in rat. Int J Neuropsychopharmacol 2013;16:849–56.

SECTION 3

Clinical Conditions Affecting Pain and Consciousness

Pain Processing in Psychiatric and Neurological Disorders Affecting Consciousness

CHAPTER 10

Pain and Nociception in Disorders of Consciousness

Camille Chatelle, Steven Laureys, and Athena Demertzi

PAIN ASSESSMENT IN NONCOMMUNICATING PATIENTS

Pain is utterly personal and intimate. Officially, it has been defined as the "unpleasant sensory and emotional experience associated with real or potential tissue damage" [30]. Currently, we know that pain results from an interaction between the sensory characteristics of a stimulus and the state of the nervous system based on past experiences and emotional processes of the body at the time of stimulation [35]. Thus, healthy subjects might experience significant pain-related suffering from a relatively low-level noxious stimulation if they believe the implications are ominous, interminable, and beyond their control.

As with other conscious experiences, pain needs to be communicated in order to be assigned to a person. In cases of severely brain-injured noncommunicating patients, conscious perception of pain is classically inferred from motor responses to noxious stimulation. This is because by definition neither patients in an unresponsive wakefulness syndrome (also known as the vegetative state, VS/UWS [37]) nor patients in a minimally conscious state (MCS [23]) are able to functionally communicate their experiences. Indeed, patients in VS/UWS are in a condition of preserved wakefulness with absent voluntary interaction with the environment. Patients in MCS show discernible but fluctuating signs of awareness but also remain unable to functionally communicate with their surroundings [23]. It is therefore impossible for them to express their own feelings or to use any usual scale (such as the Visual Analog Scale) to report the presence of pain and its intensity. Interestingly, the International Association for the Study of Pain states the inability to verbally communicate does not negate the possibility that an individual is experiencing pain and is in need of appropriate pain-relieving treatment. As pain and suffering can also be present in the absence of noxious stimulation [41], how can one know whether patients in VS/UWS or in MCS experience pain?

In a recent survey around Europe, 2059 medical and paramedical professionals expressed their beliefs on possible pain perception in patients with disorders of consciousness. To the question "Do you think that patients in a minimally conscious state can feel pain?" almost all interviewed caregivers (96% of the medical doctors and 97% of the paramedical caregivers) answered positively. To the question "Do you think that patients in a vegetative state can feel pain?" 68% of the interviewed paramedical caregivers and 56% of medical doctors endorsed the statement. Interestingly, religion correlated most with health care professionals' opinions [16]. Since nearly half of the interviewed doctors express that VS/UWS patients do not feel pain, they could be expected to act accordingly by, for instance, not providing analgesic medication in these patients. These issues become even more important in cases when VS/UWS patients are agreed to be withdrawn from life-supporting treatment, such as artificial nutrition and hydration [14]. In these cases, VS/UWS patients can be left without administration of opioids or other analgesic drugs during their dying process on the grounds that they are not able to suffer from hunger and thirst [18]. More recently, we showed that health care providers' beliefs on possible pain perception in patients in VS/UWS indeed influences opinions on end of life [15]. Specifically, respondents who considered VS/UWS patients as able to feel pain supported less the withdrawal of life-sustaining therapy. For MCS, withdrawing life-supporting treatment was denied by most respondents, independently on the status of pain perception in these patients [15]. Such data show that research on attitudes of health care providers bring forth important questions about the relationship of research to clinical guidelines, the discrepancies of attitudes between health care providers and the complex relationship between pain perception and attitudes toward life-sustaining treatments. Ethical questions like these illustrate the need for closer attention to perspectives in research and in clinical care within the development of consensual approaches and guidelines, the need to understand practice variability and to minimize its impact on families, and the careful interpretation of recent neuroimaging findings and their consequences on withdrawal of life support [13].

PAIN PROCESSING IN DISORDERS OF CONSCIOUSNESS: FINDINGS FROM NEUROIMAGING AND ELECTROPHYSIOLOGICAL STUDIES

The International Association for the Study of Pain defines nociception as "an actually or potentially tissue damaging event transduced and encoded by nociceptors" [41]. The activation of peripheral nociceptors can produce pain, but nociception is not pain, which is a conscious experience. Additionally, the activation of nociceptors can trigger reflexive and autonomic responses without necessarily generating a conscious experience of pain [27, 64]. While nociception is usually necessary for pain perception [41], pain can also occur in the absence of nociception [19].

Supporting these definitions, neuroimaging studies suggest that nociception and pain are mediated by different cortical networks, together forming the "pain matrix" [29]. Nociceptive information will be transmitted from the thalamus to the cortical nociceptive network encompassing the primary and secondary somatosensory cortices, as well as the posterior insula, the so-called lateral network participating in the sensory–discriminative aspects of pain processing [40, 48]. It has been suggested that the activation of this network is not sufficient to generate the conscious experience of pain which necessitates the cingulate, anterior insula, and prefrontal cortices, the so-called medial network, which is involved in the motivational-affective and cognitive-evaluative aspects of pain processing [60].

There is now accumulating evidence that at least part of the activation of the "pain matrix" would not reflect activity that is specific for nociception or the perception of pain but would rather be involved in multimodal processing of saliency [44, 54]. Another hypothesis is that this "salience" (nonspecific) network within the pain matrix interacts with nociceptive-specific networks of the pain matrix such as the posterior insula, to generate a pain sensation attributable to the own body [20]. Although there is still no clear interpretation of the pain matrix in humans, looking at brain responses to pain could constitute a highly useful tool to help improve and objectify our understanding of pain perception in severely brain-injured patients who are unable to communicate.

For example, a study investigating the processing of noxious stimuli in 15 patients in a VS/UWS by using H_2O positron-emission tomography (PET) imaging reported an increase in metabolism in midbrain, contralateral thalamus, and primary somatosensory cortex in response to a potentially painful electrical stimulation applied to the median nerve of the wrist [38]. Additionally, primary somatosensory cortex was functionally disconnected from associative areas (i.e., secondary somatosensory cortex, bilateral posterior parietal, premotor, polysensory superior temporal, and prefrontal cortices) as compared to 15 healthy controls. These findings suggest that in patients in VS/UWS the activation of the primary cortex was isolated from higher-order associative cortices, reducing the probability that a potentially painful stimulus could be experienced in an integrated and conscious manner. Later on, it was shown that patients in MCS had a brain activation similar to healthy controls in response to noxious stimuli, encompassing not only midbrain, thalamus, and primary somatosensory cortex, but also secondary somatosensory cortex, insular, posterior parietal, as well as the posterior part of the anterior cingulate cortex [4]. This broader pattern of activation observed in the associative cortices areas and, particularly, in the anterior cingulate cortex and insula, suggests that patients in a MCS have the ability to process the unpleasant aspect of painful stimuli [60]. Similar results were reported in a recent functional MRI study where the brain of patients with disorder of consciousness (DOC) was scanned under a resting condition [12]. Among other systems, the analysis also focused on the salience network, which encompasses mainly bilateral insula and anterior cingulate cortex [59] and which has been involved in conflict monitoring, information integration, response selection, interoceptive processes [49, 66], and the emotional counterpart of pain [60]. For the salience network, a positive correlation between clinical scores measuring the level of consciousness and part of the anterior cingulate cortex was found (Fig. 10-1). Such results could account for the preserved capacities of some patients to orient their attentional resources toward environmental salient stimuli, such as noxious stimulation, corroborating previous PET data [4]. They also relate to the issue of patients experiencing spontaneous pain in the absence of external stimulation, or experiencing pain elicited by non-noxious stimuli such as neuropathic pain, which can be caused by brain damage or dysfunction [33].

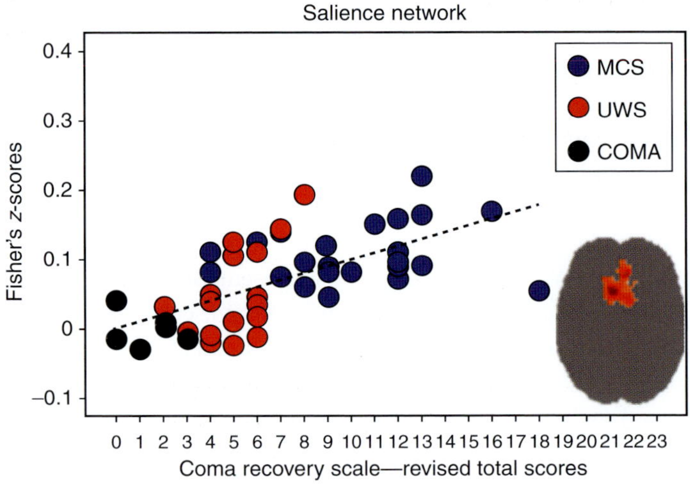

FIGURE 10-1 Potential pain perception can be studied in patients with disorders of consciousness during resting state, in the absence of external stimulation. Here, the level of consciousness in noncommunicating patients in minimally conscious state (MCS), vegetative state/unresponsive wakefulness syndrome (VS/UWS), and coma positively correlated with functional connectivity in the anterior cingulate cortex of the salience network, which has been implicated in the attentional and emotional aspects of pain. Although the subjective-emotional counterpart cannot be directly measured with this approach, these results could account for the preserved capacities of some patients to orient their attentional resources toward environmental salient stimuli, such as noxious stimulation. (Adapted from Demertzi et al. [12].)

Other studies conducted in patients in a VS/UWS showed different results. Kassubek et al. [32] studied seven anoxic patients in a VS/UWS, reporting a more widespread activity than what was reported in Laureys et al. [38] in the posterior insula/secondary somatosensory cortex, postcentral gyrus/primary somatosensory cortex, midcingulate cortex contralateral to the stimulus, and posterior insula ipsilateral to the stimulus. More recently, de Tommaso et al. [17] used nociceptive-specific laser-evoked potentials known to be related to cortical generators, such as the anterior cingulate cortex, and have reported a response (although with a longer latency) in three patients in a VS/UWS. Finally, two other studies reported an activation of both the sensory and affective pain networks (i.e., anterior cingulate cortex and/or insula) in 30% of patients in a VS/UWS in response to noxious stimulation [42] as well as pain cries [42, 68].

While these findings suggest a residual ability to perceive pain in VS/UWS, the last study also reported, in a parallel analysis, that the connectivity within the whole pain network was significantly impaired as compared with patients in a MCS [34]. Even though this supports an altered perception in patients in a VS/UWS, the activation of the affective pain network might denote the presence of residual pain perception in some of those patients. Moreover, these findings need to be interpreted with caution as many of the "pain matrix" components have been shown to be not specific to pain [43, 44, 54].

Taken together, these studies support the need of clinicians for a daily management of potential pain in every patient with DOC, independently of their clinical diagnosis at the bedside, which might be erroneous [58]. In this context, the development of tools to appropriately assess and treat pain in those patients is necessary.

BEHAVIORAL ASSESSMENT OF PAIN IN DISORDER OF CONSCIOUSNESS

Several scales have been developed and validated to detect pain in noncommunicating patients, such as newborns, patients with dementia (see Chapter 12), and sedated/intubated patients. For example, the COMFORT scale has been developed for use in young sedated patients between 0 and 3 years old [63]. It includes the observation of respiratory and motor responses, cardiac frequency, blood pressure, facial expression, agitation, and level of awakening. Each parameter is scored from 1 to 5. The total score ranges from 8 to 40, with a score between 17 and 26 indicating appropriate sedation level. To our knowledge, this is currently the sole scale that assesses oversedation, comfort, and distress in newborns and young children in intensive care. The Behavioral Pain Scale (BPS [47]) and the Critical Care Pain Observation Tool (CCPOT [22]) have been developed for noncommunicating and sedated adult patients in intensive care. The BPS assesses facial expression, movements of the upper limbs, and the compliance to mechanical ventilation in intubated adults. Each parameter is scored from 1 to 4. The total score ranges from 4 to 12. The CCPOT includes the facial expression, body movements, muscle tension, and compliance with the ventilator/vocalization. Its total score ranges from 0 to 8. Several studies have shown the reliability and validity of these scales for use in intensive care adult patients [3, 53]. Additionally, a recent study also suggested that the CCPOT would be more sensitive to pain than the BPS when comparing score changes between a nonpainful and a painful condition [53]. Recently, a new scale has also been proposed for ventilated critically ill and noncommunicating patients, the *scale of behavior indicators of pain* (Escala de Conductas Indicadoras de Dolor: ESCID). A good concurrent validity with the BPS and a good internal consistency of the scale were reported in a previous study [36].

Nevertheless, only a few scales have been developed to assess pain in patients with DOC until recently [57]. Among them, the Nociception Coma Scale (NCS [57]) was developed in 2010 to specifically assess nociception and pain in patients with DOC in acute and chronic setting. The NCS is based on preexisting pain scales validated in noncommunicating patients with advanced dementia and newborns. The first version of the scale consisted of four subscales assessing motor, verbal, visual responses, and facial expression. Initially, breathing responses were also assessed but later discarded due to the difficulty to objectively assess breathing patterns in patients not benefiting from respiratory monitoring devices [56]. In addition, previous studies have shown that physiological parameters seem insufficiently sensitive for pain assessment [21, 26]. Stress, medication, medical complications, and brain lesions affecting autonomic functions can influence these parameters and bias the assessment as well.

A first study including 48 patients from intensive care, neurology/neurosurgery units, rehabilitation centers, and nursing homes reported a good interrater reliability and good concurrent validity for the NCS total scores and subscores when compared to other scale developed for noncommunicating patients (e.g., the neonatal infant pain scale [39], the pain assessment in advanced dementia scale [65]). A second study on 64 patients investigated the sensitivity of the NCS by comparing NCS scores observed at rest, in response to a non-noxious stimulus (i.e., tap on the shoulders) and a noxious stimulus (i.e., nail bed pressure [9]). Results showed that NCS total scores as well as motor, verbal, and facial subscores were significantly higher in response to a noxious stimulus than at rest or in response to a non-noxious stimulus, reflecting the good sensitivity of the scale. However, no difference could be observed between noxious and non-noxious conditions for the visual subscores, suggesting that this subscale was not specific to nociception. A modified version of the scale excluding the visual subscale, the Nociception Coma Scale—revised (NCS-R, see Table 10-1) [9], was therefore proposed.

The NCS-R is meant to be administered in all patients who are in a VS/UWS or in a MCS, especially those who present a documented potential pain (e.g., polytraumatic

TABLE 10-1 The Nociception Coma Scale—Revised

Motor Responses

3—Localization to painful stimulation

2—Flexion withdrawal

1—Abnormal posturing

0—None/flaccid

Verbal Responses

3—Verbalization (intelligible)

2—Vocalization

1—Groaning

0—None

Facial Responses

3—Cry

2—Grimace

1—Oral reflexive movement/startle response

0—None

injuries, decubitus ulcers, severe spasticity, wounds, or arthralgia). A particular attention should be given to patients with spasticity as it is a frequent condition in chronic DOC. Indeed, a recent study showed that 89% (58/65) of patients who were in a chronic DOC demonstrated signs of spasticity (modified Ashworth Scale, MAS $\geq$ 1), including 60% (39/65) qualified with severe spasticity (MAS $\geq$ 3). In addition, the severity of spasticity was correlated to NCS-R scores (i.e., likely to reflect nociception or pain), highlighting the importance of pain management in noncommunicating patients after severe brain injury [62].

Any information about preexisting pain (e.g., osteoarthritis, rheumatoid arthritis) is helpful before starting using the scale. The NCS-R should be scored at rest and during cares in order to observe the spontaneous responses presented by the patient (preferably assessed with eyes opened) before the potentially painful care and/or stimulating a potentially painful area. Behavioral responses observed before and during the care and/or stimulation will be scored according to the NCS-R guidelines. Spontaneous behaviors at rest can also be taken into considerations. However, these responses could be unrelated to pain (e.g., pathologic activation of subcortical areas leading to constant but not appropriate cries [45]) and should therefore be replicated in a pain-related condition (i.e., mobilization/palpation). The highest scores obtained for each subscale are summed to obtain a total score ranging from 0 to 9. In case of a documented cause of potential pain, the NCS-R should be administered before and after analgesic treatment.

It is essential to assess simultaneously the patient's level of consciousness in order to avoid overmedication. Indeed, it is likely that the administration of sedating analgesics will decrease the presence of pain behaviors but also the patient's responsiveness as those medications may have an impact on alertness and vigilance in patients with severe brain injury. On the other hand, the presence of untreated pain could reduce already limited attentional resources, and prevent the patient from interacting with his or her surroundings and showing sign of consciousness. Indeed, a recent study reported an improvement of consciousness when administering analgesic treatment to a brain-injured patient suffering from severe spasticity [62]. A good balance remains therefore to be found between undertreatment and overtreatment by revising pain treatment regularly. Considerations should be given to nonsedating medications or to medications with reversible effects whenever there is question of medication effects versus ongoing deterioration of neurological status.

In this context, the NCS-R may constitute a helpful instrument for monitoring pain behavior on a daily basis. In the absence of documented conditions likely to produce pain, a sudden increase of the NCS-R total score independent from an improvement in the level of consciousness can alert the clinician of the potential presence of pain/underlying medical complication. Additional investigations may then be performed to identify its origin/localization (e.g., by using mobilization/palpation/CT scan).

In a recent study looking at the clinical validity of the scale, 39 patients with potentially painful conditions (e.g., due to fractures or spasticity) were assessed during nursing cares before and after the administration of an analgesic treatment tailored to each patient's clinical status [8]. The Glasgow coma scale (GCS) was also used before and during treatment in order to observe fluctuations in consciousness. A decrease in the NCS-R total scores and subscores was reported during treatment when compared to the scores observed before treatment. Interestingly, no difference between the GCS total scores obtained before versus during treatment was observed suggesting a good balance between decrease in pain and preserved level of consciousness. More precisely, 20 patients showed a decrease in the NCS-R scores with no decrease of the level of consciousness (i.e., GCS scores). Finally, 5 of these 20 patients showed higher signs of consciousness (i.e., increase in GCS scores) following the analgesic treatment as compared with before, suggesting that the presence of pain may have compromised the ability of the patient to respond at bedside (also see reference [62]). The fact that 59% of the patients included in the study (23 of 39) did not have any analgesic treatment prior to the assessment also underlines the crucial need for an appropriate management of pain in this population.

The COMFORT, the BPS, the CCPOT, and the ESCID were first developed for patients in the acute setting (including sedation and ventilation), and all of the scales presented here include observation of the motor response and facial expression. However, studies quantifying facial expression (i.e., grimace) in patients with DOC are currently lacking. This is even more of a problem in case of severe spasticity [62] or oral response limited by trachea/anarthria, where the use of motor or verbal responses may be limited and facial expression is sometimes the only remaining communicative means that can be used in this population. Even if grimacing is considered as an indicator of pain, the Multi-Society Task Force on PVS did not consider it as a necessary sign of conscious perception as they can occur reflexively through subcortical pathways in the thalamus and limbic system [45]. Patients showing no sign of consciousness except grimaces to nociceptive stimuli can therefore be diagnosed as being in VS/UWS. Nevertheless, very few studies have investigated such behavior in conscious (MCS) versus nonconscious (VS/UWS) patients. Recently, Schnakers et al. [55] investigated the frequency of grimace in DOC. They reported that grimaces were more frequently displayed in response to nociceptive stimuli than in response to non-nociceptive stimuli in both MCS and VS/UWS patients (i.e., 48% vs. 4% for VS/UWS and 65% vs. 3% for MCS, respectively). However, grimace to pain was not observed more frequently in MCS than in VS/UWS patients.

A recent neuroimaging study investigated the correlation between the NCS-R score and brain areas involved in the "pain matrix" network [10]. Using 18-fluorodeoxyglucose PET scan, a significant correlation was observed between NCS-R total scores and brain metabolism in the posterior part of the anterior cingulate cortex. Those results suggest that the NCS-R is at least partially related to the activity in one cortical area involved in pain processing and hence may constitute an appropriate behavioral tool to assess, monitor, and treat nociception and pain in noncommunicating patients with DOC. However, as highlighted earlier, what is crucial to lead to a fully conscious experience of pain is more the connectivity between different areas involved in pain processing than the singulate area alone, which are not necessarily specific to pain processing. Therefore, these results should be interpreted with caution and cannot be used to affirm that the NCS-R is a sensitive tool to assess subjective pain and not only nociception.

Future studies should better investigate the presence of target behaviors (e.g., grimaces) in the detection and treatment of pain in this population. It would also be useful to conduct more studies comparing changes in the scores when analgesics/potential pain condition is administered in a double-blind placebo/control study, in order to control that the observed changes were only associated with the treatment/condition. Finally, there is an urgent need for a better understanding of response to analgesic treatment in this population for short and long-term pain management.

FUTURE PERSPECTIVES

The presence of pain in patients with DOC is a real challenge to clinicians. Several studies have investigated whether these patients are able to process pain in a conscious manner, including subjective suffering [4, 38, 42]. Clinicians who deal with DOC patients should therefore be concerned about nociception, regardless of the patient's subjective experience. The presence of nociception may also help caregivers to detect medical complications, such as undiagnosed fractures, kidney stones, urinary tract infection. In this context, a method assessing the presence of nociception through behavioral (e.g., facial grimaces, moaning, restless movement) and/or physiologic (e.g., rise in heart rate or blood pressure, dilation of pupils) responses should not rely on the patient's state of consciousness.

Behavioral response to nociception is complex, and includes autonomic and reflexive responses generally displayed in various ways by VS/UWS and MCS patients (i.e., facial grimacing, moaning, producing tears, increases in tonic posturing, and thrashing limb movements [45]). Currently, the NCS-R is the only measure of nociception and pain developed specifically for patients with DOC and which has been validated. However, this tool may have limitations for use to accurately assess solely nociception in this population. First, the highest number of points that can be scored depends on the patient's state of consciousness (i.e., localization to pain, appropriate cries, and intelligible verbalization). Second, it has a relatively small point range, particularly for responses that are considered to be reflexes, and therefore of interest for assessing nociception. In this context, it may be useful to develop a measurement tool with a wider range of items to maximize sensitivity to the intensity of nociception, taking into account the limited examination time. Finally, clinicians using the NCS-R should be careful when interpreting the findings as "agitation," which may be confounded with a recovery of consciousness. Indeed, patients beginning to regain consciousness can display new spontaneous responses and agitated behaviors that may involve facial grimacing, moaning, or limb movements, for example [2], which would increase the scores observed at the NCS-R. While it is believed that the presence of nociceptive stimuli can prompt outbursts of agitation, it is also believed that agitation can appear as a primary syndrome related to brain injury, in the absence of noxious stimulation. For that reason, repetitive assessments in different condition (no noxious vs. noxious) are needed to be able to better define the presence of pain and the potential source.

In addition to behavioral responses, physiological responses to pain (e.g., heart rate, respiration, pupil dilation) are other indicators that may be of interest for assessing pain in DOC. Following a painful stimulation, breathing becomes irregular or faster, blood pressure and heart rate increase, and oxygen saturation decreases. These indicators are included in some of the validated scales for noncommunicative patients such as the COMFORT. In research, intracranial pressure, skin conductance, and heart rate are the most used indicators [28]. Some studies suggested that changes in the heart rate were associated with the subjective pain unpleasantness but not with the pain intensity [50, 51] or could be used as an indicator of inadequate analgesia [31]. On the other hand, other studies reported that vital signs (heart rate, respiration) did not correlate significantly with self-reports of pain or unpleasantness and should thus not be used as indicators of pain in the nonverbal critically ill [21, 22, 24, 52].

Pupil response to pain (noradrenergic circuits) is a complex sympathetically mediated response that involves defensive supraspinal processing in the central autonomic network [6, 7, 46], and it is associated with conscious processing [67] and subjective pain in healthy volunteers. However, few studies have been investigating pupil response in brain injured patients [61] and little is known about the variety of centrally acting drugs with potential anticholinergic or sympathomimetic effects.

Finally, in hospitalized patients, a variation of vital responses can be observed following homeostatic changes and certain medications, leading experts to recommend avoiding the use of these measures as pain indicators [1, 25]. These measures may also be disturbed by factors other than pain, such as stress, restlessness, hunger, and should therefore, if used, always be interpreted with caution [52].

Even though it is crucial to have tools for detecting and treating acute pain, another challenge in the future will be to better understand and manage neuropathic pain in patients with DOC. This would include the development or adaptation of existing scales currently validated for assessing acute pain. Indeed, it has been shown that the prevalence of chronic pain is high after a traumatic brain injury (as 50% of patients with mild to moderate injury report recurrent headaches) or after a nontraumatic brain injury (as thalamic or cortical stroke may lead to chronic pain), as well as in presence of recurrent bedsores, severe spasticity or uncomfortable deformities [5]. Future work will hopefully aim at developing guidelines regarding the type of treatment to implement in order to manage and treat pain/nociception in patients with DOC.

CONCLUSIONS

In both acute and chronic stages of DOC following a severe brain injury, several conditions are likely to induce pain, especially during care and mobilization [11]. The possibility of preserved pain perception capacities highlighted by neuroimaging studies in patients in a MCS and in some patients in a VS/UWS supports the idea that these individuals need analgesic treatment and monitoring. The NCS-R is the first tool developed to assess nociception and pain in patients with DOC in both acute and chronic stage. It is based on a rapid, standardized, and sensitive scale, which can be easily implemented in acute and subacute units for assessing acute pain. Other scales also showed their interest for assessing sedated and or intubated patients in the intensive care setting. Additional investigations are needed to develop a complete battery of valid and sensitive measures for clinicians to efficiently detect and treat nociception and pain (both acute and neuropathic pain) in patients with severe brain injury. Finally, clinical guidelines regarding prevention and treatments of pain in DOC need to be developed.

REFERENCES

1. Barr J, Fraser GL, Puntillo K, Ely EW, Gelinas C, Dasta JF, Davidson JE, Devlin JW, Kress JP, Joffe AM, et al. Clinical practice guidelines for the management of pain, agitation, and delirium in adult patients in the intensive care unit. Crit Care Med 2013;41(1):263–306.
2. Bogner JA, Corrigan JD, Fugate L, Mysiw WJ, Clinchot D. Role of agitation in prediction of outcomes after traumatic brain injury. Am J Phys Med Rehabil 2001;80(9):636–44.
3. Boitor M, Fiola JL, Gelinas C. Validation of the critical-care pain observation tool and vital signs in relation to the sensory and affective components of pain during mediastinal tube removal in postoperative cardiac surgery intensive care unit adults. J Cardiovasc Nurs 2015; Epub Mar 30.
4. Boly M, Faymonville ME, Schnakers C, Peigneux P, Lambermont B, Phillips C, Lancellotti P, Luxen A, Lamy M, Moonen G, et al. Perception of pain in the minimally conscious state with PET activation: an observational study. Lancet Neurol 2008;7(11):1013–20.
5. Borsook D. Neurological diseases and pain. Brain 2012;135(Pt 2):320–44.
6. Chapman CR, Bradshaw DH, Donaldson GW, Jacobson RC, Nakamura Y. Central noradrenergic mechanisms and the acute stress response during painful stimulation. J Psychopharmacol 2014;28(12):1135–42.
7. Chapman CR, Oka S, Bradshaw DH, Jacobson RC, Donaldson GW. Phasic pupil dilation response to noxious stimulation in normal volunteers: relationship to brain evoked potentials and pain report. Psychophysiology 1999;36(1):44–52.
8. Chatelle C, De Val MD, Catano A, Chaskis C, Seeldrayers P, Laureys S, Biston P, Schnakers C. Is the nociception coma scale-revised a useful clinical tool for managing pain in patients with disorders of consciousness? Clin J Pain 2015; Epub May 28.
9. Chatelle C, Majerus S, Whyte J, Laureys S, Schnakers C. A sensitive scale to assess nociceptive pain in patients with disorders of consciousness. J Neurol Neurosurg Psychiatry 2012;83(12):1233–7.
10. Chatelle C, Thibaut A, Bruno MA, Boly M, Bernard C, Hustinx R, Schnakers C, Laureys S. Nociception coma scale-revised scores correlate with metabolism in the anterior cingulate cortex. Neurorehabil Neural Repair 2014;28(2):149–52.
11. Chatelle C, Thibaut A, Whyte J, De Val MD, Laureys S, Schnakers C. Pain issues in disorders of consciousness. Brain Inj 2014;28(9):1202–8.
12. Demertzi A, Antonopoulos G, Heine L, Voss HU, Crone JS, de Los Angeles C, Bahri MA, Di Perri R, Gomez F, Vanhaudenhuyse A, et al. Intrinsic functional connectivity differentiates minimally conscious from unresponsive patients. Brain 2015;138:2619–31.

13. Demertzi A, Jox RJ, Racine E, Laureys S. A European survey on attitudes towards pain and end-of-life issues in locked-in syndrome. Brain Inj 2014;28(9):1209–15.

14. Demertzi A, Ledoux D, Bruno M-A, Vanhaudenhuyse A, Gosseries O, Soddu A, Schnakers C, Moonen G, Laureys S. Attitudes towards end-of-life issues in disorders of consciousness: a European survey. J Neurol 2011;258(6):1058–65.

15. Demertzi A, Racine E, Bruno M-A, Ledoux D, Gosseries O, Vanhaudenhuyse A, Thonnard M, Soddu A, Moonen G, Laureys S. Pain perception in disorders of consciousness: neuroscience, clinical care, and ethics in dialogue. Neuroethics 2013;6(1):37–50.

16. Demertzi A, Schnakers C, Ledoux D, Chatelle C, Bruno M-A, Vanhaudenhuyse A, Boly M, Moonen G, Laureys S. Different beliefs about pain perception in the vegetative and minimally conscious states: a European survey of medical and paramedical professionals. Prog Brain Res 2009;177:329–38.

17. de Tommaso M, Navarro J, Ricci K, Lorenzo M, Lanzillotti C, Colonna F, Resta M, Lancioni G, Livrea P. Pain in prolonged disorders of consciousness: laser evoked potentials findings in patients with vegetative and minimally conscious states. Brain Inj 2013;27(7–8):962–72.

18. Fins JJ. Affirming the right to care, preserving the right to die: disorders of consciousness and neuroethics after Schiavo. Palliat Support Care 2006;4(2):169–78.

19. Flor H, Nikolajsen L, Staehelin Jensen T. Phantom limb pain: a case of maladaptive CNS plasticity? Nat Rev Neurosci 2006;7(11):873–81.

20. Garcia-Larrea L, Peyron R. Pain matrices and neuropathic pain matrices: a review. Pain 2013;154(suppl 1):S29–S43.

21. Gélinas C, Arbour C. Behavioral and physiologic indicators during a nociceptive procedure in conscious and unconscious mechanically ventilated adults: similar or different? J Crit Care 2009;24(4):628.e7–17.

22. Gelinas C, Johnston C. Pain assessment in the critically ill ventilated adult: validation of the Critical-Care Pain Observation Tool and physiologic indicators. Clin J Pain 2007;23(6):497–505.

23. Giacino J, Ashwal S, Childs N, Cranford R, Jennett B, Katz D, Kelly J, Rosenberg J, Whyte J, Zafonte R. The minimally conscious state: definition and diagnostic criteria. Neurology 2002;58(3):349–53.

24. Halliburton JR. Awareness during general anesthesia: new technology for an old problem. CRNA 1998;9(2):39–43.

25. Herr K, Coyne PJ, Key T, Manworen R, McCaffery M, Merkel S, Kelly JP, Wild L. Pain assessment in the nonverbal patient: position statement with clinical practice recommendations. Pain Manag Nurs 2006;7(2):44–52.

26. Herr K, Coyne PJ, McCaffery M, Manworren R, Merkel S. Pain assessment in the patient unable to self-report: position statement with clinical practice recommendations. Pain Manag Nurs 2011;12(4):230–50.
27. Hofbauer RK, Fiset P, Plourde G, Backman SB, Bushnell MC. Dose-dependent effects of propofol on the central processing of thermal pain. Anesthesiology 2004;100(2):386–94.
28. Hummel P, van Dijk M. Pain assessment: current status and challenges. Semin Fetal Neonatal Med 2006;11:237–45.
29. Ingvar M. Pain and functional imaging. Philos Trans R Soc Lond B Biol Sci 1999;354(1387):1347–58.
30. International Association for the Study of Pain. Classification of chronic pain: descriptions of chronic pain syndromes and definitions of pain terms. Task force on taxonomy. Seattle, WA: IASP Press; 1994.
31. Jeanne M, Logier R, De Jonckheere J, Tavernier B. Heart rate variability during total intravenous anesthesia: effects of nociception and analgesia. Auton Neurosci 2009;147(1–2):91–6.
32. Kassubek J, Juengling FD, Elsa T, Spreerc J, Herpersa M, Krauseb T, Moserb E, Lücking CH. Activation of a residual cortical network during painful stimulation in long-term postanoxic vegetative state: a $^{15}O–H_2O$ PET study. J Neurol Sci 2003;212:85–91.
33. Kim CE, Kim YK, Chung G, Jeong JM, Lee DS, Kim J, Kim SJ. Large-scale plastic changes of the brain network in an animal model of neuropathic pain. Neuroimage 2014;98:203–15.
34. Kotchoubey B, Merz S, Lang S, Markl A, Muller F, Yu T, Schwarzbauer C. Global functional connectivity reveals highly significant differences between the vegetative and the minimally conscious state. J Neurol 2013;260(4):975–83.
35. Kupers R. Is the placebo powerless? N Engl J Med 2001;345(17):1278–9.
36. Latorre Marco I, Solis Muñoz M, Falero Ruiz T, Larrasquitu Sanchez A, Romay Perez AB, Millan Santos I. Validation of the scale of behavior indicators of pain (ESCID) in critically ill, non-communicative patients under mechanical ventilation: results of the ESCID scale [in Spanish]. Enferm Intensiva 2011;22(1):3–12.
37. Laureys S, Celesia GG, Cohadon F, Lavrijsen J, Leon-Carrion J, Sannita WG, Sazbon L, Schmutzhard E, von Wild KR, Zeman A, Dolce G. Unresponsive wakefulness syndrome: a new name for the vegetative state or apallic syndrome. BMC Med 2010;8:68.
38. Laureys S, Faymonville M, Peigneux P, Damas P, Lambermont B, Del Fiore G, Degueldre C, Aerts J, Luxen A, Franck G. Cortical processing of noxious somatosensory stimuli in the persistent vegetative state. Neuroimage 2002;17(2):732–41.

39. Lawrence J, Alcock D, McGrath P, Kay J, MacMurray SB, Dulberg C. The development of a tool to assess neonatal pain. Neonatal Netw 1993;12(6):59–66.

40. Lockwood PL, Iannetti GD, Haggard P. Transcranial magnetic stimulation over human secondary somatosensory cortex disrupts perception of pain intensity. Cortex 2012;49(8):2201–9.

41. Loeser JD, Treede RD. The Kyoto protocol of IASP basic pain terminology. Pain 2008;137(3):473–77.

42. Markl A, Yu T, Vogel D, Muller F, Kotchoubey B, Lang S. Brain processing of pain in patients with unresponsive wakefulness syndrome. Brain Behav 2013;3(2):95–103.

43. Moulton EA, Pendse G, Becerra LR, Borsook D. BOLD responses in somatosensory cortices better reflect heat sensation than pain. J Neurosci 2012;32(17):6024–31.

44. Mouraux A, Diukova A, Lee MC, Wise RG, Iannetti GD. A multisensory investigation of the functional significance of the "pain matrix." Neuroimage 2011;54(3):2237–49.

45. The Multi-Society Task Force on PVS. Medical aspects of the persistent vegetative state. N Engl J Med 1994;330(21):1499–508.

46. Oka S, Chapman CR, Kim B, Nakajima I, Shimizu O, Oi Y. Pupil dilation response to noxious stimulation: effect of varying nitrous oxide concentration. Clin Neurophysiol 2007;118(9):2016–24.

47. Payen JF, Bru O, Bosson JL, Lagrasta A, Novel E, Deschaux L, Lavagne P, Jacquot C. Assessing pain in critically ill sedated patients using a behavioral pain scale. Crit Care Med 2001;29(12):2258–63.

48. Ploner M, Gross J, Timmermann L, Schnitzler A. Cortical representation of first and second pain sensation in humans. Proc Natl Acad Sci U S A 2002;99(19):12444–8.

49. Ploner M, Lee MC, Wiech K, Bingel U, Tracey I. Prestimulus functional connectivity determines pain perception in humans. Proc Natl Acad Sci U S A 2010;107(1):355–60.

50. Rainville P, Bao QVH, Chrétien P. Pain-related emotions modulate experimental pain perception and autonomic responses. Pain 2005;118(3):306–18.

51. Rainville P, Carrier B, Hofbauer RK, Bushnell MC, Duncan GH. Dissociation of sensory and affective dimensions of pain using hypnotic modulation. Pain 1999;82:159–71.

52. Ranger M, Johnston CC, Anand KJS. Current controversies regarding pain assessment in neonates. Semin Perinatol 2007;31:283–8.

53. Rijkenberg S, Stilma W, Endeman H, Bosman RJ, Oudemans-van Straaten HM. Pain measurement in mechanically ventilated critically ill patients: Behavioral Pain Scale versus Critical-Care Pain Observation Tool. J Crit Care 2015;30(1):167–72.

54. Ronga I, Valentini E, Mouraux A, Iannetti GD. Novelty is not enough: laser-evoked potentials are determined by stimulus saliency, not absolute novelty. J Neurophysiol 2013;109(3):692–701.

55. Schnakers C, Chatelle C, Demertzi A, Majerus S, Laureys S. What about pain in disorders of consciousness? AAPS J 2012;14(3):437–44.

56. Schnakers C, Chatelle C, Majerus S, Gosseries O, De Val M, Laureys S. Assessment and detection of pain in noncommunicative severely brain-injured patients. Expert Rev Neurother 2010;10(11):1725–31.

57. Schnakers C, Chatelle C, Vanhaudenhuyse A, Majerus S, Ledoux D, Boly M, Bruno MA, Boveroux P, Demertzi A, Moonen G, Laureys S. The Nociception Coma Scale: a new tool to assess nociception in disorders of consciousness. Pain 2010;148(2):215–9.

58. Schnakers C, Vanhaudenhuyse A, Giacino J, Ventura M, Boly M, Majerus S, Moonen G, Laureys S. Diagnostic accuracy of the vegetative and minimally conscious state: clinical consensus versus standardized neurobehavioral assessment. BMC Neurol 2009;9(1):35.

59. Seeley WW, Menon V, Schatzberg AF, Keller J, Glover GH, Kenna H, Reiss AL, Greicius MD. Dissociable intrinsic connectivity networks for salience processing and executive control. J Neurosci 2007;27(9):2349–56.

60. Shackman AJ, Salomons TV, Slagter HA, Fox AS, Winter JJ, Davidson RJ. The integration of negative affect, pain and cognitive control in the cingulate cortex. Nat Rev Neurosci 2011;12(3):154–67.

61. Stoll J, Chatelle C, Carter O, Koch C, Laureys S, Einhauser W. Pupil responses allow communication in locked-in syndrome patients. Curr Biol 2013;23(15):R647–R648.

62. Thibaut A, Chatelle C, Wannez S, Deltombe T, Stender J, Schnakers C, Laureys S, Gosseries O. Spasticity in disorders of consciousness: a behavioral study. Eur J Phys Rehabil Med 2015;51:389–97.

63. van Dijk M, Peters WB, van Deventer P, Tibboel D. The COMFORT behavior scale: a tool for assessing pain and sedation in infants. Am J Nurs 2005;105(1):33–35, 37.

64. Wall PD, McMahon SB, Koltzenburg M. Wall and Melzack's textbook of pain. Philadelphia, PA: Elsevier/Churchill Livingstone; 2006.

65. Warden V, Hurley AC, Volicer L. Development and psychometric evaluation of the Pain Assessment in Advanced Dementia (PAINAD) scale. J Am Med Dir Assoc 2003;4(1):9–15.

66. Wiech K, Lin CS, Brodersen KH, Bingel U, Ploner M, Tracey I. Anterior insula integrates information about salience into perceptual decisions about pain. J Neurosci 2010;30(48):16324–31.

67. Yang LL, Niemann CU, Larson MD. Mechanism of pupillary reflex dilation in awake volunteers and in organ donors. Anesthesiology 2003;99(6):1281–6.

68. Yu T, Lang S, Vogel D, Markl A, Muller F, Kotchoubey B. Patients with unresponsive wakefulness syndrome respond to the pain cries of other people. Neurology 2013;80(4):345–52.

CHAPTER 11

Pain and Consciousness in Infants

Ruth E. Grunau, Manon Ranger, and Hugo Lagercrantz

In the late 20th century, the advent of high-technology neonatal intensive care and the tremendous increase in survival of tiny premature (preterm) and very sick newborns changed the prevalence of painful procedures in neonates tremendously. Infants born very preterm (23–32 weeks gestational age [GA]), 2–4 months before their due date, undergo on average 10 invasive procedures per day for weeks to months during hospitalization in the neonatal intensive care unit (NICU). Moreover, in developed countries, healthy infants born at full-term receive a routine injection of vitamin K in the delivery room, blood taken for metabolic screening about 48 hours after delivery, as well as over 15 immunization vaccines during the first 18 months of life. Questions emerge regarding the extent to which preterm- and term-born neonates are capable of experiencing pain, and whether they are conscious of pain and form memories of pain this early in life.

Evidence from human and animal studies has established that tactile sensitivity is *greater* in immature than in mature organisms [9]. Furthermore, very preterm neonates are at the greatest risk for long-term adverse effects of frequent procedural pain exposure [10]. During the fetal period of the late second and the third trimesters of pregnancy, the human brain undergoes rapid development of the cytoarchitecture. In infants born very preterm, brain development occurs during the stressful period in the NICU outside the protective intrauterine environment. During this developmental process, regional connectivity of networks begins, and the emergence of consciousness is underway. In this chapter, we consider infant pain and consciousness within the framework of the developing brain.

THE RISE OF CONSCIOUSNESS

Consciousness has been viewed as "awareness of the body, oneself and the outside world" ([16], p. 300). It is important to distinguish between states of consciousness as various levels of sleep or wakefulness versus the *content* of consciousness [17]. Memory is a crucial component of consciousness. Habituation, which provides evidence of short-term conditioning and thereby "biological memory", has been demonstrated in the human fetus from around 22–23 weeks of gestation (see reference [16]). Memory is present early since newborns recognize voices heard in utero, as well as their mother's breast milk odor (see reference [17]). Language is also an important component of human consciousness. Infants born 2–3 months preterm can distinguish spoken syllables [20]. Furthermore, infants are able to integrate sensory signals from different modalities, such as olfaction and hearing. Studies of visual and auditory sensory systems provide evidence of capacity for conditioning and thereby learning and memory in human neonates. Thus, although still developing, conscious perception is already present in infancy [15]. Moreover, human newborns, including the very preterm neonate, display specific facial expressions of apparent distress, disgust, and pleasure. However, whether this should be regarded as signs of consciousness can be questioned (see reference [16]). Thus, taken together, in the context of the relatively mature brain of the full-term infant, some degree of conscious awareness may play a role in the pain experience; however, experimental support for this is difficult if not impossible to obtain in the preverbal infant [16]. Even more challenging is the question of when consciousness may begin in the very preterm infant in the NICU environment. To be fully conscious is to be capable of reflecting on the past and planning for the future, which does not apply to the newborn infant—preterm or full-term.

Examination of the extent to which consciousness may be present across early human development, especially prior to term equivalent age, requires consideration of neuroanatomical changes, as well as whether the "fetus" is inside or outside the protective intrauterine environment.

IS FETAL PAIN LIKELY?

To address the capacity of the fetus to experience pain sensation at any given GA of development, it is essential to distinguish between the immature preterm neonate in the NICU and the fetus within the protective intrauterine environment, because there are specific differences between these environments that are important for pain [21]. In utero, the fetus is surrounded by the amniotic fluid and exposed to high levels of endogenous neuroinhibitors produced in the fetoplacental unit, such as adenosine and pregnanolone. Moreover, together with low oxygen levels, the fetus is in a continuous sleep-like state, oscillating between rapid-eye-movement (active sleep) and non–rapid-eye-movement (quiet sleep) sleep states. Fetal behaviors resembling wakefulness are related to changes between these sleep states rather than suggesting wakefulness. For all these reasons, it is unlikely that the fetus is conscious of pain in utero, even after 24 weeks gestation, when neuroanatomically capable of pain processing [21].

Even at the same GA, and thereby the same degree of brain development, since the fetal and NICU environments are distinctly different, the potential for conscious awareness of pain is not comparable in utero versus in the NICU. In the NICU, the fetus born very preterm is in a developmentally unexpected environment, lacking the protection as described above. Therefore, findings from studies showing behavioral, autonomic, and hormonal responses, as well as changes in hemodynamic and electrophysiological brain activity, to invasive procedures in preterm neonates in the NICU, cannot be generalized to fetal pain experience in utero. A systematic review of the evidence concluded that fetal pain is unlikely before the third trimester [19].

NOCICEPTION AND PAIN

The distinction between nociception and pain is crucial when considering the role of consciousness. Nociception is the activation of specialized systems of detection of noxious stimuli, from peripheral sensory neurons, which transduce these stimuli into electrical signals that are transmitted through the spinal cord, to be relayed to subcortical brain structures and ultimately to higher cortical centers. "Nociception" evokes a reflex response to protect against a noxious stimulus, whereas "pain" has both sensory and emotional components, as well as cognitive aspects of appraisal, requiring consciousness. The International Association for the Study of Pain (IASP) defined pain as "an unpleasant sensory and emotional experience associated with actual or potential tissue damage, or described in terms of such damage" and further that "pain is always subjective. Each individual learns the application of the word through experiences related to pain" ([22], p. 250). However, the IASP definition excludes the possibility of pain in infants, animals, as well as adults with limited language capacity such as the cognitively impaired, and further that pain is perceived by infants on first occurrence rather than learned [2]. For infants and nonhuman animals, it is difficult, if even possible, to know whether a conscious emotional pain experience has occurred.

The phylogenetic origin of consciousness is under debate, and is addressed elsewhere in this volume (see Chapter 15). Among the criteria for ascribing pain to animals is the concept of argument by analogy, which applies equally well to human infants who also cannot verbally express pain. This is the principle that if a nonverbal human or animal responds in a way similar to humans who can report pain verbally, then the capacity for experiencing pain should be assumed. A set of criteria has been advanced to judge the potential to experience pain in animals, including the ability to experience sensations, physiological changes, and protective motor behaviors to noxious stimuli, avoidance learning, as well as demonstration of higher cognitive ability [7]. Based on argument by analogy, given that human infants react to invasive procedures with behavioral, autonomic, hormonal, electrophysiological, and neurovascular changes, it is now recognized that at some level infants *perceive* pain, starting at the time of clear viability outside the womb around 24 weeks gestation. Furthermore, facial behaviors suggest emotional responses accompanying pain. However, the question remains to what extent newborns can consciously experience pain.

EMERGENCE OF NOCICEPTIVE REACTIVITY

Tactile responses are the earliest sensations, evident around 9–12 weeks of fetal life; however, this is reflex reactivity. Nociception involves a balance of endogenous excitatory and inhibitory processes [9]. In both humans and rodents, the immature nervous system is highly responsive to tactile and noxious stimulation, mediated at the spinal cord level. Ontogenetically, excitatory mechanisms precede capacity to dampen, and in humans, modulatory influences appear around term-equivalent age [9]. This has distinct implications for enhanced sensitivity in human infants born very preterm and in immature rat pups. Modulation of excitation through dampening mechanisms develops around term-equivalent age. Particularly during vaginal delivery the sensitivity to pain is decreased possibly induced by the surge of oxytocin [24], which induces GABA-related inhibition. Thus, infants born vaginally seem to react less to the injection of vitamin K after birth as compared with infants delivered by C-section [4].

Facial expressions similar to those seen in more mature infants during procedures have been observed in preterm infants at 25 weeks gestation age, but there is considerable variability in occurrence of facial grimacing at very low GAs. Moreover, these facial reactions are not always present in the presence of clear nociceptive cortical activation [12]. While facial responses suggest an emotional reaction to pain, these may be largely reflexive in the very immature infant. Alternatively, due to the relatively well-developed subcortical components of the limbic system, an emotional response may be possible. The lack of facial grimace in some infants may be due to the fact that a sick tiny highly stressed newborn may not have the energy reserves to mount a clear facial response.

Analogous to responses in adults, in immature infants, nociceptive reactivity is evident behaviorally, physiologically, and hormonally, suggesting that pain is perceived from the earliest stages of human viability, around 24 weeks GA. Thus, these preterm infants are probably conscious about pain but more so at a basic level. While the sensations and emotions related to pain appear to be present given the facial expressions of preterm and full-term neonates, the evaluative capacity to reflect on pain and place this experience in context develops far later.

MEMORY FOR PAIN?

It is challenging to deduce memory for pain from the biobehavioral pain responses of very preterm infants undergoing neonatal intensive care; however, some longitudinal studies suggest a "biological" memory for pain, although whether conscious awareness is involved cannot be known. In very preterm infants at 32 weeks postmenstrual age, while infants were hospitalized in the NICU, facial, cardiac, and cortisol (stress hormone) responses were lower in infants born at an earlier GAs compared to infants born closer to 32 weeks, suggesting dampening of the response to pain over time in the NICU (see reference [10]). In contrast, *lower* threshold (higher sensitivity) to touch on the heel "primed" from repeated heel lances for blood sampling during the NICU stay was described in very preterm infants during the first year of life, compared to term-born controls [1]. However, local hypersensitivity or central sensitization can be induced at a cellular level, and does not provide evidence of awareness or memory for pain.

Infants born extremely preterm (micropremies < 26 weeks gestation), thereby repeatedly exposed to many medical procedures over a prolonged period of neonatal intensive care, displayed an altered pattern of facial behavior during a painful procedure at 8 months corrected age for prematurity [11]. In that study, the extremely preterm infants displayed a faster facial behavioral reaction to a finger lance (which was a "pain naïve" site) followed by faster dampening of their facial response, compared to full-term infants. This very quick behavioral reaction then suppression, which was a different pattern from that of the full-term infants, suggested the micropremies "remembered" pain from months earlier. Interestingly, their peak behavioral response did not differ from the more mature infants; it was their pattern of quicker reactivity and then dampening that suggested "memory" for pain. Moreover, boys born full-term, who underwent neonatal circumcision, showed greater reactivity to a subsequent immunization injection also suggested biological "memory" for pain, especially since the accentuating effect was reduced in those boys who had received topical analgesia prior to circumcision [23]. However, in all these studies—whether preterm or full-term neonates—altered responses appear to be a form of inherent "biological memory" that do not imply processing at a conscious level. It is more likely that aversive conditioning is involved, especially in the context of repeated pain stimulation, rather than evidence of an effect of conscious awareness or memory for pain.

CONSCIOUSNESS AND BRAIN DEVELOPMENT

Brain Development

In the late second and third trimesters of fetal life, the period when the very preterm neonate born at 24–32 weeks gestation is in the NICU, the developing brain undergoes major changes in cytoarchitecture and development of functional networks.

Repeated procedural pain exposure in very preterm neonates takes place during this critical time of rapid brain development. Synaptic connections are being formed, activity-dependent selective cell death (apoptosis) shapes the developing brain, and integrated cortical networks are becoming established (see reference [18]). These processes are affected by developmentally unexpected stimulation. Moreover, electrophysiological evidence suggests that acute pain induces diffuse brain activation across multiple regions in preterm neonates [8]; thus, these neurologically immature infants are the most susceptible to long-term effects of pain.

The cerebral cortex is postulated to be the main site for consciousness (see reference [18]). Therefore, human consciousness cannot emerge until the connections from the thalamus to the cortex have been established, which only begin around 24 weeks of human gestation. Thalamocortical connections are not fully established until the subplate is resolved, around term-equivalent age [14] (see Fig. 11-1). Thus, after about 24 weeks GA pain stimuli may begin to be processed at a cortical level. However, subcortical limbic structures involved in processing of emotion develop earlier; thus, some degree of awareness of aversive experience may be possible before the process of thalamocortical connectivity is well underway. Given the lack of

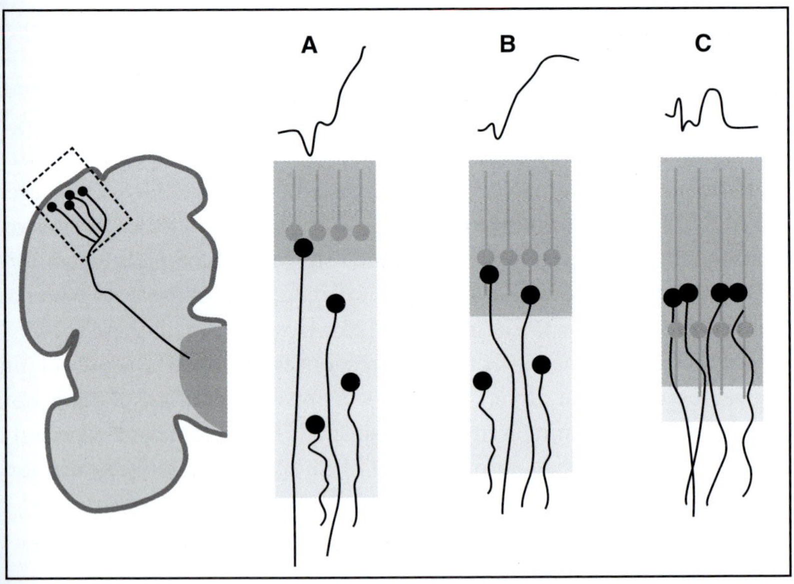

FIGURE 11-1 Maturation of thalamocortical connections and somatosensory-evoked potentials. In early preterm infants (<24 gestational weeks) the neurons from the sensory organs terminate in the subplate (the waiting zone) **(A)**. After 24 weeks they start to make connections in the cortical layer **(B)** and reach the final destination at term **(C)**. This is also reflected by the patterns of spontaneous activity transients and somatosensory-evoked potentials. (Original figure by Vanhatalo modified by Lagercrantz [16].)

thalamocortical connections before 24 weeks gestation, it is unlikely that preterm infants born before this can experience consciousness [16]. Importantly, cortico-cortical connections are essential for the emergence of networks subserving the complex integrated sensory, emotional, and cognitive pain experience, and these begin to develop close to term-equivalent age.

Spontaneous Brain Activity

Low-frequency intrinsic spontaneous brain activity is evident in the human electroencephalogram (EEG), when no external stimulation is taking place. In adults, this spontaneous resting activity corresponds to the uncensored thinking related to random episodic memory, retrieving past experiences, reflecting on current experience, and planning for the future. Resting-state networks, that is, the default mode network that includes temporal, parietal, and anterior prefrontal cortices begin to develop early, and have been identified in preterm and full-term infants. This spontaneous resting state activity has been proposed to correspond to "the stream of consciousness" (see reference [16]).

Evoked Activity

In adults, cortical networks activated during pain involve thalamus, posterior and anterior insulae, secondary somatosensory cortex, anterior cingulate cortex, and the periaqueductal gray matter [5]. Moreover, this large network is comprised of multiple interacting pain matrices. These imaging studies reveal a complex network of responsive regional brain activity that underlies the multidimensional nature of pain in the mature human. Characterization of pain networks in infants has received little attention so far. Importantly, magnetic resonance imaging (MRI) of children born very prematurely at age 11–16 years, during quantitative testing of sensory thresholds, revealed that adolescents born preterm showed significantly greater BOLD signal than full-term controls in the primary somatosensory cortex, anterior cingulate cortex, and insula [13]. In that study, the exaggerated brain response was pain-specific and was not observed during nonpainful warmth stimulation. Clearly experiential factors in the individual's life course and environmental context that inform the full complex multidimensional experience of the adolescent or adult have not yet emerged in the early developing human. Yet, differences in threshold to temperature in micropremies compared to full-term adolescents at this age have been largely accounted for by exposure to neonatal surgery, rather than prematurity per se. Therefore, a lot remains to be learned about the potential for long-term changes to pain processing in this population.

Recently Hartley and Slater [12] summarized the literature on nociceptive-evoked brain activity in newborn infants. Using near-infrared spectroscopy (NIRS), studies have shown increases in hemoglobin oxygen concentration over central regions following acute noxious stimulation. EEG recordings in full-term infants show a specific localized somatosensory response to noxious stimulation, but not to tactile stimulation; thus, these responses are nociceptive-specific. In contrast, in preterm newborns before 35 weeks gestation, both tactile- and noxious stimuli-evoked nonspecific delta brush activity widespread throughout the cortex [8, 12]. In preterms, this lack of a mature localized response, with diffuse activation across the cortex, suggests increased vulnerability to external stimulation. As Hartley and Slater conclude, since cortical activation is a fundamental component of pain processing well-established in adults, observations that even the very preterm newborns manifest cortical responses to noxious stimuli is of clear importance. In summary, evidence of evoked activity suggests that infants process pain.

Long-term Effects of Early Pain Exposure: Is Consciousness Required?

Frequent procedural pain in the very preterm neonate during the period of hospitalization in the NICU is associated with altered brain development over and above other clinical risk factors of prematurity, thereby contributing to poorer neurodevelopment [6, 10, 25]. Importantly, the greatest effect is seen in extremely preterm infants [6], who have the least mature brain development at the time of pain exposure, suggesting that consciousness is not involved in long-term effects of neonatal procedural pain on altered brain development. Rather, it is the immaturity of the developing brain that renders it most vulnerable to repeated procedures, due to immature autoregulation of cerebral blood flow, the developmental window for vulnerability of the developing white matter to excitotoxic damage [3], and the widespread generalized electrocortical response to nociceptive stimulation seen in the preterm brain [8]. Alterations to brain development do not depend on memory, awareness, or consciousness. Arguments that more fully developed brain cytoarchitecture is required for pain perception imply that prior pain exposures have little importance, whereas the evidence suggests that the more immature the brain, the more vulnerable it is to perturbations of stress and repeated painful procedures.

CONCLUSIONS

The emphasis on pain as a learned psychological phenomenon, which works well in understanding complexities of pain in adults, actually undermines the importance of pain in the least-mature humans. Advances in neuroimaging techniques have significantly improved our understanding of sensory, emotional, and cognitive processing in the brain. These techniques will be powerful in exploring tactile and nociceptive processing in the infant brain. However, neurovascular and electrophysiological responses to nociceptive stimulation do not necessarily inform us about the subjective feelings experienced by the individual. Consciousness probably develops gradually, and as with other developmental processes. Certainly neonates outside the womb, given their advanced development of the subcortical limbic system, are likely to experience emotions to some extent, during the establishment of thalamocortical and cortico-cortical connections and brain networks. This immature form of consciousness likely gradually progresses across infancy. While we would not question that young children have the capacity for conscious experience, they cannot yet place pain into a cognitive framework the way an adult can contextualize injury. Rather than an "all-or-none" phenomenon, consciousness emerges gradually in the human neonate outside the protective intrauterine environment. Early pain consciousness likely evolves over time, eventually integrating pain experience and family history, to become the adult complex pain experience.

ACKNOWLEDGMENTS

Dr. Grunau's research program is supported by grants from the Canadian Institute of Health Research (CIHR) grants MOP86489 and MOP79262, Eunice Kennedy Shriver Institute of Child Health and Human Development (NICHD/NIH) grant R01 HD039783, and she holds a Senior Scientist salary award from the Child and Family Research Institute. Dr. Ranger is supported by CIHR and Quebec Research Funds—health postdoctoral fellowships. Dr. Lagercrantz's research program is supported by the European Union 7th Framework grant no. 223767.

REFERENCES

1. Allegaert K, Devlieger H, Bulckaert D, Naulaers G, Casaer P, Tibboel D. Variability in pain expression characteristics in former preterm infants. J Perinat Med 2005;33:442–8.
2. Anand KJ, Craig KD. New perspectives on the definition of pain. Pain 1996;67:3–6.
3. Back SA, Miller SP. Brain injury in premature neonates: a primary cerebral dysmaturation disorder? Ann Neurol 2014;75:469–86.
4. Bergqvist LL, Katz-Salamon M, Hertegard S, Anand KJ, Lagercrantz H. Mode of delivery modulates physiological and behavioral responses to neonatal pain. J Perinatol 2009;29(1):44–50.
5. Denk F, McMahon SB, Tracey I. Pain vulnerability: a neurobiological perspective. Nat Neurosci 2014;17:192–200.

6. Doesburg SM, Moiseev A, Herdman AT, Ribary U, Grunau RE. Region-specific slowing of alpha oscillations is associated with visual-perceptual abilities in children born very preterm. Front Hum Neurosci 2013;7:791.
7. Elwood RW. Pain and suffering in invertebrates? ILAR J 2011;52:175–84.
8. Fabrizi L, Slater R, Worley A, Meek J, Boyd S, Olhede S, Fitzgerald M. A shift in sensory processing that enables the developing human brain to discriminate touch from pain. Curr Biol 2011;21:1552–8.
9. Fitzgerald M. The development of nociceptive circuits. Nat Rev Neurosci 2005;6:507–20.
10. Grunau RE. Neonatal pain in very preterm infants: long-term effects on brain, neurodevelopment and pain reactivity. Rambam Maimonides Med J 2013;4(4):e0025.
11. Grunau RE, Oberlander TF, Whitfield MF, Fitzgerald C, Morison SJ, Saul JP. Pain reactivity in former extremely low birth weight infants at corrected age 8 months compared with term born controls. Infant Behav Dev 2001;24:41–55.
12. Hartley C, Slater R. Neurophysiological measures of nociceptive brain activity in the newborn infant—the next steps. Acta Paediatr 2014;103:238–42.
13. Hohmeister J, Kroll A, Wollgarten-Hadamek I, Zohsel K, Demirakca S, Flor H, Hermann C. Cerebral processing of pain in school-aged children with neonatal nociceptive input: an exploratory fMRI study. Pain 2010;150:257–67.
14. Kostovic I, Judas M. The development of the subplate and thalamocortical connections in the human foetal brain. Acta Paediatr 2010;99:1119–27.
15. Kouider S, Stahlhut C, Gelskov SV, Barbosa LS, Dutat M, de Gardelle V, Christophe A, Dehaene S, Dehaene-Lambertz G. A neural marker of perceptual consciousness in infants. Science 2013;340:376–80.
16. Lagercrantz H. The emergence of consciousness: science and ethics. Semin Fetal Neonatal Med 2014;19:300–5.
17. Lagercrantz H, Changeux JP. The emergence of human consciousness: from fetal to neonatal life. Pediatr Res 2009(65):255–60.
18. Lagercrantz H, Hanson MA, Ment LR, Peebles DM. The newborn brain: neuroscience and clinical applications. Cambridge: Cambridge University Press; 2010.
19. Lee SJ, Ralston HJ, Drey EA, Partridge JC, Rosen MA. Fetal pain: a systematic multidisciplinary review of the evidence. JAMA 2005;294:947–54.
20. Mahmoudzadeh M, Dehaene-Lambertz G, Fournier M, Kongolo G, Goudjil S, Dubois J, Grebe R, Wallois F. Syllabic discrimination in premature human infants prior to complete formation of cortical layers. Proc Natl Acad Sci U S A 2013;110:4846–51.

21. Mellor DJ, Diesch TJ, Gunn AJ, Bennet L. The importance of "awareness" for understanding fetal pain. Brain Res Brain Res Rev 2005;49:455–71.
22. Merskey H. The need of a taxonomy. Pain 1979;6:247–54.
23. Taddio A, Katz J, Ilersich AL, Koren G. Effect of neonatal circumcision on pain response during subsequent routine vaccination. Lancet 1997;349:599–603.
24. Tyzio R, Cossart R, Khalilov I, Minlebaev M, Hübner CA, Represa A, Ben-Ari Y, Khazipov R. Maternal oxytocin triggers a transient inhibitory switch in GABA signaling in the fetal brain during delivery. Science 2006;314(5806):1788–92.
25. Vinall J, Miller SP, Bjornson BH, Fitzpatrick KP, Poskitt KJ, Brant R, Synnes AR, Cepeda IL, Grunau RE. Invasive procedures in preterm children: brain and cognitive development at school age. Pediatrics 2014;133(3):412–21.

CHAPTER 12

Recognizing Pain in Dementia

Thomas Hadjistavropoulos

Dementia is a condition that impairs consciousness (e.g., by causing fluctuations in attention and awareness) [10]. With the aging of the world population, the number of dementia cases has been increasing significantly. Specifically, a scientific group working for Alzheimer's Disease International [3], the international federation of Alzheimer associations, was projecting the total number of cases around the world to be 35.6 million in 2010 and to rise to 65.7 million in 2030. Compounding the problem, painful conditions are very common in dementia populations, with pain-prevalence estimates as high as 50–80% of seniors residing in long-term care facilities [14].

The undertreatment of pain in people with dementia has been documented in both the United States and Canada [17, 36]. This undertreatment has been attributed, at least in part, to dementia patients' difficulty communicating the pain experience due to the cognitive and linguistic impairments caused by the illness [24]. The communication difficulty, in turn, reduces the probability of pain being reported. Favoring this explanation, people with dementia have been shown to present with increased nonverbal pain displays (at least during acute-phasic exacerbations of musculoskeletal pain) relative to their cognitively intact counterparts [39]. Such behavioral reactivity may be due to confusion caused by a more limited understanding of the painful situation.

Despite neurobiological changes that accompany dementia, there is no convincing evidence that dementia causes reductions in clinical pain-related suffering [24, 38, 39]. Nonetheless, psychophysical studies conducted in the experimental laboratory have considered the possibility of detectable differences in pain threshold in older people with and without dementia. Such research has demonstrated a small increase in pain threshold in dementia populations particularly for thermal stimuli [11, 22, 23, 33, 41], although the results for other stimulus modalities have been less consistent [42, 51].

Several studies have associated lower pain tolerance with aging, suggesting increased vulnerability to pain among older adults [25, 41]. Findings concerning possible decreases in pain tolerance as a function of dementing illness have been quite inconsistent [11, 23, 33]. It is difficult to reconcile these inconsistencies, but it appears, from examination of the available studies, that variations in degree/type of dementia may be partially responsible for the differences across investigations [25].

In an effort to better understand the pain experience in dementia, research involving evoked potentials has also been conducted. Some results show differences in components of somatosensory-evoked potentials between patients with and without dementia and suggest possible abnormalities in pain perception among those with severe dementia [59]. Moreover, although not pain specific, autonomic age-related changes in response to painful stimulation have been found in older persons with and without dementia (e.g., heart rate changes). That is, at least some of these autonomic responses (e.g., evoked heart rate responses) seem to be somewhat attenuated in older adults in general [49]. Nonetheless, it has also been suggested that there may be further attenuation of such autonomic responses in certain dementia subtypes, although this possibility requires further investigation [49]. When it comes to the examination of autonomic reactivity in the clinical assessment of pain, a limitation is that such reactivity is not pain-specific. This lack of specificity complicates pain assessment and detection.

CONSCIOUSNESS, PAIN, AND PERSONHOOD IN DEMENTIA

Related to the issue of consciousness in seniors with dementia, who suffer from pain, is the notion of personhood. Personhood has been defined as a standing or status that is bestowed upon one human being, by others, in the social context of human relationships [37]. Personhood implies recognition, respect, and trust [37]. Recent research suggests that people with dementia may be perceived by others as having reduced personhood and that perceptions of reduced personhood incorporate aspects of consciousness (i.e., perceptions that people with severe dementia "are no longer persons because they do not think or reason logically") [32]. Related to these findings, some research evidence is suggesting that, when dementia patients are perceived as having reduced personhood (which incorporates perceptions of reduced consciousness), the quality of pain management offered by health care staff could be compromised (e.g., reduced likelihood that an analgesic will be administered) [32]. To overcome this problem, pain care approaches for dementia patients have begun to emphasize not only standardized pain evaluation and management but also person-centered care designed to enhance staff perceptions of patient personhood [21]. Enhanced staff perceptions of patient personhood could foster a better understanding of the pain experience through consideration of the whole person ("I will care for Mr. S who is a war hero and a kind man who suffers from pain" as opposed to "I will treat the broken hip in Room 5.").

PAIN ASSESSMENT IN DEMENTIA

The assessment of pain can be based on self-report as well as on the observation of pain-related behaviors. Self-report and nonverbal expressions of pain vary with respect to the extent that they each rely on cognitive executive mediation versus reflexive automaticity (see reference [24] for a discussion). Specifically, the self-report of pain relies heavily on cognitive executive mediation and voluntary control. As such, it necessitates cognitive capability that allows for comprehension of the question, ability to evaluate one's own pain experience, and ability to express it, usually verbally. In contrast, nonverbal pain behaviors tend to be more reflexive (e.g., reflexive withdrawal of limb) and less subject to voluntary control. Given their reduced reliance on cognitive executive mediation, nonverbal responses are less likely to be affected by the presence of dementia than is self-report and would, therefore, be an extremely important target for assessment in this population. Nonetheless, although nonverbal pain expression is generally preserved in dementia, it tends to be more ambiguous than verbal report and, therefore, more difficult for observers to interpret correctly [24].

Related to difficulties in effectively recognizing pain among older patients with limited ability to communicate is that the ambiguity of nonverbal signs of pain leads to frequent misattribution. For example, pain can lead to increases in aggressive behavior [16] and clinicians often attribute such behavior to psychiatric disturbance rather than to pain. As a result, patients with pain may be treated with psychiatric rather than analgesic medication [8], increasing unnecessary polypharmacy as well as the risk of serious side effects, including death, associated with use of certain psychiatric medications in frail older adults [9]. To avoid such problems and potentially decrease unnecessary polypharmacy [27] effective pain assessment is necessary. In fact, a reduction in benzodiazepine use has been found among dementia patients who were assessed regularly with a research physician being involved in communicating pain assessment results to the patients' prescribing physicians [27].

It is important to emphasize that the assessment of pain should be multidimensional and not limited to the investigation of pain intensity. That is, a comprehensive pain assessment should take into account the patient's clinical and psychosocial history, psychological and physical comorbidities, functional capabilities, coping skills, social supports, past/current treatment, caregiver reports, and other related dimensions. This chapter focuses primarily on the assessment of pain intensity, which is only one of several dimensions that clinicians should be evaluating. The interested reader is referred to work of an international consensus group for a detailed description of all dimensions of pain assessment [26]. Given the negative impact that pain tends to have on patient mood, for example, specialized tools exist that can assess depression and various dimensions of quality of life in patients who suffer from both dementia and chronic pain [2, 50].

Assessing Pain in Dementia Using Self-Report

The clinical literature suggests that most people with mild to moderate dementia, with severity often estimated using the Mini Mental Status Examination (MMSE) [19], are capable of providing some form of valid self-report of pain whereas people with more severe dementia are less likely to provide it [26]. That is, mild to moderate dementia patients' pain scores appear to increase as a function of the extent to which the stimulus or situation is believed to be painful. Chibnall and Tait [15] showed that older adults with dementia, who had an average MMSE [19] score of at least 18 (out of a possible 30), which falls within the upper range of moderate impairment [48], tended to be able to provide valid responses to the 21-point box scale [34]. More recently, Lukas et al. [47] showed that at least 90% of seniors with mild to moderate cognitive impairments are able to complete verbal rating scales (i.e., scales that involve words ranging from "no pain" to "extremely painful," with each word corresponding to a numeric rating). Similarly, Lukas et al. [47] showed that 57.5% of adults with moderate dementia could use an 11-point numeric rating scale, with higher numbers corresponding to higher pain ratings. This suggests that it would be important for clinicians assessing pain in seniors with dementia to attempt a variety of different self-report formats. Scherder and Bouma [53] described a brief protocol that they used to evaluate dementia patients' ability to comprehend a self-report scale. Their approach involves, for example, asking patients to point to the scale, to point to the part of the scale that would correspond to "no pain," to point to the part of the scale that would correspond to very intense pain, etc. Such an approach might be helpful to implement prior to using unidimensional pain scales with patients suffering from dementia.

It has been suggested [24], based on the preexisting literature [15, 58], that a rule of thumb would be that seniors with MMSE scores of 18 or greater would likely be able to provide valid self-report of pain but those with scores of lower than 13 would be less likely to be able. It is important to note, however, that existing national and international clinical guidelines stress the importance of attempting self-report with all dementia patients [26] because there are individuals with low MMSE scores who are capable of providing valid reports. The guidelines also suggest that the self-report of pain be supplemented with results of a well-validated observational tool [26].

Assessing Pain in Dementia Using Nonverbal Expressions

The American Geriatrics Society [4, 5] has determined that several domains are important to evaluate when conducting assessments of nonverbal pain behavior in dementia patients. These domains are shown on Table 12-1.

A variety of observational tools have been developed in recent years to assess pain in populations with dementia. Table 12-2 contains a list of some of the most cited tools. A more detailed list of tools can be found in a recently published review [25]. Some of

TABLE 12-1 **Nonverbal Pain Assessment Domains Deemed Important by the American Geriatrics Society [4]**
Facial expressions (e.g., grimacing)
Verbalizations and vocalizations (e.g., crying, grunting)
Body movements (e.g., rubbing the affected area, limping)
Changes in interpersonal interactions (e.g., not wanting to interact with others)
Changes in activity patterns or routines (e.g., reduced level of activity)
Mental status changes

TABLE 12-2 **Useful Information for Clinicians Interested in Assessing Pain in Dementia Patients**
Major Practice Guideline Documents
American Geriatrics Society (2002) [4]
American Medical Directors' Association Pain Management Guideline (2012) [6]
Australian Pain Society (2005) [7]
The British National guideline for assessment of pain in older people (2007) [52]
International interdisciplinary consensus statement on pain assessment in older persons (2007) [26]
Expert consensus recommendations for use of behavioral assessment tools in the nursing home (2010) [30]
Task force of the American Society for Pain Management Nursing (2006) [31]
Transforming pain management in long-term care (2009) [28]
Selected Observational Pain Assessment Tools for Older Adults with Dementia
Abbey pain scale [1]
DOLOPLUS-2 [56, 57]
Non-Communicative Patient's Pain Assessment Instrument (NOPPAIN) [54]
Pain Assessment Checklist for Seniors with Limited Ability to Communicate (PACLSAC and PACSLAC-II) [13, 20, 61]
Pain Assessment in Advanced Dementia (PAINAD) [55, 61]

these assessment instruments have been shown in several studies and reviews of the literature to be valid and useful [13, 30, 43, 60, 61]. Among the most recommended tools are the Pain Assessment in Advanced Dementia [55], the Abbey Pain Scale [1], the DOLOPLUS-2 [56, 57], as well as the Pain Assessment Checklist for Seniors with Limited Ability to Communicate (PACSLAC and PACSLAC-II; see Fig. 12-1) [13, 20]. The various tools differ in length and with respect to the extent to which they cover all of the nonverbal behavior domains deemed important by the American Geriatrics Society. Many of these tools have been shown to discriminate pain from non–pain-related states [13, 43]. Use of these tools to systematize observation seems important especially in light of research, suggesting that caregivers sometimes disregard nonverbal cues when they estimate pain in seniors with dementia [18]. Such cues may be disregarded possibly because our culture is so heavily reliant on language that, in the absence of verbal report (providing linguistic context), nonverbal responses may be perceived as less salient or may be attributed to states other than pain.

The Doloplus-2 was developed in France and was one of the first tools of this kind [56]. At the time of this writing, an English translation of the scale was available at www.doloplus.com/travaux/travaux6.php. The tool consists of five somatic (e.g., protection of sore areas, sleep patterns), six psychosocial (e.g., communication), and two psychomotor (i.e., washing/dressing and mobility) items that are scored along 0–3 scales, with the anchor for each of the scales being clearly defined. The psychometric properties of the Doloplus-2 are satisfactory but, in a clinical investigation of three scales (i.e., the PACSLAC, the PAINAD, and the Doloplus-2), participating nurses found the Doloplus-2 to be less clinically useful [61], possibly because the Doloplus-2 relies on prior knowledge of the patient.

The Abbey Scale consists of only six items (e.g., facial expression, change in body language, physiological change, physical change) rated from 0 to 3, and the PAINAD consists of five items (e.g., breathing, negative vocalization, facial expression) rated from 0 to 2. Both the Abbey Scale and the PAINAD have been shown to have good psychometric properties, although [25, 61] their coverage of the nonverbal pain assessment domains recommended by the American Geriatrics Society is more limited than that of the PACSLAC scales.

The most recent version of the PACSLAC, the PACSLAC-II [13] is a comprehensive tool that covers all of the domains deemed important by the American Geriatrics Society and contains 31 items (e.g., "a specific sound for pain [e.g., 'ow, ouch']," "clenched fist," "limping"). The tool has been shown to have strong psychometric properties and in psychometric investigation accounted for more variance in differentiating pain from nonpain states than other commonly used pain assessment tools for dementia populations [13].

One key issue concerns the sensitivity of pain behaviors in observational tools. Pain in persons with dementia can result in behavioral disturbance and even delirium [16]. Delirium is a transient altered state of consciousness involving a disturbance of

Pain Assessment Checklist for Seniors with Limited Ability to Communicate-II (PACSLAC-II)	
Date of Assessment: _______________ Time: __________	Check If Present
Check if present	
Facial Expressions	
1. Grimacing	
2. Tighter face	
3. Pain expression	
4. Increased eye movement	
5. Wincing	
6. Opening mouth	
7. Creasing forehead	
8. Lowered eyebrows or frowning	
9. Raised cheeks, narrowing of the eyes, or squinting	
10. Wrinkled nose and raised upper lip	
11. Eyes closing	
Verbalizations and Vocalizations	
12. Crying	
13. A specific sound for pain (e.g., "ow," "ouch")	
14. Moaning and groaning	
15. Grunting	
16. Gasping or breathing loudly	
Body Movements	
17. Flinching or pulling away	
18. Thrashing	
19. Refusing to move	
20. Moving slow	
21. Guarding sore area	
22. Rubbing or holding sore area	
23. Limping	
24. Clenched fist	
25. Going into foetal position	
26. Stiff or rigid	
27. Shaking or trembling	
Changes in Interpersonal Interactions	
28. Not wanting to be touched	
29. Not allowing people near	
Changes in Activity Patterns or Routines	
30. Decreased activity	
Mental Status Changes	
31. Are there mental status changes that are due to pain *and* are not explained by another condition (e.g., delirium due to medication)?	
TOTAL SCORE (Add up checkmarks)	

FIGURE 12-1 Pain Assessment Checklist for Seniors with Limited Ability to Communicate-II (PACSLAC-II). The subscale names on the PACSLAC-II represent the pain assessment domains recommended by the American Geriatrics Society (2002).

attention and awareness. Delirium also affects judgment [12]. Given the association of pain with behavioral disturbance and delirium, assessment tools include items (e.g., aggression) that may be due to pain but are not specific to pain [29]. Lints-Martindale et al. [43] studied the impact of excluding these types of items (i.e., items most likely to overlap with delirium) from pain assessment tools. They concluded that elimination of those items from assessment tools such as the PACSLAC and the PAINAD did not affect much the ability of the tools to discriminate pain-related from non–pain-related states in that particular investigation. More research is needed to further investigate this issue. It is important to mention, however, that Chan et al. [13] developed the PACSLAC-II in part on the strength of the Lints-Martindale et al. findings. That is, the PACSLAC-II, which is much shorter than the PACSLAC, excluded items most likely to overlap with delirium and effectively discriminated between pain and nonpain states.

Work completed wordwide has resulted in translations of various observational tools designed for the assessment of pain in dementia. Translations and research on translations of many observational tools are now available in a variety of languages including, but not limited to, Dutch, Italian, Spanish, Japanese, Portuguese, French, Chinese, and German (see reference [25] for review).

Relation of Self-Report and Nonverbal Pain Assessment in Dementia

Labus et al. [40] considered the relationship between self-report and observational measures of pain in cognitively intact samples and concluded that these do not always overlap. Specifically, in a meta-analytic investigation they found that the average association between self-reported pain intensity and observations of pain behavior is moderately positive ($r = 0.26$) and that a significant relationship is more likely to be found when global observations of behavior and acute (as opposed to chronic pain) are considered. It is probable that, at high intensities, the correlation between pain and nonverbal expressions would increase. Nonetheless, Labus et al. concluded that the relatively low association between self-reported pain and observed pain behaviors demonstrates that self-report and nonverbal responses tap different aspects of the pain experience. The former may be more subject to situational and demand characteristics than the latter which are more likely to tap more immediate and phasic responses to painful stimulation. With this in mind, we can consider the association between nonverbal pain behaviors and self-report in patients with dementia who are capable of responding to questions. The findings concerning this issue are not perfectly consistent across studies. Some studies have failed to find a significant association. For example, Lints-Martindale et al. [43] did not find an association between self-reported pain and a variety of observational measures (e.g., PACSLAC, PAINAD) used to assess movement-exacerbated musculoskeletal pain in older long-term care residents with dementia (average MMSE score of 5.35). In contrast, Lukas et al. [46] found significant associations between the PAINAD, the Abbey, and the Non-Communicative Patient's Pain Assessment Instrument (NOPPAIN) scales with self-report in participants with cognitive impairments (with average MMSE scores of 13.6). Similarly, Kaasalainen et al. [35] found a high association between self-reported pain and PACSLAC scores in a mixed sample of long-term care residents that included individuals with and without dementia. Differences among the findings of such studies are likely due to sample differences with the Lints-Martindale et al. sample, for example, having MMSE scores that were much lower than those of Lukas et al. The strong possibility that self-reported pain and scores on observational tools tap nonperfectly overlapping aspects of the pain experience underscores the need for using both self-report and observational indices of pain, when possible.

Guidelines for Assessing Pain in Dementia and Limited Ability to Communicate

A wide variety of consensus and/or guideline documents [4, 7, 26, 30] provide clinical guidance on how to assess pain in dementia. The reader is referred to the guideline documents for more detailed information. Generally, adopting an individualized approach to assessment is important [6, 26, 52]. That is, it is recommended that pain be assessed on a regular basis (e.g., at least once a week [28]) with the clinician observing the patient's pattern of scores. A sudden change in a patient's pattern of scores may be indicative of a change in pain level and would warrant further investigation. Such regular assessments should be occurring under similar circumstances if the scores are to be meaningfully compared across situations (e.g., during a standardized set of movements). Comparing scores before and after the administration of analgesics is useful [26, 31]. Moreover, assessment during movement is more likely to elicit pain behaviors than is assessment during rest [26, 31].

Although some have argued that it is beneficial to establish cutoff scores for observational assessment tools for seniors with dementia, this approach is not without its criticism. That is, scores on observational tools are affected by a variety of variables, including duration of observation (i.e., longer periods of observation would typically result in higher scores), the nature of the situation being observed (e.g., rest vs. movement), and individual differences among patients (e.g., a patient who is ambulatory has a broader repertoire of pain behaviors that he or she could potentially display, such as limping, as compared to a patient who is not ambulatory). Given such variables, it may be more constructive to employ an individualized approach to assessment as described above (comparing each patient with his or her own scores over time) than attempting to apply the same cutoff score to all patients.

FUTURE DIRECTIONS

Computerized vision systems have been applied to the detection/recognition of pain behaviors [44, 45], but work toward the application of such systems among seniors with dementia is more limited. Nonetheless, our group has begun investigations aimed toward the identification of optimal computerized algorithms and hardware requirements that could lead to the development of affordable systems capable of recognizing pain behaviors in long-term care facilities. Such vision systems could increase assessment efficiencies and improve care in light of staff shortages that result in adequate and potentially continuous pain assessment among seniors with dementia. Such an approach could also increase our understanding of the pain experience of the other adult with severe dementia because the current empirical knowledge base primarily consists of information obtained during distinct and very limited periods of observations. In contrast, a computerized vision system approach would allow for the collection of pain expression information on a continuous and long-term basis, allowing the systematic investigation of fluctuations in pain responses.

CONCLUSION

Pain is a subjective experience, and, in severe dementia, it is especially difficult to fully comprehend the patient's pain-related suffering because of the communication barriers that result from the neurological condition. Given dementia patients' increased behavioral responses to painful situations, clinically significant suffering does not appear to diminish as a function of dementing illness [24]. Nonetheless, despite inconsistencies in the literature, some studies have suggested the possibility that severe dementia is associated with an attenuation in certain physiological responses to noxious stimulation, [59] as well as possible increases in pain thresholds particularly for thermal stimuli [25]. Although it is probable that the neurobiological changes that accompany dementia affect aspects of pain perception, the manner in which this occurs (i.e., impact on pain perception) is poorly understood. To address challenges in understanding the pain experience of the patient with dementia and severe limitations in ability to communicate, clinically useful observational pain assessment tools have been developed [25]. The utility of such specialized tools is likely to be maximized with increased training of health care staff as well as through adoption of person-centered patient care.

ACKNOWLEDGMENTS

The author acknowledges the support of the (University of Regina) Chair in Aging and Health that was made possible through the contributions of an anonymous donor with matching funds from the University of Regina. The author also declares that he is one of the copyright holders of the Pain Assessment Checklist for Seniors with Limited Ability to Communicate (PACSLAC scales) that is discussed, along with others, in this chapter. The author has no financial interest in the PACSLAC scales.

REFERENCES

1. Abbey J, Piller N, De Bellis A, Esterman A, Parker D, Giles L, Lowcay B. The Abbey pain scale: a 1-minute numerical indicator for people with end-stage dementia. Int J Palliat Nurs 2004;10:6–13.
2. Alexopoulos GS, Abrams RC, Young RC, Shamoian CA. Cornell scale for depression in dementia. Biol Psychiatry 1988;23:271–84.
3. Alzheimer's Disease International. World Alzheimer report 2009: Executive summary; 2009. Available at: https://www.alz.co.uk/research/files/WorldAlzheimerReport-ExecutiveSummary.pdf.
4. American Geriatrics Society (AGS). The management of persistent pain in older persons. J Am Geriatr Soc 2002;50:S205–S224.
5. American Geriatrics Society (AGS). Pharmacological management of pain: recommendations from the American Geriatrics Society Guidelines on the management of persistent pain in older persons. J Am Geriatr Soc 2009;57:1331–46.
6. American Medical Directors Association (AMDA). Pain management in the long term care setting. Columbia, MD: American Medical Directors Association (AMDA); 2012.
7. Australian Pain Society. Pain in residential aged care facilities: management strategies. North Sydney: Australian Pain Society; 2005.
8. Balfour JE, O'Rourke N. Older adults with Alzheimer disease, comorbid arthritis and prescription of psychotropic medications. Pain Res Manag 2003;8:198–204.
9. Ballard C, Hanney ML, Theodoulou M, Douglas S, McShane R, Kossakowski K, Gill R, Juszczak E, Yu L. The dementia antipsychotic withdrawal trial (DART-AD): long-term follow-up of a randomised placebo-controlled trial. Lancet Neurol 2009;8:151–7.
10. Ballard CG, Court JA, Piggott M, Johnson M, O'Brien J, McKeith I, Holmes C, Lantos P, Jaros E, Perry R, Perry E. Disturbances of consciousness in dementia with Lewy bodies associated with alteration in nicotinic receptor binding in the temporal cortex. Conscious Cogn 2002;11:461–74.
11. Benedetti F, Vighetti S, Ricco C, Lagna E, Bergamasco B, Pinessi L, Rainero I. Pain threshold and tolerance in Alzheimer's disease. Pain 1999;80:377–82.
12. Bhat R, Rockwood K. Delirium as a disorder of consciousness. J Neurol Neurosurg Psychiatry 2007;78:1167–70.

13. Chan S, Hadjistavropoulos T, Williams J. Evidence-based development and initial validation of the Pain Assessment Checklist for Seniors with Limited Ability to Communicate-II (PACSLAC-II). Clin J Pain 2014;30:816–24.
14. Charlton JE. Core curriculum for professional education in pain. Seattle, WA: IASP Press; 2005.
15. Chibnall JT, Tait RC. Pain assessment in cognitively impaired and unimpaired older adults: a comparison of four scales. Pain 2001;92:173–86.
16. Cipher DJ, Clifford PA, Roper KD. Behavioral manifestations of pain in the demented elderly. J Am Med Dir Assoc 2006;7:355–65.
17. de Souto Barreto P, Lapeyre-Mestre M, Vellas B, Rolland Y. Potential underuse of analgesics for recognized pain in nursing home residents with dementia: a cross-sectional study. Pain 2013;154:2427–31.
18. Eritz H, Hadjistavropoulos T. Do informal caregivers consider non-verbal behavior when they assess pain in people with dementia? J Pain 2011;12:331–9.
19. Folstein MF, Folstein SE, McHugh PR. "Mini-mental state": a practical method for grading the cognitive state of patients for the clinician. J Psychiatr Res 1975;12:189–98.
20. Fuchs-Lacelle S, Hadjistavropoulos T. Development and preliminary validation of the pain assessment checklist for seniors with limited ability to communicate (PACSLAC). Pain Manag Nurs 2004;5:37–49.
21. Ghandehari OO, Hadjistavropoulos T, Williams J, Thorpe L, Alfano DP, Dal Bello-Haas V, Malloy DC, Martin RR, Rahaman O, Zwakhalen SM, et al. A controlled investigation of continuing pain education for long-term care staff. Pain Res Manag 2013;18:11–8.
22. Gibson SJ, Farrell M. A review of age differences in the neurophysiology of nociception and the perceptual experience of pain. Clin J Pain 2004;20:227–39.
23. Gibson SJ, Voukelatos X, Ames D, Flicker L, Helme RD. An examination of pain perception and cerebral event-related potentials following carbon dioxide laser stimulation in patients with Alzheimer's disease and age-matched control volunteers. Pain Res Manag 2001;6:126–32.
24. Hadjistavropoulos T, Breau L, Craig KD. Pain assessment in adults and children with limited ability to communicate. In: Turk DC, Melzack R, editors. Handbook of pain assessment. New York, NY: Guilford Press; 2011. pp. 260–80.
25. Hadjistavropoulos T, Herr K, Prkachin K, Craig K, Gibson S, Lukas L, Smith J. Pain assessment in older adults with dementia. Lancet Neurol 2014;13:1216–27.
26. Hadjistavropoulos T, Herr K, Turk DC, Fine PG, Dworkin RH, Helme R, Jackson K, Parmelee PA, Rudy TE, Lynn Beattie B, et al. An interdisciplinary expert consensus statement on assessment of pain in older persons. Clin J Pain 2007;23:S1–S43.

27. Hadjistavropoulos T, Kaasalainen S, Williams J, Zacharias R. Improving pain assessment practices and outcomes in long-term care facilities: a mixed methods investigation. Pain Manag Nurs 2014;15:748–59.

28. Hadjistavropoulos T, Marchildon GP, Fine PG, Herr K, Palley HA, Kaasalainen S, Béland F. Transforming long-term care pain management in North America: the policy-clinical interface. Pain Med 2009;10:506–20.

29. Hadjistavropoulos T, Voyer P, Sharpe D, Verreault R, Aubin M. Assessing pain in dementia patients with comorbid delirium and depression. Pain Manag Nurs 2008;9:48–54.

30. Herr K, Bursch H, Ersek M, Miller LL, Swafford K. Use of pain-behavioral assessment tools in the nursing home: expert consensus recommendations for practice. J Gerontol Nurs 2010;36:18–31.

31. Herr K, Coyne PJ, Key T, Manworren R, McCaffery M, Merkel S, Pelosi-Kelly J, Wild L. Pain assessment in the nonverbal patient: position statement with clinical practice recommendations. Pain Manag Nurs 2006;7:44–52.

32. Hunter PV, Hadjistavropoulos T, Smythe WE, Mallow DC, Kaasalainen S, Williams J. The Personhood in Dementia Questionnaire (PDQ): establishing an association between beliefs about personhood and health providers' approaches to person-centred care. J Aging Stud 2013;27:276–87.

33. Jensen-Dahm C, Werner MU, Dahl JB, Jensen TS, Ballegaard M, Hejl AM, Waldemar G. Quantitative sensory testing and pain tolerance in patients with mild to moderate Alzheimer disease compared to healthy control subjects. Pain 2014;155:1439–45.

34. Jensen MP, Miller L, Fisher LD. Assessment of pain during medical procedures: a comparison of three scales. Clin J Pain 1998;14:343–9.

35. Kaasalainen S, Akhtar-Danesh N, Hadjistavropoulos T, Zwakhalen S, Verreault R. A comparison between behavioral and verbal report pain assessment tools for use with residents in long term care. Pain Manag Nurs 2013;14:e106–e114.

36. Kaasalainen S, Middleton J, Knezacek S, Hartley T, Stewart N, Ife C, Robinson L. Pain and cognitive status in the institutionalized elderly: perceptions & interventions. J Gerontol Nurs 1998;24:24–31; quiz 50–1.

37. Kitwood T. Dementia reconsidered: the person comes first. Philadelphia, PA: Open University Press; 1997.

38. Kunz M, Mylius V, Scharmann S, Schepelman K, Lautenbacher S. Influence of dementia on multiple components of pain. Eur J Pain 2009;13:317–25.

39. Kunz M, Scharmann S, Hemmeter U, Schepelmann K, Lautenbacher S. The facial expression of pain in patients with dementia. Pain 2007;133:221–8.

40. Labus JS, Keefe FJ, Jensen MP. Self-reports of pain intensity and direct observations of pain behavior: when are they correlated? Pain 2003;102:109–24.

41. Lautenbacher S. Experimental approaches in the study of pain in the elderly. Pain Med 2012;13(suppl 2):S44–S50.
42. Lautenbacher S, Kunz M, Strate P, Nielsen J, Arendt-Nielsen L. Age effects on pain thresholds, temporal summation and spatial summation of heat and pressure pain. Pain 2005;115:410–8.
43. Lints-Martindale AC, Hadjistavropoulos T, Lix LM, Thorpe L. A comparative investigation of observational pain assessment tools for older adults with dementia. Clin J Pain 2012;28:226–37.
44. Littlewort GC, Bartlett MS, Lee K. Faces of pain: automated measurement of spontaneousall facial expressions of genuine and posed pain. Proceedings of the 9th International Conference on Multimodal Interfaces (ICMI). Nagoya, Aichi, Japan: ACM; 2007. pp. 15–21.
45. Lucey P, Cohn J, Lucey S, Matthews I, Sridharan S, Prkachin KM. Automatically detecting pain using facial actions. IEEE Trans Syst Man Cybern B Cybern 2011;41:664–74.
46. Lukas A, Barber JB, Johnson P, Gibson SJ. Observer-rated pain assessment instruments improve both the detection of pain and the evaluation of pain intensity in people with dementia. Eur J Pain 2013;17:1558–68.
47. Lukas A, Niederecker T, Günther I, Mayer B, Nikolaus T. Self-and proxy report for the assessment of pain in patients with and without cognitive impairment. Z Gerontol Geriatr 2013;46:214–21.
48. Perneczky R, Wagenpfeil S, Komossa K, Grimmer T, Diehl J, Kurz A. Mapping scores onto stages: mini-mental state examination and clinical dementia rating. Am J Geriatr Psychiatry 2006;14:139–44.
49. Plooij B, Swaab D, Scherder E. Autonomic responses to pain in aging and dementia. Rev Neurosci 2011;22:583–9.
50. Rabins PV, Kasper JD, Kleinman L, Black BS, Patrick D. Concepts and methods in the development of the ADRQL: an instrument for assessing health-related quality of life in persons with Alzheimer's disease. J Ment Health Aging 1999;5:33–48.
51. Riley JL, Cruz-Almeida Y, Glover TL, King CD, Goodin BR, Sibille KT, Bartley EJ, Herbert MS, Sotolongo A, Fessler BJ, et al. Age and race effects on pain sensitivity and modulation among middle-aged and older adults. J Pain 2013;15:272–82.
52. Royal College of Physicians, British Geriatrics Society and British Pain Society. The assessment of pain in older people: National guidelines. London: Royal College of Physicians; 2007.
53. Scherder EJ, Bouma A. Visual analogue scales for pain assessment in Alzheimer's disease. Gerontology 2000;46:47–53.

54. Snow AL, Weber JB, O'Malley KJ, Cody M, Beck C, Bruera E, Ashton C, Kunik ME. NOPPAIN: a nursing assistant-administered pain assessment instrument for use in dementia. Dement Geriatr Cogn Disord 2004;17:240–6.

55. Warden V, Hurley AC, Volicer L. Development and psychometric evaluation of the Pain Assessment in Advanced Dementia (PAINAD) scale. J Am Med Dir Assoc 2003;4:9–15.

56. Wary B, Doloplus C. DOLOPLUS 2, une échelle pour évaluer la douleur. Soins Gerontol 1999;19:25–7.

57. Wary B, Serbouti S, Doloplus C. Validation d'une échelle d'évaluation comportementale de la douleur chez la personne âgée. Douleurs 2001;2:35–8.

58. Weiner D, Peterson B, Ladd K, McConnell E, Keefe F. Pain in nursing home residents: an exploration of prevalence, staff perspectives, and practical aspects of measurement. Clin J Pain 1999;15:92–101.

59. Yamamoto M, Kachi T, Igata A. Pain-related somatosensory evoked potentials in dementia. J Neurol Sci 1996;137:117–9.

60. Zwakhalen SMG, Hamers JPH, Abu-Saad H, Berger MPF. Pain in elderly people with severe dementia: a systematic review of behavioural pain assessment tools. BMC Geriatr 2006;6:3–3.

61. Zwakhalen SMG, Hamers JPH, Berger MPF. The psychometric quality and clinical usefulness of three pain assessment tools for elderly people with dementia. Pain 2006;126:210–20.

CHAPTER 13

Out of Sight but Not Out of Mind: The Role of Vision in Pain Perception

Vanessa Harrar, Sophie Vandenbroucke, Hocine Slimani, Maurice Ptito, and Ron Kupers

When we are first taught about the senses, we learn that they function independently and that eyes are for vision, ears are for hearing, and skin is for touch. However, the senses do not work independently. A growing body of research has demonstrated that our perception of the world is multisensory and that information from individual senses is most often combined before reaching awareness. A classic audiovisual illusion occurs when a ventriloquist speaks without lip movements while moving a puppet's mouth vigorously, which causes the illusion that the sound comes from the puppet's mouth [1]. In this chapter, we will investigate how vision can affect our sense of touch and pain, and more specifically, how viewing the body affects the perception of painful tactile or thermal stimuli.

Even though audiovisual and audio–tactile integration have been well investigated, the interactions between vision and pain have received comparatively little attention. The first experimental evidence that vision may affect pain processing came from the pioneering studies by Zubek and colleagues [51] in the early 1960s, and we had to wait until recently for a real breakthrough in the interest in the role of vision in pain perception. In recent years, a number of well-controlled laboratory studies were published on the effects of visual information on thermal pain perception and on the role of visual input in pain empathy and vicarious responses to pain. At the same time, studies assessed the effect of manipulating visual input to treat some forms of clinical pain.

PAIN FRAMEWORK AND PATHWAYS

According to a crude but still vivid biomedical model, pain is a direct representation of noxious sensorial input—that is, physiological damage. In this model, a direct and unchangeable relationship exists between the experience of pain and a particular sensory input. However, since the late 20th century, the biomedical model has been replaced by a biopsychosocial one that provides a more thorough explanation for the human pain experience [29]. While pain has specific sensory and perceptual characteristics, the biopsychosocial model claims that there is no absolute congruency between pain and tissue damage [9]; a person may have tissue damage without feeling pain, and pain can occur in the absence of tissue damage [7]. The psychological state of mind also appears to affect pain perception since certain mental health conditions are more prevalent in chronic pain patients compared to the general population [5]. Thus, psychological and social factors, in addition to biological factors, are crucial to fully understand pain [9]. The effects of vision on pain perception are likely mediated by these psychological and social factors. The shift from the biomedical to the biopsychosocial perspective has fostered new research on how vision affects pain perception, and has supported nonmedical alternative treatments to pain relief rooted in these lines of research.

The International Association for the Study of Pain (IASP) defined pain as "an unpleasant sensory and emotional experience associated with actual or potential tissue damage, or described in terms of such damage" ([28], p. 210). Nociceptive stimuli trigger activity in an extensive cortical network, including somatosensory, insular, and cingulate areas, as well as prefrontal and parietal areas, the so-called pain matrix. The pain matrix is traditionally considered as the conglomerate of brain areas whose neural activity is associated with the sensory and affective processing of a nociceptive stimulus that elicits a painful percept [22]. However, recent experiments revealed that non-nociceptive stimuli, provided that they are salient, can elicit cortical responses with a spatial configuration very similar, although not identical, to that of the pain matrix [30], and that the intensity of a painful stimulus is not linearly represented in the pain matrix [4, 15]. The "new" view of the pain matrix suggests that its functional significance is adaptive—the purpose of pain is to elicit action from the organism: fight or flight. Legrain and colleagues [22] suggest that the "pain matrix" is a cortical network with a more basic function of detecting events that threaten the body's integrity, regardless of the sensory channel through which they are conveyed (Fig. 13-1). The pain matrix is viewed as a neural network that includes a combination of detection, orienting attention toward, and reacting to, the occurrence of salient sensory events. The emphasis is no longer on the quality of the sensation elicited by the noxious stimulus but on the *action* prompted by the occurrence of potential threats. This view remains controversial though, as there is recent evidence that γ-band activity in primary somatosensory cortex correlates with subjective pain reports independent of saliency [52].

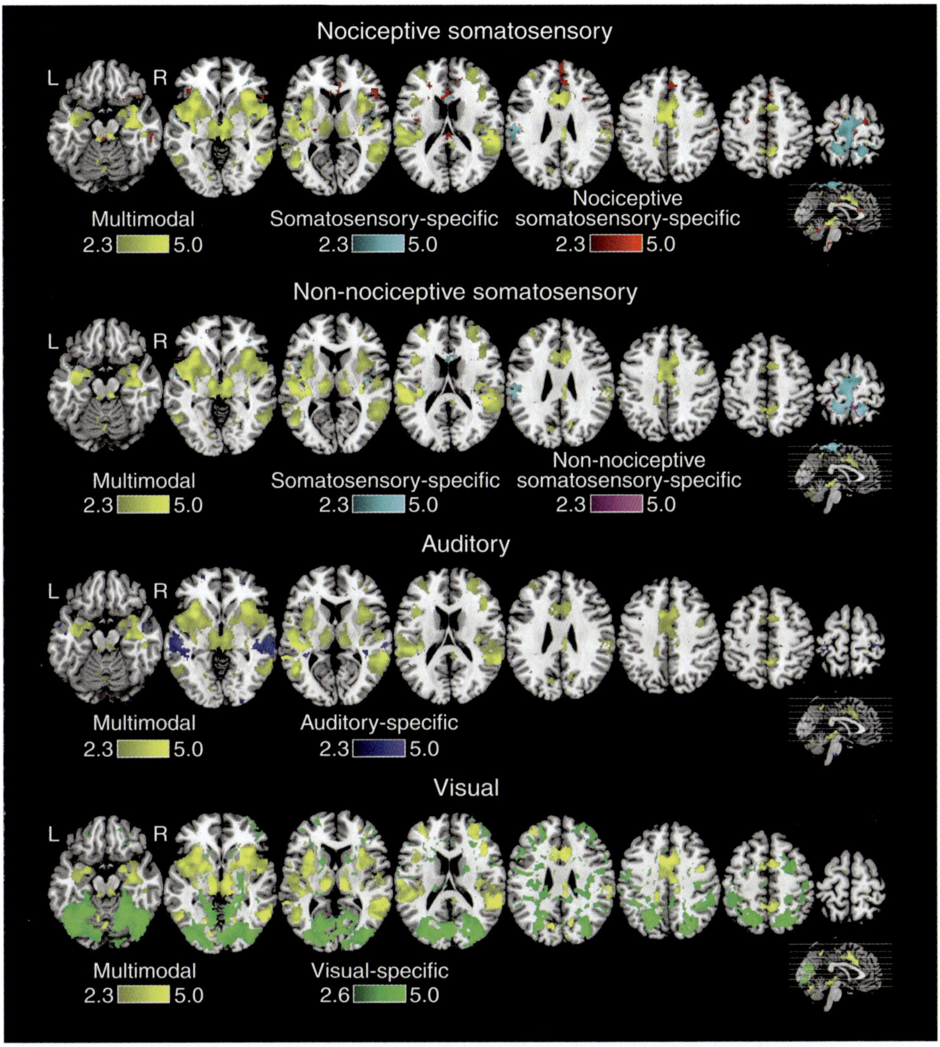

FIGURE 13-1 Modality-specific and multimodal brain responses in response to nociceptive, non-nociceptive somatosensory, auditory, and visual stimulation. Brain areas displaying a significant activation to all four types of sensory stimuli are shown in yellow. Voxels displaying selective activation to nociceptive and non-nociceptive somatosensory stimulation are shown in cyan. Voxels displaying significant activation only to nociceptive somatosensory stimuli are shown in red. Non-nociceptive somatosensory-specific, auditory-specific, and visual-specific voxels are shown in purple, blue, and green, respectively. (Adapted from Mouraux et al. [30] with permission.)

THE ROLE OF VISION IN SOMATOSENSORY PERCEPTION IN SIGHTED INDIVIDUALS

When information is transmitted to the brain through multiple senses, there are significant performance benefits in terms of speed and accuracy [42]. The effects are enhanced when different sensory stimuli are presented in a spatially and temporally congruent manner.

Visual–Tactile Integration

The multisensory benefits of visual–tactile integration have been repeatedly demonstrated. People are more likely to detect a near-threshold tactile stimulus when it is presented concurrently with a visual stimulus, compared to when it is presented alone [19]. Even if the visual stimulus is entirely task-irrelevant, it can enhance the detection of a tactile stimulus. Serino et al. [38] showed enhanced detection of subthreshold tactile stimuli on observers' faces when they saw a face being touched by hands rather than a face being merely approached by hands. Even when the visual stimulus, the forearm, was both uninformative and irrelevant to the task, performance benefited, suggesting that vision is able to focus tactile attention and to modulate somatosensory cortical activity [43].

Visual Information of One's Own Body Modulates Pain

Similar to the effects of vision on touch, pain perception is also modulated by specific visual information. As many of us have probably already experienced, after banging our knee the perception of pain can be minimized or exacerbated, depending on whether the knee looks normal or injured. This anecdotal observation has been confirmed in controlled studies reporting that viewing an undamaged body part can have an analgesic effect [23]. This "visually induced analgesia" suggests an interplay between the brain's pain network and a posterior network for body perception, which modulates the experience of pain. Mancini and colleagues [25] further explored the relationship between pain and body perception by artificially distorting the image of the hand so that it appeared excessively larger or smaller than usual. When participants gazed toward the distorted reflection of their hands while receiving a noxious thermal stimulus, their experience of pain was inversely correlated with the relative size of their hands: enlarging the hand had an analgesic effect, whereas reducing its size resulted in increased pain ratings [25]. Interestingly, the analgesic effect of vision is strongly linked to embodiment; the magnitude of the effect is positively correlated with the belief that the hand is one's own [25].

Neural networks involved in body image overlap considerably with the pain matrix, making these regions (especially the posterior parietal and somatosensory cortices) possible candidates for involvement in visual analgesia [24]. Neuroimaging studies have shown that extensive areas of the posterior parietal and inferotemporal cortices are involved in body representation, including the extrastriate body area, the fusiform body area, and have revealed a topographic map of viewed body parts throughout the visual cortex [6, 31, 33]. Interestingly, Longo et al. [24] reported that activity within parts of the pain matrix, like the primary somatosensory and the operculoinsular cortices, show reduced activity to a noxious heat stimulus when viewing the body compared to viewing an object. These authors further reported an increased functional coupling between the posterior parietal nodes of the visual body network and areas of the cortical pain network during viewing of the stimulated hand, compared to viewing an object. This finding suggests that multisensory interactions involving the perception of one's own body underlie visual analgesia [12]. However, the perception of one's own body is not directly linked to visual analgesic effects because opposite effects are reported when we view other people's bodies in pain. Reports of vicarious pain demonstrate a relationship between observed and experienced pain [2, 48].

Visual analgesia may seem somewhat paradoxical as one would rather expect that directed attention would lead to enhanced pain responses [34]. Indeed, not all studies have replicated the visual analgesic effect. In fact, Valentini and colleagues [47] found no analgesic effect when seeing the hand in a normal position. Instead, these authors reported that viewing the hand in a crossed position had an analgesic effect compared to viewing the hand in its hemispace, or viewing an object placed in the contralateral space, suggesting that proprioceptive information can modulate pain perception. Another recent study also failed to replicate the visual analgesic effect [44]. These authors compared the effects of direct versus mirror vision of the stimulated hand or an object on nociceptive and non-nociceptive stimuli, while measuring event-related potentials (ERPs). Results showed that looking at the hand compared to an object did not modulate the subjective pain perception; however, it reduced the magnitude of the nociceptive N240 wave, and enhanced the magnitude of the non-nociceptive P200. The results of these two recent studies question both the robustness and the ubiquity of visual analgesia. Skin color can also affect pain responses. Inflamed or injured skin tends to be red, whereas a more bluish skin color is typically associated with cold skin. When painful thermal stimuli are applied to a red patch of skin on an embodied virtual arm, participants have lower thresholds for pain compared to when the embodied arm is blue [26]. An increased pain perception is also observed when a painful stimulus is felt at the same time as viewing a hand being pricked with a needle, compared to viewing a hand poked with a Q-tip [13]. Unlike the visual analgesic effect, this increased pain response is associated with reduced α-band activity in the posterior cingulate cortex and fusiform gyrus [14].

Visual Information of Someone Else' Body Modulates Visual-Nociceptive Integration

Seeing another person in pain makes people more sensitive to pain [17], whereas observing a stoic person's lack of response to pain can inhibit the experience of pain in the observer [46]. Several factors, in particular empathy, facilitate or interfere with somatosensation as a result of observing someone in pain. Empathy is generally defined as the capacity to understand and respond to the unique affective experiences of another person [11]. Although empathy for a co-fellow's pain and pain in one's own body are perceived differently, they are represented very similarly in the brain [17, 39].

Associative learning plays an important role in explaining whether a stimulus is perceived as painful or not. During our lives, we learn to associate the visual images of our wounds with pain. Thus, through classical conditioning, seeing injuries (such as others bleeding) may induce the conditioned autonomic response to pain. The conditioned response to painful images, such as images of people in pain, can then modulate one's own pain perception [36]. The association has been demonstrated through a conditioning paradigm in the laboratory study conducted by Wunsch and colleagues [50]. They found that painful and nonpainful thermal stimuli were perceived as more intense and more unpleasant when they were immediately preceded by one of the conditioned aversive stimuli (e.g., an image of a mutilated body), compared to the same tactile stimulation preceded by one of the images that were used in the neutral or positive conditioning sequences.

Vicarious Pain or "I Feel Your Pain"

Vicarious somatosensory experiences occur when one has a sensation of pain, or more often a "tingling," without being touched at all, after observing another in pain. In contrast to empathic pain, where a tactile stimulus is perceived as more unpleasant when empathy is activated, vicarious pain is a tactile or nociceptive sensation without any direct input to the skin. Vicarious pain sensations have been reported both in patients and in healthy control populations.

Vicarious pain intense enough to be problematic has only been reported in patients with a history of intense, traumatic pain [2]. Since phantom pain is often triggered by thinking about, observing, or inferring that another person is in pain, it is often categorized as a vicarious pain [10]. Thus, the population with the highest number of vicarious pain reports are amputees with phantom pain [10]. Indeed, memories from painful experiences appear to play a role in determining where on the body the vicarious pain is felt [18].

Normal individuals without a history of trauma also sometimes report sensations simply from observing others in pain, without any stimulation to the skin [48].

Vicarious "pain" is fairly weak and low in intensity, and does not resemble the pain that is actually felt. Roughly 30% of a normal population will report low-intensity vicarious sensations, labeled as "tingling," from looking at images and video clips depicting painful events [32]. When looking at painful scenes, vicarious pain responders have stronger activation of emotional (insular cortex) and sensory (i.e., secondary somatosensory cortex) brain regions associated with pain, compared to people who do not report such sensations [32].

Fitzgibbon and colleagues [8] proposed that vicarious sensations are caused by a dysfunctional mirror neuron system that causes the perceptual state to exceed threshold, leading to consciously experienced sensations. They further speculate that the painful and/or traumatic history of amputees may be the catalyst for the disinhibition of the mirror system for pain and touch.

PAIN PERCEPTION IN THE ABSENCE OF VISION

After reviewing the now extensive evidence demonstrating that visual information influences pain perception, the question then becomes how does blindness, either from birth or acquired later in life, affect pain processing? It has been well documented that the loss of one sense is sometimes compensated by improved development in the remaining senses. Numerous studies have shown that congenitally blind individuals demonstrate compensatory plasticity for their lack of vision with more efficient auditory, tactile, and even olfactory senses (see reference [21] for a recent review). Even after only 1 week of complete visual deprivation, induced with blindfolding, otherwise normal people increase their tactile and thermal acuity [51]. This blindfolding also caused a drop in heat pain thresholds, indicating that a lack of vision may induce hypersensitivity to pain. Vision, when present, can signal potential threats to the body, for example, a red-hot stove. In the absence of this warning function, blind individuals might instead adopt a chronic state of hypervigilance as a way to avoid tissue injury.

In our pioneering study of pain and temperature perception in congenital blindness, we demonstrated that blind subjects had significantly lower heat pain and cold pain thresholds than matched controls [41]. Further, while congenitally blind people did not differ from matched controls in terms of their ability to detect innocuous warmth and cold, they rated suprathreshold heat stimuli as significantly more painful than their sighted counterparts. Results of pain questionnaires further revealed that blind subjects were more anxious about pain (Fig. 13-2). These findings were replicated in a cohort of blind and sighted control subjects from another ethnic background [41]. We demonstrated that hypersensitivity to pain is not culturally based, and is specific to noxious thermal stimulation, rather than to thermal stimulation in general. Taken together with findings of augmented responses to threatening

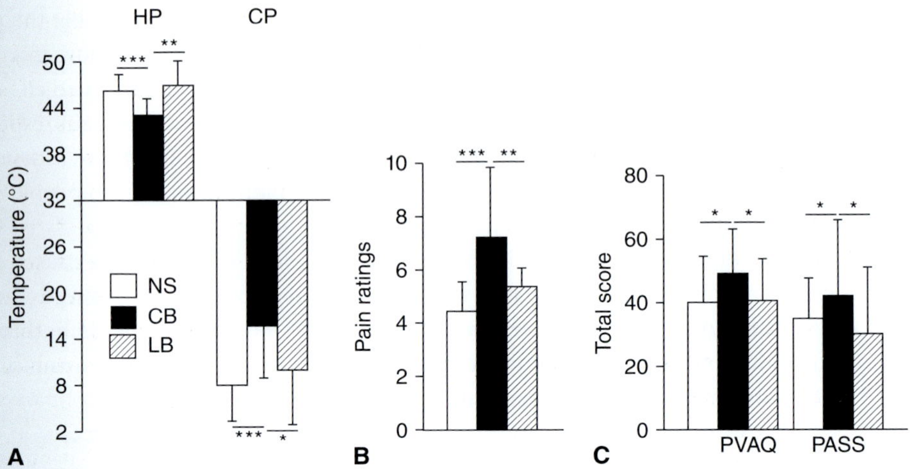

FIGURE 13-2 Pain sensitivity in normally sighted (NS), late blind (LB), and congenitally blind (CB) subjects. **A:** CB have lower heat pain (HP) and cold pain (CP) thresholds compared to NS and LB. **B:** CB rate suprathreshold nociceptive stimuli as more painful than NS and LB. **C:** Unlike NS and LB, CB score higher on the Pain Vigilance and Awareness Questionnaire (PVAQ) and the Pain Anxiety Symptoms Scale (PASS). Error bars represent standard errors. $*P < 0.05$, $**P < 0.01$, $***P < 0.001$. (Adapted from Slimani et al. [40] with permission.)

auditory stimuli in blind subjects [20], these data provided compelling evidence that congenitally blind individuals are more attentive to signals of external threats.

In order to determine if the hypersensitivity to threatening stimuli arises from a compensatory neural plasticity that is rooted in the critical period of development, we compared the pain sensitivity in early and late blind people. In fact, data from late blind subjects was very similarly to that of sighted individuals, including both responses to painful heat stimuli, and questionnaires assessing awareness and anxiety toward pain [40]. This suggests that visual deprivation per se does not determine the development of pain hypersensitivity—the time at which the visual system is deprived is equally important.

In a third study, we tried to disentangle the individual roles of Aδ- and C-fiber activation in the pain hypersensitivity of congenitally blind people. Due to the difference in conduction velocity of the Aδ- and C-fiber sets, pain is often referred to as a double-alarm system, in which the first and second alarms are mediated by the fast-conducting Aδ-fibers and the slow-conducting C-fibers, respectively [35]. Consequently, reaction times to ultrafast, highly synchronized nociceptive radiant heat are distributed in a bimodal manner, whereby the first part of the distribution represents responses to Aδ-fiber activation, and the second part is caused by responses to the slower-conducting C-fibers [3]. We therefore measured reaction times to brief nociceptive radiant heat stimuli, applied by a CO_2 laser, thereby taking advantage of the anatomophysiological organization of the nociceptive system. Results showed that congenitally blind participants detected more C-fiber–mediated stimuli and with faster reaction times compared to sighted controls [Slimani, Plaghki, Ptito, & Kupers, 2015, manuscript submitted for publication]. Analysis of the reaction times indicated that the faster response times in the congenitally blind participants were due to a more efficient central processing of C-fiber–mediated sensations.

Two competing hypotheses have been proposed to explain pain hypersensitivity, following congenital blindness [40, 41]. According to the first hypothesis, the pain hypersensitivity reflects cross-modal plasticity of brain circuits as a result of a lack of visual input. Thus, due the lack of inhibitory effects of vision on pain perception (c.f. visual analgesia), early visual deprivation rewires the brain circuitry, causing increased sensitivity to nociceptive inputs [23, 24, 51]. According to the second hypothesis, the pain hypersensitivity is the result of a hypervigilance to threatening stimuli in congenitally blind individuals. This more integrative interpretation of the pain hypersensitivity can also account for the observations that congenitally blind individuals show increased responses to auditory threats [20] and are better at identifying body odors with a negative emotional valence [16]. This interpretation is also in line with the view that stimulus salience detection is one of the basic functions of the pain matrix, regardless of the sensory channel through which the stimuli are conveyed. Indeed, as shown in recent brain imaging studies, salient visual and noxious stimuli activate a partly overlapping cortical network [30], supporting the hypothesis that there is an intricate integration of vision and pain processing.

VISION-BASED TREATMENT OF CHRONIC PAIN CONDITIONS

While the causes and underlying mechanisms of pain remain elusive, research reviewed here clarifies that vision plays an important role in signaling, monitoring, exciting, or inhibiting pain signals. Our increased understanding of the integration of vision and pain has been used to reduce pain and improve people's quality of life.

Pioneering but largely anecdotal work has shown that simply seeing unharmed limbs can reduce the feeling of pain in amputated patients with phantom limb pain [37]. In much the same way that viewing the body can reduce acute pain [23], viewing the body can also reduce chronic pain. In the mirror-box setup, amputees view a reflection of their unaffected limb in the anatomical position of their amputated limb. Phantom limb patients perceive their body to be intact and that they have regrown their amputated limb (which is really only a reflection of their healthy limb), and that it is unharmed. Simply seeing an intact unharmed limb in the place of their phantom significantly reduced phantom limb pain, and sometimes even removed it completely after a few hours of visual exposure with the mirror box [37].

Unfortunately, no rigorously controlled studies have been carried out on the effect of mirror therapy in large cohorts of phantom limb patients.

Mirror-box therapy is inexpensive, simple, versatile, and in contrast with medication therapy, devoid of adverse effects. Consequently, clinicians have tried to extend its use to other chronic pain conditions that are hard to treat, including complex regional pain syndrome [27] and lower back pain [49]. As for phantom limb pain, few well-controlled studies have been carried out; a recent critical review concluded that there is no conclusive evidence that mirror box therapy works for complex regional pain syndrome [45]. Even though it is still controversial, using mirrors and visual cues as a way to reduce pain is a minimal risk treatment program. It can be done at home, it is inexpensive, and there are no negative side effects. Keeping in mind that chronic pain keeps people out of the workforce, there is an economic as well as a social benefit to continued research into the effects of vision on pain, and alternative treatments to pain relief that capitalize on the multisensory nature of pain.

CONCLUSION

We have reviewed the evidence for the role of vision in pain perception in sighted and blind individuals. This overview demonstrates that the perception of pain is inextricably linked to vision. Vision of one's own intact body can have an analgesic effect, while vision of another person in pain can increase one's own pain sensitivity; empathy appears to play a role in the latter condition. The loss of vision at an early age induces a hypersensitivity to pain that may have evolved as a way to keep safe in the absence of visual warning signals. Clinical therapies that have capitalised on the relationship between vision and pain include the mirror box for treating phantom pain, but so far there is only anecdotal evidence in support of its effectiveness. It remains to be seen what further clinical therapies for pain management will be developed that exploit the automatic integration of pain and vision.

REFERENCES

1. Alais D, Burr D. The ventriloquist effect results from near-optimal bimodal integration. Curr Biol 2004;14(3):257–62.
2. Bradshaw JL, Mattingley JB. Allodynia: a sensory analogue of motor mirror neurons in a hyperaesthetic patient reporting instantaneous discomfort to another's perceived sudden minor injury? J Neurol Neurosurg Psychiatry 2001;70(1):135–6.
3. Churyukanov M, Plaghki L, Legrain V, Mouraux A. Thermal detection thresholds of Adelta- and C-fibre afferents activated by brief CO_2 laser pulses applied onto the human hairy skin. PLoS One 2012;7(4):e35817.

4. Clark JA, Brown CA, Jones AK, El-Deredy W. Dissociating nociceptive modulation by the duration of pain anticipation from unpredictability in the timing of pain. Clin Neurophysiol 2008;119(12):2870–8.
5. Demyttenaere K, Bruffaerts R, Lee S, Posada-Villa J, Kovess V, Angermeyer MC, Levinson D, de Girolamo G, Nakane H, Mneimneh Z, et al. Mental disorders among persons with chronic back or neck pain: results from the World Mental Health Surveys. Pain 2007;129(3):332–42.
6. Downing PE, Jiang Y, Shuman M, Kanwisher N. A cortical area selective for visual processing of the human body. Science 2001;293(5539):2470–3.
7. Fernandez E, Turk DC. Sensory and affective components of pain: separation and synthesis. Psychol Bull 1992;112(2):205-217.
8. Fitzgibbon BM, Giummarra MJ, Georgiou-Karistianis N, Enticott PG, Bradshaw JL. Shared pain: from empathy to synaesthesia. Neurosci Biobehav Rev 2010;34(4):500–12.
9. Gatchel RJ, Peng YB, Peters ML, Fuchs PN, Turk DC. The biopsychosocial approach to chronic pain: scientific advances and future directions. Psychol Bull 2007;133(4):581–624.
10. Giummarra MJ, Fitzgibbon BM, Chou M, Gibson SJ, Georgiou-Karistianis N, Bradshaw JL. Synaesthetic phantom sensations in an upper limb amputee. Proceedings of the 12th World Congress on Pain. Glasgow; 2008.
11. Goubert L, Craig KD, Vervoort T, Morley S, Sullivan MJ, de CWAC, Cano A, Crombez G. Facing others in pain: the effects of empathy. Pain 2005;118(3):285–8.
12. Haggard P, Iannetti GD, Longo MR. Spatial sensory organization and body representation in pain perception. Curr Biol 2013;23(4):R164–R176.
13. Höfle M, Hauck M, Engel AK, Senkowski D. Viewing a needle pricking a hand that you perceive as yours enhances unpleasantness of pain. Pain 2012;153(5):1074–81.
14. Höfle M, Pomper U, Hauck M, Engel AK, Senkowski D. Spectral signatures of viewing a needle approaching one's body when anticipating pain. Eur J Neurosci 2013;38(7):3089–98.
15. Iannetti GD, Hughes NP, Lee MC, Mouraux A. Determinants of laser-evoked EEG responses: pain perception or stimulus saliency? J Neurophysiol 2008;100(2):815–28.
16. Iversen KD, Ptito M, Moller P, Kupers R. Enhanced chemosensory detection of negative emotions in congenital blindness. Neural Plast 2015;2015:469750.
17. Jackson PL, Meltzoff AN, Decety J. How do we perceive the pain of others? A window into the neural processes involved in empathy. Neuroimage 2005;24(3):771–9.
18. Ji RR, Kohno T, Moore KA, Woolf CJ. Central sensitization and LTP: do pain and memory share similar mechanisms? Trends Neurosci 2003;26(12):696–705.

19. Johnson RM, Burton PC, Ro T. Visually induced feelings of touch. Brain Res 2006;1073–1074:398–406.

20. Klinge C, Roder B, Buchel C. Increased amygdala activation to emotional auditory stimuli in the blind. Brain 2010;133(Pt 6):1729–36.

21. Kupers R, Ptito M. Compensatory plasticity and cross-modal reorganization following early visual deprivation. Neurosci Biobehav Rev 2014;41:36–52.

22. Legrain V, Iannetti GD, Plaghki L, Mouraux A. The pain matrix reloaded: a salience detection system for the body. Prog Neurobiol 2011;93(1):111–24.

23. Longo MR, Betti V, Aglioti SM, Haggard P. Visually induced analgesia: seeing the body reduces pain. J Neurosci 2009;29(39):12125–30.

24. Longo MR, Iannetti GD, Mancini F, Driver J, Haggard P. Linking pain and the body: neural correlates of visually induced analgesia. J Neurosci 2012;32(8):2601–7.

25. Mancini F, Longo MR, Kammers MP, Haggard P. Visual distortion of body size modulates pain perception. Psychol Sci 2011;22(3):325–30.

26. Martini M, Perez-Marcos D, Sanchez-Vives MV. What color is my arm? Changes in skin color of an embodied virtual arm modulates pain threshold. Front Hum Neurosci 2013;7:438.

27. McCabe CS, Haigh RC, Ring EF, Halligan PW, Wall PD, Blake DR. A controlled pilot study of the utility of mirror visual feedback in the treatment of complex regional pain syndrome (type 1). Rheumatology 2003;42(1):97–101.

28. Mersky H, Bodguk N. Task force on taxonomy of the international association for the study of pain: classification of chronic pain, description of chronic pain syndromes and definition of pain terms. Seattle, WA: IASP Press; 1994.

29. Morley S, Vlaeyen JW. 50 years on, Henry Beecher's "measurement of subjective responses." Pain 2010;150(2):211–2.

30. Mouraux A, Diukova A, Lee MC, Wise RG, Iannetti GD. A multisensory investigation of the functional significance of the "pain matrix." Neuroimage 2011;54(3):2237–49.

31. Orlov T, Makin TR, Zohary E. Topographic representation of the human body in the occipitotemporal cortex. Neuron 2010;68(3):586–600.

32. Osborn J, Derbyshire SW. Pain sensation evoked by observing injury in others. Pain 2010;148(2):268–74.

33. Peelen MV, Downing PE. Selectivity for the human body in the fusiform gyrus. J Neurophysiol 2005;93(1):603–8.

34. Peyron R, Garcia-Larrea L, Gregoire MC, Costes N, Convers P, Lavenne F, Mauguiere F, Michel D, Laurent B. Haemodynamic brain responses to acute pain in humans: sensory and attentional networks. Brain 1999;122 (Pt 9):1765–80.

35. Plaghki L, Decruynaere C, Van Dooren P, Le Bars D. The fine tuning of pain thresholds: a sophisticated double alarm system. PLoS One 2010;5(4):e10269.

36. Rainville P, Bao QV, Chretien P. Pain-related emotions modulate experimental pain perception and autonomic responses. Pain 2005;118(3):306–18.

37. Ramachandran VS, Hirstein W. The perception of phantom limbs. The D. O. Hebb lecture. Brain 1998;121 (Pt 9):1603–30.

38. Serino A, Pizzoferrato F, Làdavas E. Viewing a face (especially one's own face) being touched enhances tactile perception on the face. Psychol Sci 2008;19(5):434–8.

39. Singer T, Seymour B, O'Doherty J, Kaube H, Dolan RJ, Frith CD. Empathy for pain involves the affective but not sensory components of pain. Science 2004;303(5661):1157–62.

40. Slimani H, Danti S, Ptito M, Kupers R. Pain perception is increased in congenital but not late onset blindness. PLoS One 2014;9(9):e107281.

41. Slimani H, Danti S, Ricciardi E, Pietrini P, Ptito M, Kupers R. Hypersensitivity to pain in congenital blindness. Pain 2013;154(10):1973–8.

42. Stein BE, London N, Wilkinson LK, Price DD. Enhancement of perceived visual intensity by auditory stimuli: a psychophysical analysis. J Cogn Neurosci 1996;8(6):497–506.

43. Taylor-Clarke M, Kennett S, Haggard P. Vision modulates somatosensory cortical processing. Curr Biol 2002;12(3):233–6.

44. Torta DM, Legrain V, Mouraux A. Looking at the hand modulates the brain responses to nociceptive and non-nociceptive somatosensory stimuli but does not necessarily modulate their perception. Psychophysiology 2015;52(8):1010–8.

45. Torta DM, Legrain V, Rossetti Y, Mouraux A. Prisms for pain. Can visuo-motor rehabilitation strategies alleviate chronic pain? Eur J Pain 2015; Epub Jun 11. doi: 10.1002/ejp.723.

46. Turkat ID, Guise BJ, Carter KM. The effects of vicarious experience on pain termination and work avoidance: a replication. Behav Res Ther 1983;21(5):491–3.

47. Valentini E, Koch K, Aglioti SM. Seeing one's own painful hand positioned in the contralateral space reduces subjective reports of pain and modulates laser evoked potentials. J Pain 2015;16(6):499–507.

48. Vandenbroucke S, Crombez G, Loeys T, Goubert L. Observing another in pain facilitates vicarious experiences and modulates somatosensory experiences. Front Hum Neurosci 2014;8:631.

49. Wand BM, Tulloch VM, George PJ, Smith AJ, Goucke R, O'Connell NE, Moseley GL. Seeing it helps: movement-related back pain is reduced by visualization of the back during movement. Clin J Pain 2012;28(7):602–8.

50. Wunsch A, Philippot P, Plaghki L. Affective associative learning modifies the sensory perception of nociceptive stimuli without participant's awareness. Pain 2003;102(1–2):27–38.

51. Zubek JP, Flye J, Aftanas M. Cutaneous sensitivity after prolonged visual deprivation. Science 1964;144(3626):1591–3.

52. Zhang ZG, Hu L, Hung YS, Mouraux A, Iannetti GD. Gamma-band oscillations in the primary somatosensory cortex—a direct and obligatory correlate of subjective pain intensity. J Neurosci 2012;32:7429–38.

SECTION 4

Behind and Beyond the Consciousness of Pain

CHAPTER 14

Attention, Emotions, and Pain

Luis Garcia-Larrea and Philip L. Jackson

Pain is recognized as a complex experience composed of multiple interacting components, of which both cognitive and motivational dimensions are acknowledged as essential elements. These dimensions contribute to the contextual modulations of pain and to making this experience conscious. Common knowledge is that identical noxious stimuli can elicit very diverse subjective impressions as a function of the attention devoted to them, or the emotional state in which the subject is feeling them. Such perceptual modulations are not trivial; they can transform the sensation from clearly unpleasant to barely noticeable and from slightly painful to almost unbearable. In this chapter, we summarize research that focuses on the attentional and emotional modulation of pain percepts, their associated brain responses, and their interaction.

ATTENTION TO PAIN

Attention: Matricial versus Vectorial Components

The attentional capacities of the human brain are multifaceted and terms such as "alertness," "awareness," "vigilance," or "selective attention" are commonly used to describe particular aspects of this conceptual construct. An intuitive dichotomy separates a *basic attentional state,* which allows becoming aware of the external world and processing sensory events, from a *selective attention* capacity that privileges certain information and filters out other. Marcel Mesulam [59] proposed the notions of "matricial" and "vectorial" components to distinguish these two aspects. The "matrix" function relates to concepts such as arousal, alertness, and vigilance level, and regulates overall processing capacity, focusing power, and resistance to interference. The "vector" or channel function, on the other hand, regulates the *direction* and target of attention in relevant behavioral spaces—bodily, extrapersonal, mnemonic, semantic, etc. The overall attention capacities at any moment are a composite of these two aspects. Other chapters in this book analyze pain in relation with the matricial facets of attention, such as sleep, coma, and other altered states of consciousness; here we will mainly focus on the directional ("vectorial") aspects of attention.

"Top-Down" Attentional Modulation: From Common Sense to Physiology

It has been known for millenaries that directing attention toward or away from a noxious stimulus can profoundly modify pain sensation.* Formalization and quantification of this effect, however, were not available until psychophysical techniques allowed precise control of both the sensory input and stimulus-response functions [56, 61]. These studies confirmed that focusing attention on noxious stimuli made them be perceived as more intense *and* more unpleasant than directing attention elsewhere. Moreover, when confronted to several concurrent sensory stimuli, subjects tended to direct their attention preferentially toward those that are painful [61]. Thus, unless an individual actively directs his attention away from a painful stimulus, that stimulus will dominate over other nonpainful ones—a phenomenon often observed in the clinics.

In parallel, several groups were investigating the cerebral events underlying these behavioral effects, both regarding pain and general somatosensory perception. In the early 1980s, it was shown that actively attending to a somatic stimulus (electric shock) entailed a significant enhancement of brain responses to this stimulus, relative to those in response to nonattended identical shocks [19]. The centroparietal topography and early latency (30–40 ms) of this effect suggested that it was generated within the primary somatosensory cortex (S1), reflecting increased "sensory gain" of attended stimuli before they could reach conscious analysis ([26], Fig. 14-1). Attentional effects at longer latencies yielded a more complex picture, combining activity changes in S1, S2 posterior parietal, and cingulate cortices, but most of them at latencies preceding, rather than following conscious stimulus detection [27].

Early nociceptive responses (triggered by laser pulses) were also enhanced when stimuli were selectively attended, and depressed when the subject was distracted from the pain [29, 47]. In the case of pain, the earliest attentional changes concerned responses from the operculoinsular cortex [47, 84], in accordance with the predominant projections of spinothalamic afferents to this region [21]. Positron-emission tomography (PET), and functional magnetic resonance imaging (fMRI) confirmed the enhanced activation of operculoinsular cortex during deliberate attention toward a

---

* Marcus Aurelius (160 CE): "the pain is not due to the thing itself but to your own estimate of it; and this you have the power to revoke at any moment" (*Meditations.* Book VIII).

Top-down attentional effects:
Spatial attention changes early activity in sensory (S1–S2) networks

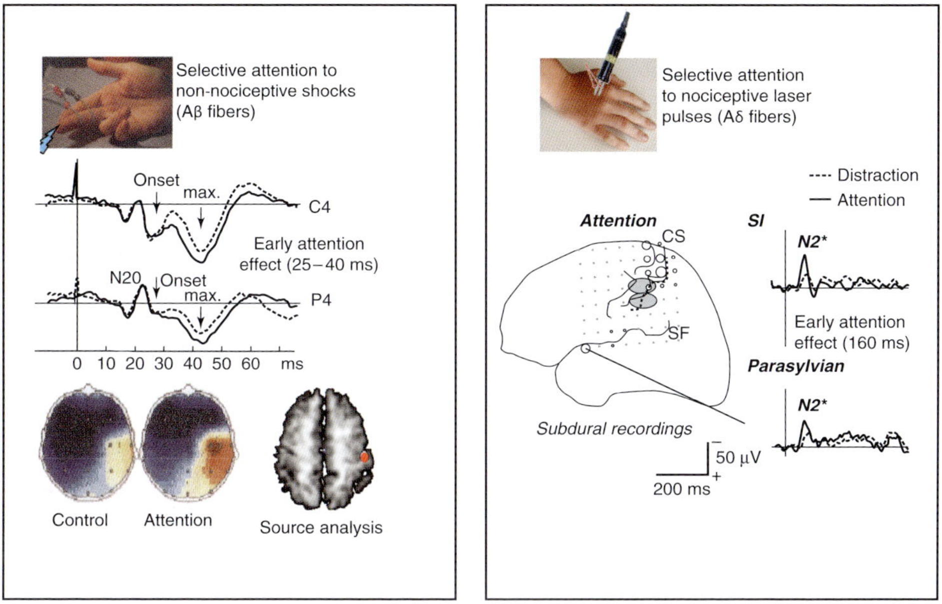

FIGURE 14-1 Attention effects on early somatosensory responses in humans. **Left panel:** Attention spatially directed toward one hand enhances early somatosensory responses to all stimuli addressed to this same hand. The attention effect involves sensory networks in areas BA1-2 of S1, in the crown of the postcentral gyrus, at 25–50 ms poststimulus. **Right panel:** Selective attention to the hand stimulated by nociceptive inputs (delivered via a laser beam) also enhances the earliest sensory responses from S1 and S2, recorded from subdural electrodes. Note that the earliest somatosensory responses to non-noxious (Aβ) input arises exclusively from S1 **(left panel)**, while in case of nociceptive Aδ-spinothalamic input **(right panel)** sensory responses are simultaneous in S1 and the opercular (parasylvian) cortex, including S2. (Data from Garcia-Larrea et al. [26] and Ohara et al. [64], reproduced with permission.)

painful stimulus [1, 68]. Attentional changes in S1 responses were small and not precisely described until some years later, probably due to the small contribution of S1 to specific noxious processing; such changes were shown using intracranial subdural recordings [64] and then PET [43]. Consistent with the parallel processing of spinothalamic inputs in several sensory areas, attentional changes in S1 and opercular-insular cortex responses had a very simultaneous timing ([64], and see Fig. 14-1).

Attention-related changes in the processing of noxious stimuli are not restricted to sensory cortices: associative, multimodal, and supramodal regions also change their activity patterns under conditions in which attention is modulated. In 1999, Peyron et al. [68] used PET to show that selective attention to pain stimuli entailed changes in a widely distributed cortico-subcortical network, including thalamus and sensory areas, but also the anterior cingulate (ACC), posterior parietal (PPC), and dorsal prefrontal (DLPFC) cortices (Fig. 14-2). Distraction from pain was shown to reduce the activity of these areas, in correlation with a decrease in subjective pain reports, but distraction also showed enhanced responses in regions involved in descending pain control, in particular the perigenual cingulate (pgACC), orbitofrontal cortex (OFC), and periaqueductal gray (PAG) matter [91, 96]. By the turn of the century it had become clear that (i) attended and unattended noxious stimuli were processed differently in sensory areas, (ii) that this occurred *before* the generation of a perceptual representation of the stimulus, and (iii) that these early effects triggered subsequent changes in higher-order areas subserving conscious perception. Since the decision to attend is deliberate, such mechanisms are defined as "top-down," whereby an a priori resolution to direct attention, triggered by high-order networks, influences lower-level sensory responsiveness and amplify sensory transmission. The enhanced output from sensory cortices influences in turn associative and multimodal evaluative networks, hence modulating the perception of the painful event. The use of attention/distraction procedures to control pain is being increasingly adapted to clinical settings, in particular with the advent of virtual reality procedures [33].†

A Paradoxical Analgesic Effect of Sustained Attention?

While attending to a noxious stimulus most often tends to enhance pain sensations, it can also, under certain circumstances, *minimize* pain-related perceptions. This most often relates to the unpleasantness of the pain stimulus (i.e., the pain-related "suffering"), rather than the perception of its intensity. For instance, the emotional distress reported during the cold pressor test (immersing the hand in ice-cold water) decreased when subjects attended deliberately to their bodily sensations throughout the test [50, 56], and this was found to be more effective to alleviate pain than distraction procedures [41]. These surprising effects, demonstrated more than 20 years ago, may be relevant to understand a number of recent coping strategies and therapies for chronic pain, which are based more on analysis and acceptance of pain characteristics than on simple distraction from them [57]. For instance, recent research is putting much emphasis on "meditation-like" techniques of pain control that are not based on distraction, but rather on deliberate focusing on the moment-to-moment characteristics of bodily events (see Chapter 8). Functional imaging techniques in subjects receiving painful stimuli while practicing such techniques have provided novel and

† A particular situation that remains hardly understood concerns the effect of observation of the body part being stimulated, which has been reported to enhance sensations [40, 60], or decrease pain [53], or still have differential effects depending on the position of the observed region [93]. Differences might be rooted on the distractive or attractive effects of visual focusing, but controlled studies contrasting different experimental settings are still lacking.

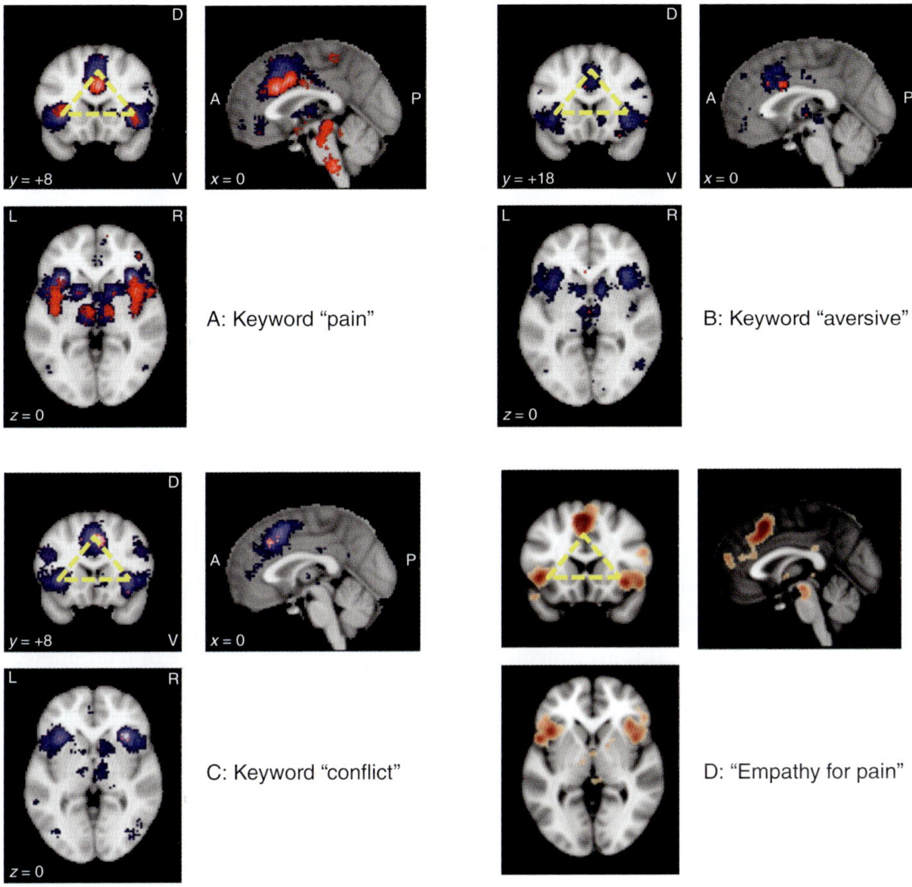

FIGURE 14-2 Joint activations of the dorsal part of the anterior cingulate cortex (ACC) and the anterior part of the insula cortex (AI), known to be multimodal hubs receiving input from sensory and limbic systems, have been associated with a number of different processes. **Panel A**: activations for "pain" are quite robust as shown by term-based meta-analyses using Neurosynth (www.neurosynth.org; 420 studies, 20,123 activations, threshold = 5). Note that both forward *(red)* and reverse *(blue)* inference algorithms show the typical "triangle" activation patterns (**top left panel; yellow)**. **Panels B and C**: the ACC-AI "triangle" is found for several other keywords implicating emotional relevance, including "aversive" (192 studies, 6602 activations, threshold = 5) and "conflict" (273 studies, 9092 activations, threshold = 5), and is also observed during "empathy for pain"/vicarious pain paradigms (**Panel D**: modified from: www.neurovault.org; image 12017; original study by Bzdok et al., Brain Struct Funct 2012). Not surprisingly, these two areas show important functional connectivity (**Panel E**: www.neurosynth.org; resting-state data of 1000 studies; seed placed at 0, 20, 26), supporting the numerous data sets showing that they respond as a functional unit. A, anterior; P, posterior; D, dorsal; V, ventral; L, Left; R, right.

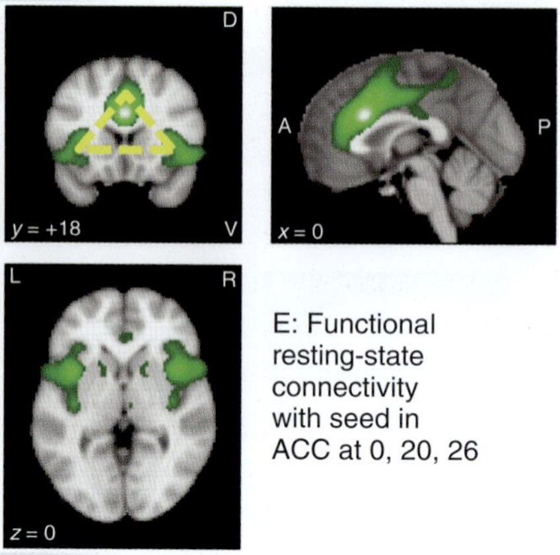

FIGURE 14-2 *(continued)*

intriguing data. Notably, while sensory responses to painful stimuli were enhanced in sensory cortices (S1, S2, posterior insula), as expected from a sustained attention condition, reduced activity was observed in high-order executive, evaluative, and emotion-related areas such as the dorsolateral prefrontal cortex (DLPFC), the amygdala, and the hippocampus, concomitant with a significant decrease in pain unpleasantness [32, 54]. These results indicate that it is possible to develop "peculiar" states of attention to body events which, instead of inducing a joint increase of sensory and evaluative networks (as is common in selective attention) are on the contrary able to *dissociate* them, setting up a state of increased sensory, but decreased executive and affective processing and prompting a reduction in the unpleasantness of the pain experience. Such dissociation is reminding of that observed during altered states of consciousness such as hypnosis ([75], and see Chapter 7), and of the dissociation between sensory and evaluative networks induced by emotional stimuli, discussed below in this chapter.

Anticipation Can Be Analgesic or Hyperalgesic

Anticipation and selective attention are tightly associated, anticipation relating strictly to the period when pain is expected but not yet present. Apart from such phenomenological considerations, the mechanisms involved in attention to, and anticipation of, pain largely overlap, and single unit experiments often found it difficult to disclose whether neural responses were associated with the animal's attention toward or with anticipation of a noxious stimulus [78].

Experiments that selectively manipulate pain anticipation allow assessing brain activity in the absence of actual pain, and hence can dissociate anticipative responses from those involved when a nociceptive stimulus is present. Regions activated during anticipation of pain involve the ACC, anterior insula, and even somatosensory areas, at sites only slightly different from those activated during the processing of actual pain [10, 72]. The electrophysiological concomitants of anticipatory processes (a slow negative potential termed "contingent negative variation") were also found to involve generators in the mid- and rostral ACC, dorsolateral frontal, and sensory cortices [6]. The magnitude of anticipatory responses increases when the anticipated stimulus is of noxious or aversive nature, and prestimulus negativity to noxious stimuli also increases when they are actively anticipated [46].

Networks involved in pain anticipation and pain processing partially overlap: in humans most sensory and cingulate regions activated during pain anticipation were also activated by somatosensory stimulation [73], and in the macaque half of ACC neurons activated during anticipation of a noxious stimulus were also activated in response to the actual stimulus [42]. Also, in close relation with what occurs during selective attention, anticipation of a noxious stimulus enhances activity within primary somatosensory areas, as if "preactivating" them before stimulus occurrence [73, 74].

Anticipation of pain can either exacerbate or decrease the pain experience, the result greatly depending on the predictable/unpredictable nature of the expected pain stimulus, and the control the subject can exert onto it. In rodents, stimuli predicting with certainty a noxious stimulus consistently decrease the pain behaviors (reviewed in reference [70]), and similar effects have been shown in humans, including in clinical settings, where reliable information about the characteristics of the approaching stimuli decreases clinical pain (reviewed in reference [90]). In animal experiments, anticipation-related analgesia has been linked to a "fear response," involving activation of the rostralmost cingulate cortex and upper brain stem structures (PAG) triggering descending pain control. The rostral ACC is indeed recruited in humans during pain anticipation [10, 72] and, in many other contexts, its activation has been shown to correlate *negatively* with perceived pain [67, 73, 74, 96]. Therefore, *certainty and cognitive control* of the anticipated stimulus may trigger analgesic mechanisms through a *common final descending pathway*, which is also activated during other analgesic situations including the "freezing" reaction [24], active distraction [91], placebo analgesia, [66] and even neurostimulation procedures of pain control [67]. The neurochemical mediation of anticipation-related analgesia has been suggested to be opioidergic in the short-term, while non-opioidergic systems may activate after extended exposure [51]. Besides fear-related analgesia, sophisticated processes of cognitive control are certainly also active in humans, in whom interaction between high-order cognition and emotional drives are ever present [63].

In contrast with the above, anticipation of aversive stimuli that are *unpredictable* (i.e., of unknown intensity or aggressiveness) tends to *enhance* the painful experience [70, 71]. Uncertain expectation of a painful stimulus can amplify perceived unpleasantness and brain responses even to *nonpainful* stimuli [83]. This effect has been mostly associated with anticipatory anxiety, which enhances pain ratings and participates to clinical pain chronification. Brain networks activated during the expectation of certain *versus* uncertain pain events may be partly different: uncertain expectancy inducing anxiety has been associated with the ventromedial prefrontal cortex, hippocampal formation, and ventral striatum [34, 38, 70]. Results diverge regarding the *direction* of changes (i.e., activation *vs.* deactivation) in these areas, and it has been suggested that enhanced activity in ventromedial prefrontal cortex appears when uncertainty regards the *type* of upcoming stimulus (e.g., painful or not), whereas activity tends to abate when uncertainty concerns the *intensity* of the expected stimulus [70]. Such conceptual constructions appear, however, somewhat optimistic regarding the capacities of ventromedial prefrontal networks to "calibrate" the characteristics of upcoming stimuli. A simpler explanation suggests that the magnitude of ventromedial frontal activation during anticipation relates to the *intensity* of anticipatory anxiety [81]. This explanation appears more parsimonious, and consistent with the role of ventromedial prefrontal cortex in the control of emotions (see reference [63]). Activity in ventromedial frontal networks during anticipation might therefore reflect a "hard-wired" reaction that restrains the anxiety state.

The Other Way Round: Automatic ("Bottom-Up") Orienting to Pain

Any intruding or behaviorally relevant sensory stimuli can drive attention without any previous deliberate decision from the subject. Such stimulus-driven, automatic mode of attention is known as "ascending" or "bottom-up." It reflects the orienting component of the arousal reaction (c.f. Chapters 1 and 2 in this Volume) and its adaptive value for survival is evident, as failure to orient to crucial stimuli may lead to serious damage or death.

The immediate behavioral relevance of painful stimuli makes them intrinsically attention-capturing. When confronted to several concurrent sensory stimuli, subjects tend to direct attention preferentially toward that of highest intrusiveness [48], and this enhances the subjective perception of intensity and unpleasantness [61]. Importantly, the intruding effects of pain are decreased when the noxious stimuli is delivered while subjects are engaged in a concurrent demanding task [64], which entails decrease in its subjective intensity (an effect known for centuries, and used therapeutically both by folk and academic medicine). It has been argued that enhanced bottom-up orienting, together with failure to modulate noxious perception by cognitive control, may contribute to chronification of pain syndromes such as migraine [15].

Intruding painful stimuli induce rapid shifts of orienting systems involving mid and anterior cingulate (MCC, ACC), partly reflected in positive-polarity waves culminating about 400 ms following nociceptor activation [48]. Functional imaging has suggested that the *specific* regions within the ACC mediating deliberate (top-down) and automatic (bottom-up) attention may not be the same. Peyron et al. [68]

compared the ACC responses during sustained attention to thermal painful stimuli, *versus* those obtained when a distracted subject was occasionally disrupted by unpredictable painful stimuli. The ACC sectors activated during sustained attention corresponded to rostral area BA32, while disrupting painful stimuli activated a more caudal and posterior ACC region (area BA24). Similar results were reported using a different setting by Davis et al. [14] who compared ACC activity while subjects received occasional painful stimuli *versus* a sustained attention task of word generation. Again, the ACC loci activation were confined to BA24 in response to (intruding) painful stimuli, but more rostral and superior (BA32) during the sustained attentional task, underscoring the functional bias of posterior sections of the ACC (BA24 and MCC) as systems mediating bottom-up orienting reactions.

Back to Real Life: Bottom-Up and Top-Down Mechanism Acting Together

While experimental settings may allow to disentangle the system structure underlying top-down and bottom-up mechanisms, real-life conditions most often engage both systems, the resulting experience stemming from their coordinated or opposed activity. Any unexpected pain stimuli will drive automatically attention to the body region affected (bottom-up), but this will also induce a top-down reaction of deliberate orienting toward the same region, via frontoparietal descending influences that will increase the sensory gain of primary areas and possibly also the thalamus [39], hence promoting arousal and anticipation toward potential new stimuli. The corollary is that in real situations bottom-up and top-down systems continuously interact, and that the resulting perception can only be predicted by adequately combining the joint contribution of ascending and descending systems. The fact that different modes of anticipation and sustained attention can lead to dissimilar, sometimes opposite experiential consequences explains why attention-based pain modulations are so difficult to reproduce consistently in the clinics. Notwithstanding such difficulties, attention/distraction procedures to control pain have proved useful in different clinical settings, in particular with the recent advent of virtual reality techniques [33].

EMOTION AND SOCIAL CONTEXT INFLUENCES ON PAIN

Reviewing the growing literature on emotion and the experience of pain quickly underlines the intricacy of pain as a conscious experience. Not only can emotions triggered through different modalities lead to hyper- or hypoalgesia, but the emotional component of pain can also interact with the full range of attentional processes discussed earlier. Pain and emotion interaction at the experiential level is underpinned by interaction also at the cerebral level, as they share similar brain networks. The neural regions and networks specialized in the processing of emotional stimuli include notably the limbic and reward systems, which are also involved in cognitive-driven learning and conditioning. Although the joint contributions of these systems are often congruent, varying levels of attention and affect during pain may lead to opposing interactions and unexpected experiences.

As for pain, different brain networks with distinct functional roles tap into many of the same regions [28]. The motivational/affective/reappraisal component involving orbitofrontal, pgACC, and anterolateral prefrontal cortices is the most likely to interact with the limbic and the reward systems. Pinpointing how emotions can affect pain in different ways is a step toward acknowledging it as an experience that reaches far beyond nociception, and even far beyond immediate perceptions. Proper decoding and management of pain, an intruder in people's consciousness, requires the appreciation of the full extent of this experience.

Similarly to the matricial versus vectorial distinction drawn about attention, affect can be divided into "mood" versus "discrete emotions." Mood is the underlying affective state of an individual that emerges from a multitude of sources of information from past, present, and future events. Mood is related to traits and thus considered more stable, changing within a larger time window than discrete emotions, and typically assessed by subjective self-reported measures. Discrete emotions on the other hand are more rapidly changeable and often triggered by one specific source (although their expression will also be mood-dependent). Discrete emotions are thus more easily addressed in an experimental setting and will be reviewed here. In the clinic, however, consideration to both is warranted in the context of pain.

The relationship between emotions and pain experience is not linear, not always specific, nor absolute. However, patterns emerge from the literature indicating that some types of emotional stimuli tend to increase the level of pain reported by individuals, while others generally decrease it. Most studies showing the effect of emotions on pain have relied on the valence continuum model whereby any emotion can be situated somewhere between positive (appetitive) and negative (aversive) experiences. Pain would be situated on the negative end of this continuum. Thus, receiving stimuli perceived as positive (pleasant) will tend to decrease concomitant pain (hypoalgesia), while stimuli perceived as negative (unpleasant) will increase the level of pain (hyperalgesia). There have been, however, some contradictory findings, and the effects do not seem to be symmetrical, with negative emotions being more consistently effective than positive emotions in modulating pain.

Emotional Stimuli and Acute Pain

A few research groups have investigated the effect of *unpleasant* odors on pain, and generally find an increase in the pain ratings for both intensity and unpleasantness [99, 100], while *pleasant* odors seem to affect more pain unpleasantness than intensity [98, 99]. Increased activity in ACC and insula has been proposed as the cerebral basis of hyperalgesic effects, while the ventral striatum and its descending inhibitory influences via the PAG might play a role in the hypoalgesia effect of pleasant odors [98]. Olfactory stimuli can also modulate spinal nociception (amplitude of the withdrawal reflex) in the predicted direction [2].

In healthy subjects, pleasant music can decrease the reported pain to controlled nociceptive stimuli [80]. The impact of music on pain appears to be modulated both in cerebrum and spinal cord, as suggested by electrophysiological and fMRI evidence that descending pain pathways are modulated by music down to the spinal cord gray matter [20, 79]. On clinical grounds, listening to pleasant music decreased very slightly postoperatory pain [7], and a randomized controlled study on its effects during labor showed reduced pain and anxiety reports, lower needs for postdelivery analgesia, and reduced physiological responses of both mother and baby [87]. A recent meta-analysis showed that, although exerting a positive effect on pain and anxiety levels during endoscopies, listening to music did not reduce the amount of analgesia needed, nor was useful in colpo- or bronchoscopy [102]. Music can therefore have physiological effects reaching beyond the actual subjective experience, but its clinical impact remains limited.

Individual or gender-related differences can crucially influence the effect of emotional input. Rhudy and Meagher [76] exposed participants to loud unpleasant noise bursts prior to receiving a noxious stimulus and found that while women showed the expected fear response, which produced hypoalgesia, men's response was more characteristic of surprise (hence of arousal) and had the effect of *increasing* pain reactivity. Fear is such a salient emotion rooted in the amygdala and other subcortical structures that its effects on pain are likely akin to the gating effect observed for touch, and may predominate over any other possible outcome. On the side of confounding factors, it is also essential to note that most emotion-driven analgesic therapies induce arousal, as well as attention/distraction effects analogous to those discussed in the previous section. Indeed, a number of studies, especially in clinical settings, failed to control for levels of attention or arousal when testing the effect of emotional stimuli on pain. Such effects are often difficult if not impossible to disentangle from the effect of emotion per se, to the point that it has been suggested that the main beneficial effect of emotion-induced procedures is to divert the patients' attention from unpleasant experiences and future interventions [65].

Of all modalities, visual stimuli have been the most frequently used to examine affect-related changes in pain experience. Some studies have shown emotion pictures during nociceptive stimulation and, most specifically, some studies showed *pain-related visual stimuli* during painful stimulations. Meagher and collaborators [58] reported that seeing slides evoking negative emotions such as fear or disgust can decrease pain intensity and unpleasantness thresholds as compared with neutral pictures, while some stimuli categorized as pleasant (erotic pictures) increased the thresholds in healthy male (but not female) participants—an example of how gender differences may be important confounders. This seminal study set the stage for many others, and also raised a number of important issues that allowed refining further work. For instance, the lack of control of arousal and attention appeared clearly as an important confounder, since unpleasant pictures are commonly more arousing than neutral images. Also, while both "fear" and "disgust" stimuli similarly changed pain thresholds, only the latter decreased the pain tolerance in the cold-pressor test, suggesting a potential dissociation between determining subjective thresholds (immediate assessment of current experience of intensity or unpleasantness) and the decision/action of moving away from an aversive situation (tolerance). Even "vicarious" emotion elicited through observation of facial expressions can suffice to modulate pain, and Bayet and collaborators [3] showed that viewing sad human faces led to higher pain reports to thermal stimulation compared to happy and neutral faces. Importantly, this effect was the same whether the participant's attention was focused on the face or on the pain stimulation. In general, positive stimuli are less efficient than negative input at modulating pain; however, even if the observation of positive facial expressions is not sufficient to reduce pain, it might enhance the strength of a placebo analgesia [94], thereby opening the door to novel hypotheses on the indirect uses of positive emotional stimuli in the management of pain.

Seeing Pain Changes the Brain

Inspired by the seminal work of Ken Craig [13] on the effect of seeing other people in pain during a pain experiment, several groups launched a series of studies meant at measuring changes in behavior, subjective feelings, and/or brain activity caused by the observation of pain in others. The initial research question of this endeavor was whether seeing pain and feeling pain would tap into the same neural systems. A more clinical question was to what extent seeing pain affects the pain experience.

An early answer to the first question came from concomitant studies showing that seeing images of pain [36, 62] or seeing a symbol that announces that pain is inflicted to a loved person [88] systematically activated the anterior insula and the dorsal anterior cingulate, which are often described as participating to the encoding of the affective-motivational dimension of pain.[‡] This pattern was also found in experiments using facial expressions of pain [5, 82]. The consistency of such activation pattern, along with the lack of concomitant activity in somatosensory areas, led these studies to generally conclude that the motivational rather than the sensory dimension of pain is somewhat shared between a target and an observer.

‡ The initial ascription of these studies to "pain empathy" could have contributed to the overinterpretation of these findings. Empathy, even in the context of pain, needs to take several other components into consideration, beyond the initial observation of an affective situation [11, 17, 31].

While changes in somatosensory areas during attention are the rule (see earlier sections in this chapter), the search of some equivalent somatosensory activation during the observation of pain has led to controversial results. In most published reports, the observation/imagination of pain did not lead to changes in somatosensory activation [23, 30, 36, 62, 88, 89, 92]. A few studies, on the contrary, did report somatosensory activity changes during pain observation, either in the sense of activation [9, 35, 101] or inhibition [95]. Since in some of these instances the attentional level of the participants may have changed through instructions [35, 45], different attentional levels between conditions could explain sensory modifications. Another source of "vicarious" somatosensory activation may derive from subtle contractions of body segments during observation of the same regions in pictures. Perceiving body representations can elicit covert sensorimotor processes that internally simulate the observed pattern [77], and even a very tiny activation of joint/muscle afferents can trigger significant cerebral events. In this vein, a recent meta-analysis showed that somatosensory areas were only activated during picture-based (but not abstract information-based) "empathy" paradigms [44]. It is very difficult if not impossible at this stage to determine the possible influence of attentional changes and/or micromovements as a trigger of somatosensory changes during empathy-driving experiments. Although methodological issues prevent concluding that emotional modulation per se is able to modify the activity in somatosensory cortices, they do not rule out such possibility. Demonstration of specific somatosensory effects of emotion would require thorny experiments with perfect control of any significant change in attention, arousal, and peripheral activation. Such experiments would not only be exceedingly complex, but also steer away from naturalistic conditions. In real-life situations, every emotional input triggers changes in attention and arousal, and therefore, experiential changes during the observation of pain are contingent on the obligatory *concurrence* of emotional and attentional networks (most likely including somatic areas). Trying to disentangle the two via complex laboratory experiments might not be the most productive road to understanding pain experiences, but could help to identify the internal structure of certain pathological conditions in which an isolated emotional drive may be at work.

A second problem concerns the legitimacy of considering that activity in regions of the pain matrix (PM) indicates actual bodily pain—something that quickly leads to mis-/overinterpretations. For instance, enhanced activity in the ACC and anterior insula (AI) during social exclusion experiments was considered to imply that "social pain is analogous in its neurocognitive function to physical pain" [22]. ACC and AI, however, are part of a network subserving salience detection and orienting [49], driven by the reception of any behaviorally relevant sensory input. Enhanced activity of the AI and ACC is not restricted to pain-related contexts, but is triggered by many other negative emotions (Fig. 14-2), for instance disgust [69, 103] or guilt [86]. Also *positive* stimuli, if behaviorally relevant, can be associated to changes in ACC/AI, for instance during a detection game [105] or when expecting erotic or monetary reward [85]. The amalgamation of such partial PM activations and actual physical pain can be misleading. Current knowledge indicates that the patterns of brain activation associated with the observation of pain, or the recollection of a past painful sensation, are different from those evoked by actual bodily pain, and that differences essentially concern somatosensory regions such as the posterior insula [8, 23]. Once such differences are characterized, and undue extrapolations avoided, it becomes crucial to understand the neural common ground to the internal experiences of "affliction." Such common core may underlie the distressing aspects shared by emotional and bodily aggressions, and its role appears essential to translate (or not) bodily pain into "experiential suffering."

Seeing Pain Changes the Pain Experience

Besides changing the brain activity, a number of studies have shown that viewing pain in others can enhance pain reports to a concomitant or subsequent noxious stimulus [13, 16, 30, 52, 106]—a phenomenon termed "vicarious pain" or "compassionate hyperalgesia." Two studies found that pictures depicting human pain increased pain reports to a greater extent than similarly negatively valenced images unrelated to pain [16, 30]. Various types of aversive pictures have been found to modulate the experience of pain; considering this effect as quantitatively different when the pictures are specific for human pain [30] is an appealing notion, which remains debatable. The brain areas responsible for such "vicarious" or "compassionate" pain enhancement have seldom been explored. Godinho et al. [30] reported that increased pain ratings were associated with activity in high-order areas (mainly dorsolateral prefrontal (DLPFC), posterior parietal, and orbitofrontal cortices) without participation of sensory regions, suggesting that the effect did not rely on a simple "direct sensory resonance." In support of this hypothesis, ratings of unpleasantness while viewing images of other humans in pain were modulated by concomitant cortical stimulation over the DLPFC, but not over visual or sensorimotor areas [4]. Observation of pain in others can also affect the neurophysiological response to self-pain at spinal levels, and can modify spinal reflexes and spontaneous facial pain expressions [55]. Such effects can be triggered through descending influences from OFC and pgACC, secondary to reappraisal of pain (cf. [28]). Thus, even in the absence of direct somatosensory changes, higher-order processing seems able to influence the extent to which one can apprehend the pain of another, and hence *change pain without changing nociception.*

Knowing that the experience of pain can be influenced by attention, emotion, and the social context also brings the reverse problem to mind: Does being in pain affect attentional processes, emotional responses, as well as social interactions? [104] Are actual pain and vicarious pain two points in the space of aversive body experiences? At the experiential level, they can feel similar (even very similar in some cases[§]), but they are usually immediately distinguished by the healthy individual. These two experiences share many attributes, including part of the same neural systems [12, 44], but probably not the exact same regions or neuronal pathways [37].

Taken together, the findings of the preceding sections would state that attention to pain can (*principally*) modify early sensory processing (sensory gating), while emotion-driven modulation would tend (*principally*) to modify high-level interpretation or reinterpretation of pain stimuli (pain appraisal). The change in sensory processing occurs early (<50 ms) while the change in higher-order representation occurs much later (>300 ms). Attentional and emotional modulations are thus complementary and act upon distinct yet interacting brain networks.

CONCLUSIONS AND CLINICAL IMPLICATIONS

Sensory information undergoes extensive attentional modulation as it becomes incorporated into the texture of cognition along a hierarchy of primary sensory, association, supramodal, and limbic zones of the cortex [59]. Each cortical area provides a nexus for information convergence and divergence, and reciprocal connections allow higher levels to exert top-down influence upon earlier levels of processing. The ideas summarized in this chapter insist on the continuous interaction between top-down and bottom-up processes. Sustained attention involves top-down modulation of sensory networks, which in turn entail changes in high-order processes leading to modification of conscious perception. While attention to pain tends in general to determine enhanced perception, peculiar forms of sustained attention may be analgesic, if they allow dissociation of executive activity from sensory enhancement (e.g., meditation, hypnosis). Anticipation becomes hyperalgesic only if associated with stress and anxiety, and this can participate to pain chronification. Interventions aiming at modulating abnormal anticipatory anxiety, such as cognitive and behavioral therapies of various sorts, can be therefore useful in modulating chronic pain.

The influence of affect on pain perception presents a complex pattern, with similar emotional stimuli sometimes modulating pain experiences in opposite directions. This variability likely reflects the interaction of emotional stimuli with attention and arousal, which were unfortunately seldom controlled for in early literature, but also with individual differences such as sex and gender, personality, and past experiences.

[§] Transformation of visual or auditory sensations into somatic experiences has been described as a rare condition named "vision–touch synaesthesia," which is seen as an "abnormal form of empathy" [25]. Recently, this effect has been reported to be more prevalent than previously thought [18].

Nevertheless, several points emerge with relative consistency in the literature: (i) negative emotions are more powerful in enhancing pain than are positive emotions in reducing it; (ii) being confronted with the pain of others (either though explicit images or through emotional-communicative information) is a powerful drive that enhance our own pain; (iii) all these effects are not hardwired, but context-dependent, and subject to change as a function of beliefs, affinities, etc. Consistent with this, (iv) the effects of emotions on pain involve high-order neural systems of prefrontal control, working memory, and multimodal integration, rather than rely on a simple sensory resonance. Notwithstanding the bulk of evidence for the desirable effect of positive emotions on pain, knowing more precisely what are the active ingredients of these effects will help guide their use and target the conditions and possibly the individuals for which they are better suited.

Although presented separately in this chapter and relying on partly distinct neural networks [97], attentional and emotional influences on pain in most circumstances interact. Integrating these two dimensions into pain management practice should lead to more comprehensive and somewhat "cumulative" interventions. Understanding the complex interactions between mental processes that colors our state of consciousness is important to learn more about the pain experience, which has evolved from a simple warning system to flee aversive situations to one of the driving forces behind social communication and interaction.

REFERENCES

1. Bantick SJ, Wise RG, Ploghaus A, Clare S, Smith SM, Tracey I. Imaging how attention modulates pain in humans using functional MRI. Brain 2002;125:310–9.
2. Bartolo M, Serrao M, Gamgebeli Z, Alpaidze M, Perrotta A, Padua L, Pierelli F, Nappi G, Sandrini G. Modulation of the human nociceptive flexion reflex by pleasant and unpleasant odors. Pain 2013;154:2054–9.
3. Bayet S, Bushnell MC, Schweinhart P. Emotional faces alter pain perception. Eur J Pain 2014;18:712–20.
4. Boggio PS, Zaghi S, Fregni F. Modulation of emotions associated with images of human pain using anodal transcranial direct current stimulation (tDCS). Neuropsychologia 2009;47:212–7.
5. Botvinick M, Jha A, Bylsma LM, Fabian SA, Solomon PE, Prkachin KM. Viewing facial expressions of pain engages cortical areas involved in the direct experience of pain. Neuroimage 2005;25:312–9.
6. Brunia CH. Neural aspects of anticipatory behavior. Acta Psychol (Amst) 1999;101: 213–42.

7. Cepeda MS, Carr DB, Lau J, Alvarez H. Music for pain relief. Cochrane Database Syst Rev 2006;(2):CD004843.

8. Chan AW, Baker CI. Seeing is not feeling: posterior parietal but not somatosensory cortex engagement during touch observation. J Neurosci 2015;35(4):1468–80.

9. Cheng Y, Yang CY, Lin CP, Lee PL, Decety J. The perception of pain in others suppresses somatosensory oscillations: a magnetoencephalography study. Neuroimage 2008;40:1833–40.

10. Chua P, Krams M, Toni I, Passingham R, Dolan R. A functional anatomy of anticipatory anxiety. Neuroimage 1999;9:563–71.

11. Coll MP, Grégoire M, Latimer M, Eugène F, Jackson PL. Perception of pain in others: implication for caregivers. Pain Manage 2011;1:257–65.

12. Corradi-Dell'Acqua C, Hofstetter C, Vuilleumier P. Felt and seen pain evoke the same local patterns of cortical activity in insular and cingulate cortex. J Neurosci 2011;31(49):17996–18006.

13. Craig KD, Weiss SM. Vicarious influences on pain-threshold determinations. J Pers Soc Psychol 1971;19:53–9.

14. Davis KD, Taylor SJ, Crawley AP, Wood ML, Mikulis DJ. Functional MRI of pain- and attention-related activations in the human cingulate cortex. J Neurophysiol 1997;77:3370–80.

15. De Tommaso M, Valeriani M, Guido M, Libro G, Specchio LM, Tonali P, Puca F. Abnormal brain processing of cutaneous pain in patients with chronic migraine. Pain 2003;101:25–32.

16. De Wied M, Verbaten MN. Affective pictures processing, attention, and pain tolerance. Pain 2001;90:163–72.

17. Decety J, Jackson PL. The functional architecture of human empathy. Behav Cogn Neurosci Rev 2004;3:71–100.

18. Derbyshire SW. Are mirror-sensations really synesthetic? Cogn Neurosci 2015;6(2–3):134–5.

19. Desmedt JE, Huy NT, Bourguet M. The cognitive P40, N60 and P100 components of somatosensory evoked potentials and the earliest electrical signs of sensory processing in man. Electroencephalogr Clin Neurophysiol 1983;56:272–82.

20. Dobek EC, Beynon EM, Bosma LR, Stroman WP. Music modulation of pain-related activity in the brain, brain stem, and spinal cord : a functional magnetic resonance imaging study. J Pain 2014;15:1057–68.

21. Dum RP, Levinthal DJ, Strick PL. The spinothalamic system targets motor and sensory areas in the cerebral cortex of monkeys. J Neurosci 2009;29:14223–35.

22. Eisenberger NI, Lieberman MD, Williams KD. Does rejection hurt? An fMRI study of social exclusion. Science 2003;302:290–2.
23. Fairhurst M, Fairhurst K, Berna C, Tracey I. An fMRI study exploring the overlap and differences between neural representations of physical and recalled pain. PLoS One 2012;7:e48711.
24. Fanselow, MS, Helmstetter FJ. Conditioned analgesia, defensive freezing, and benzodiazepines. Behav Neurosci 1988;102:233–43.
25. Fitzgibbon BM, Giummarra MJ, Georgiou-Karistianis N, Enticott PG, Bradshaw JL. Shared pain: from empathy to synaesthesia. Neurosci Biobehav Rev 2010;34(4):500–12.
26. Garcia-Larrea L, Bastuji H, Mauguière F. Mapping study of somatosensory evoked potentials during selective spatial attention. Electroencephalogr Clin Neurophysiol 1991;80:201–14.
27. Garcia-Larrea L, Lukaszewicz AC, Mauguière F. Somatosensory responses during selective spatial attention: the N120-to-N140 transition. Psychophysiology 1995;32:526–37.
28. Garcia-Larrea L, Peyron R. Pain matrices and neuropathic pain matrices: a review. Pain 2013;154(suppl 1):S29–S43.
29. Garcia-Larrea L, Peyron R, Laurent B, Mauguiere F. Association and dissociation between laser-evoked potentials and pain perception. Neuroreport 1997;8:3785–9.
30. Godinho F, Faillenot I, Perchet C, Frot M, Magnin M, Garcia-Larrea L. How the pain of others enhances our pain: searching the cerebral correlates of 'compassional hyperalgesia.' Eur J Pain 2012;16:748–59.
31. Goubert L, Craig KD, Vervoort T, Morley S, Sullivan MJL, de C Williams AC, Cano A, Crombez G. Facing others in pain: the effects of empathy. Pain 2005;118:285–8.
32. Grant JA, Courtemanche J, Rainville P. A non-elaborative mental stance and decoupling of executive and pain-related cortices predicts low pain sensitivity in Zen meditators. Pain 2011;152:150–6.
33. Hoffman HG, Chambers GT, Meyer WJ 3rd, Arceneaux LL, Russell WJ, Seibel EJ, Richards TL, Sharar SR, Patterson DR. Virtual reality as an adjunctive non-pharmacologic analgesic for acute burn pain during medical procedures. Ann Behav Med 2011;4:183–91.
34. Hsieh JC, Stone Elander S, Ingvar M. Anticipatory coping of pain expressed in the human anterior cingulate cortex: a positron emission tomography study. Neurosci Lett 1999;262:61–4.

35. Jackson PL, Brunet E, Meltzoff AN, Decety J. Empathy examined through the neural mechanisms involved in imagining how I feel versus how you feel pain. Neuropsychologia 2006;44:752–61.

36. Jackson PL, Meltzoff AN, Decety J. How do we perceive the pain of others? A window into the neural processes involved in empathy. Neuroimage 2005;24:771–9.

37. Jackson PL, Rainville P, Decety J. To what extent do we share the pain of others? Insight from the neural bases of pain empathy. Pain 2006;125:5–9.

38. Jensen J, McIntosh AR, Crawley AP, Mikulis DJ, Remington G, Kapur S. Direct activation of the ventral striatum in anticipation of aversive stimuli. Neuron 2003;40:1251–7.

39. Kaufman EF, Rosenquist AC. Efferent projections of the thalamic intralaminar nuclei in the cat. Brain Res 1985;335:257–79.

40. Kennett S, Taylor-Clarke M, Haggard P. Noninformative vision improves the spatial resolution of touch in humans. Curr Biol 2001;11(15):1188–91.

41. Keogh E, Mansoor L. Investigating the effects of anxiety sensitivity and coping on the perception of cold pressor pain in healthy women. Eur J Pain 2001;5(1):11–22.

42. Koyama T, Tanaka YZ, Mikami A. Nociceptive neurons in the macaque anterior cingulated activate during anticipation of pain. Neuroreport 1998;9:2663–7.

43. Kulkarni B, Bentley DE, Elliott R, Youell P, Watson A, Derbyshire SW, Frackowiak RS, Friston KJ, Jones AK. Attention to pain localization and unpleasantness discriminates the functions of the medial and lateral pain systems. Eur J Neurosci 2005;21:3133–42.

44. Lamm C, Decety J, Singer T. Meta-analytic evidence for common and distinct neural networks associated with directly experienced pain and empathy for pain. Neuroimage 2011;54(3):2492–502.

45. Lamm C, Nusbaum HC, Meltzoff AN, Decety J. What are you feeling? Using functional magnetic resonance imaging to assess the modulation of sensory and affective responses during empathy for pain. PLoS One 2007;2(12):e1292.

46. Larbig W, Elbert T, Lutzenberger W, Rockstroh B, Schnerr G, Birbaumer N. EEG and slow brain potentials during anticipation and control of painful stimulation. Electroencephalogr Clin Neurophysiol 1982;53:298–309.

47. Legrain V, Guerit JM, Bruyer R, Plaghki L. Attentional modulation of the nociceptive processing into the human brain: selective spatial attention, probability of stimulus occurrence, and target detection effects on laser evoked potentials. Pain 2002;99:21–39.

48. Legrain V, Guerit JM, Bruyer R, Plaghki L. Electrophysiological correlates of attentional orientation in humans to strong intensity deviant nociceptive stimuli, inside and outside the focus of spatial attention. Neurosci Lett 2003;339:107–10.

49. Legrain V, Iannetti GD, Plaghki L, Mouraux A. The pain matrix reloaded: a salience detection system for the body. Prog Neurobiol 2011;93(1):111–24.

50. Leventhal H, Brown D, Shacham S, Engquist G. Effects of preparatory information about sensations, threat of pain, and attention on cold pressor distress. J Pers Soc Psychol 1979;37:688–714.

51. Lichtman AH, Fanselow MS. Opioid and nonopioid conditional analgesia: the role of spinal opioid, noradrenergic, and serotonergic systems. Behav Neurosci 1991;105:687–98.

52. Loggia ML, Mogil JS, Bushnell MC. Empathy hurts: compassion for another increases both sensory and affective components of pain perception. Pain 2008;136(1–2):168–76.

53. Longo MR, Iannetti GD, Mancini F, Driver J, Haggard P. Linking pain and the body: neural correlates of visually induced analgesia. J Neurosci 2012;32(8):2601–7.

54. Lutz A, McFarlin DR, Perlman DM, Salomons TV, Davidson RJ. Altered anterior insula activation during anticipation and experience of painful stimuli in expert meditators. Neuroimage 2013;64:538–46.

55. Mailhot JP, Vachon-Presseau E, Jackson PL, Rainville P. Dispositional empathy modulates vicarious effects of dynamic pain expressions on spinal nociception, facial responses and acute pain. Eur J Neurosci 2012;35:271–8.

56. McCaul KD, Haugtvedt C. Attention, distraction, and cold-pressor pain. J Pers Soc Psychol 1982;43:154–62.

57. McCracken LM, Vowles KE. A Prospective analysis of acceptance of pain and values-based action in patients with chronic pain. Health Psychol 2008;27:215–20.

58. Meagher MW, Arnau RC, Rhudy JL. Pain and emotion: effects of affective picture modulation. Psychosom Med 2001;63(1):79–90.

59. Mesulam MM. From sensation to cognition. Brain 1998;121:1013–52.

60. Michael GA, Dupuy MA, Deleuze A, Humblot M, Simon B, Naveteur J. Interacting effects of vision and attention in perceiving spontaneous sensations arising on the hands. Exp Brain Res 2012;216(1):21–34.

61. Miron D, Duncan GH, Bushnell C. Effects of attention on the intensity and unpleasentness of thermal pain. Pain 1989;39:345–52.

62. Morrison I, Lloyd D, di Pellegrino G, Roberts N. Vicarious responses to pain in anterior cingulate cortex: is empathy a multisensory issue? Cogn Affect Behav Neurosci 2004;4:270–8.

63. Ochsner KN, Gross JJ. The cognitive control of emotions. Trends Cogn Sci 2005;9:242–9.

64. Ohara S, Crone NE, Weiss N, Vogel H, Treede RD, Lenz FA. Attention to pain is processed at multiple cortical sites in man. Exp Brain Res 2004;156:513–7.

65. Pauwels EK, Volterrani D, Mariani G, Kostkiewics M. Mozart, music and medicine. Med Princ Pract 2014;23:403–12.

66. Petrovic P, Kalso E, Petersson KM, Ingvar M. Placebo and opioid analgesia. Imaging a shared neuronal network. Science 2002;295:1737–40.

67. Peyron R, Faillenot I, Mertens P, Laurent B, Garcia-Larrea L. Motor cortex stimulation in neuropathic pain. Correlations between analgesic effect and hemodynamic changes in the brain: a PET study. Neuroimage 2007;34:310–21.

68. Peyron R, Garcia-Larrea L, Gregoire MC, Costes N, Convers P, Lavenne F, Mauguiere F, Michel D, Laurent B. Haemodynamic brain responses to acute pain in humans: sensory and attentional networks. Brain 1999;122:1765–80.

69. Phillips ML, Young AW, Senior C, Brammer M, Andrew C, Calder AJ, Bullmore ET, Perrett DI, Rowland D, Williams SC, et al. A specific neural substrate for perceiving facial expressions of disgust. Nature 1997;389:495–8.

70. Ploghaus A, Becerra L, Borras C, Borsook D. Neural circuitry underlying pain modulation: expectation, hypnosis, placebo. Trends Cogn Sci 2003;7:197–200.

71. Ploghaus A, Narain C, Beckmann CF, Clare S, Bantick S, Wise R, Matthews PM, Rawlins JN, Tracey I. Exacerbation of pain by anxiety is associated with activity in a hippocampal network. J Neurosci 2001;21:9896–903.

72. Ploghaus A, Tracey I, Gati JS, Clare S, Menon RS, Matthews PM, Rawlins JNP. Dissociating pain from its anticipation in the human brain. Science 1999;284: 1979–81.

73. Porro CA, Baraldi P, Pagnoni G, Serafini M, Facchin P, Maieron M, Nichelli P. Does anticipation of pain affect cortical nociceptive systems? J Neurosci 2002;22:3206–14.

74. Porro CA, Cettolo V, Francescato MP, Baraldi P. Temporal and intensity coding of pain in human cortex. J Neurophysiol 1998;80:3312–20.

75. Rainville P, Hofbauer RK, Bushnell MC, Duncan GH, Price DD. Hypnosis modulates activity in brain structures involved in the regulation of consciousness. J Cogn Neurosci 2002;14(6):887–901.

76. Rhudy JL, Meagher MW. Noise stress and human pain thresholds: divergent effects in men and women. J Pain 2001;2(1):57–64.

77. Rizzolatti G, Craighero L. The mirror-neuron system. Annu Rev Neurosci 2004;27:169–192.

78. Robinson CJ, Burton H. Somatic submodality distribution within the second somatosensory (SII), 7b, retroinsular, postauditory, and granular insular cortical areas of *M. fascicularis*. J Comp Neurol 1980;192:93–108.

79. Roy M, Lebuis A, Hugueville L, Peretz I, Rainville P. Spinal modulation of nociception by music. Eur J Pain 2012;16:870–7.

80. Roy M, Peretz I, Rainville P. Emotional valence contributes to music-induced analgesia. Pain 2008;134:140–7.

81. Rubio A, Van Oudenhove L, Pellissier S, Ly HG, Dupont P, de Micheaux HL, Tack J, Dantzer C, Delon-Martin C, Bonaz B. Uncertainty in anticipation of uncomfortable rectal distension is modulated by the autonomic nervous system—a fMRI study in healthy volunteers. Neuroimage 2015;107:10–22.

82. Saarela MV, Hlushchuk Y, Williams AC, Schürmann M, Kalso E, Hari R. The compassionate brain: humans detect intensity of pain from another's face. Cereb Cortex 2007;17:230–7.

83. Sawamoto N, Honda M, Okada T, Hanakawa T, Kanda M, Fukuyama H, Konishi J, Shibasaki H. Expectation of pain enhances responses to nonpainful somatosensory stimulation in the anterior cingulate cortex and parietal operculum/posterior insula: an event-related functional magnetic resonance imaging study. J Neurosci 2000;20:7438–45.

84. Schlereth T, Baumgärtner U, Magerl W, Stoeter P, Treede RD. Left-hemisphere dominance in early nociceptive processing in the human parasylvian cortex. Neuroimage 2003;20:441–54.

85. Sescousse G, Redouté J, Dreher JC. The architecture of reward value coding in the human orbitofrontal cortex. J Neurosci 2010;30(39):13095–104.

86. Shin LM, Dougherty DD, Orr SP, Pitman RK, Lasko M, Macklin ML, Alpert NM, Fischman AJ, Rauch SL. Activation of anterior paralimbic structures during guilt-related script-driven imagery. Biol Psychiatry 2000;48:43–50.

87. Simavli S, Gumus I, Kaygusuz I, Yildirim M, Usluogullari B, Kafali B. Effect of music on labor pain relief, anxiety level and postpartum analgesic requirement: a randomized controlled clinical trial. Gynecol Obstet Invest 2014;78:244–50.

88. Singer T, Seymour B, O'Doherty J, Kaube H, Dolan RJ, Frith CD. Empathy for pain involves the affective but not sensory components of pain. Science 2004;303:1157–62.

89. Singer T, Snozzi R, Bird G, Petrovic P, Silani G, Heinrichs M, Dolan RJ. Effects of oxytocin and prosocial behavior on brain responses to direct and vicariously experienced pain. Emotion 2008;8:781–91.

90. Suls J, Wan CK. Effects of sensory and procedural information on coping with stressful medical procedures and pain: a meta-analysis. J Consult Clin Psychol 1989;57:372–9.

91. Tracey I, Ploghaus A, Gati JS, Clare S, Smith S, Menon RS, Matthews PM. Imaging attentional modulation of pain in the periaqueductal gray in humans. J Neurosci 2002;22:2748–52.

92. Vachon-Presseau E, Roy M, Martel MO, Albouy G, Chen J, Budell L, Sullivan MJ, Jackson PL, Rainville P. Neural processing of sensory and emotional-communicative information associated with the perception of vicarious pain. Neuroimage 2012;63:54–62.

93. Valentini E, Koch K, Aglioti SM. Seeing one's own painful hand positioned in the contralateral space reduces subjective reports of pain and modulates laser evoked potentials. J Pain 2015;16:499–507.

94. Valentini E, Martini M, Lee M, Aglioti MS, Iannetti G. Seeing facial expressions enhances placebo analgesia. Pain 2014;155:666–73.

95. Valeriani M, Betti V, Le Pera D, De Armas L, Miliucci R, Restuccia D, Avenanti A, Aglioti SM. Seeing the pain of others while being in pain: a laser-evoked potentials study. Neuroimage 2008;40:1419–28.

96. Valet M, Sprenger T, Boecker H, Willoch F, Rummeny E, Conrad B, Erhard P, Tolle TR. Distraction modulates connectivity of the cingulo-frontal cortex and the midbrain during pain—an fMRI analysis. Pain 2004;109:399–408.

97. Villemure C, Bushnell MC. Mood influences supraspinal pain processing separately from attention. J Neurosci 2009;21;29(3):705–15.

98. Villemure C, Laferrière AC, Bushnell MC. The ventral striatum is implicated in the analgesic effect of mood changes. Pain Res Manag 2012;17:69–74.

99. Villemure C, Slotnick BM, Bushnell MC. Effects of odors on pain perception: deciphering the roles of emotion and attention. Pain 2003;106:101–8.

100. Villemure C, Wassimi S, Bennett GJ, Shir Y, Bushnell MC. Unpleasant odors increase pain processing in a patient with neuropathic pain: psychophysical and fMRI investigation. Pain 2006;120:213–20.

101. Voisin JI, Marcoux LA, Canizales DL, Mercier C, Jackson PL. I am touched by your pain: limb-specific modulation of the cortical response to a tactile stimulation during pain observation. J Pain 2011;12:1182–9.

102. Wang MC, Zhang LY, Zhang YL, Zhang YW, Xu XD, Zhang YC. Effect of music in endoscopy procedures: systematic review and meta-analysis of randomized controlled trials. Pain Med 2014;15:1786–94.

103. Wicker B, Keysers C, Plailly J, Royet JP, Gallese V, Rizzolatti G. Both of us disgusted in My insula: the common neural basis of seeing and feeling disgust. Neuron 2003;40:655–64.

104. Wieser MJ, Gerdes AB, Reicherts P, Paul P. Mutual influences of pain and emotional face processing. Front Psychol 2014;5:1160.

105. Wittmann M, van Wassenhove V, Craig AD, Paulus MP. The neural substrates of subjective time dilation. Front Hum Neurosci 2010;4:2.

106. Wunsch A, Philippot P, Plaghki L. Affective associative learning modifies the sensory perception of nociceptive stimuli without participant's awareness. Pain 2003;102:27–38.

CHAPTER 15

The Neuroevolutionary Sources of Consciousness and Affect

Jaak Panksepp

How does the brain create affective experiences such as pain? Such foundational issues for understanding the brain are also critical for understanding consciousness. A key issue is where did consciousness begin? Getting the foundations correct is essential for all higher levels of analysis. Indeed, the emergence of consciousness has an evolutionary history that can only be decoded by the study of living brain, with strict criteria for what counts as consciousness or not. The study of homologous processes in animal models will be critical for such endeavors: Any complete understanding of the diversity of "pains"—from somatic to emotional—requires animal models where the detailed neuroscientific inquiries can be pursued. Although it is still widely believed that the affective and other qualities of subjective experiences (including of course painful ones) cannot be studied in animals, one goal of this paper is to highlight how it can, thereby enriching our understanding of human psychological pain engendered by social separation (such as separation distress, loneliness, grief, as opposed to bodily/physical pains), which are especially intense among the young of most mammalian and certain avian species. The species that do not show robust emotional-pain responses to social separation are ones in which the young are born *altricial*—namely so immature that they cannot get lost on their own (for discussion, see references [28, 38]).

Indeed, it seems reasonable that consciousness initially emerged from brain systems that encoded ancestral survival values as experienced primal (inborn) affective states. From a neuroevolutionary vantage, "mental stuff" first emerged from the ability of neural networks to encode for survival values—namely, "good" and "bad" affective feelings, which were probably unconditional survival indicators: The arousal of negative feelings, such as pain, indicated the trajectories of potential destruction. All positively valenced feeling registered survival trajectories, namely, feelings of "goodness" and "badness" were "survival-codes" for approach and avoidance that regulated learning. They can be classified into diverse forms including *emotional* ones (e.g., RAGE and PANIC), *homeostatic* (e.g., HUNGER and THIRST), and various *sensory* ones (e.g., diverse externally driven passions and pleasures).

I use such capitalizations to highlight primary-process categorizations of the mind—functions that were built into the evolutionary infrastructure of mammalian brains and, no doubt, many other classes of animals. Hence, we may learn more about the neural nature of various pains and other affects, including purely psychological ones such as separation distress, by studying the brains and behaviors of other animals than human beings. That is the theoretical infrastructure for the epistemological strategies of a cross-species' "affective neuroscience" [27]. Most of the chapters of this book focus on the nature of sensory pains. Here I expand toward the nature of emotional pain, especially the "separation distress" engendered by social loss [24, 30]. This system appears to be a key motivator for fundamental learning of social bonds whether between children and their mothers, or the love between adults.

THE EVOLUTION OF CONSCIOUSNESS

There are good evolutionary reasons to suspect that valenced affective feelings—from various pains to pleasures—may have been among the earliest forms of consciousness on the face of the earth, having evolved to provide guidance for diverse behavioral survival trajectories [31]. Through the analysis of rewarding and punishing (valence) effects with Deep Brain Stimulation (DBS), it has become evident that primal affects, both "good" (rewarding) and "bad" (punishing), are coded largely by sub-neocortical systems [27, 35], which must lead one to wonder whether higher forms of consciousness were built on a basic platform of affective values [47]. We have long known that consciousness cannot be sustained without the so-called Ascending Reticular Activating System (ARAS), which abounds with rewarding and punishing brain circuitry, and those valenced states survive extensive cortical lesions [9] and perhaps even radical neodecortication (see pp. 290–293 in reference [27]), although the role of other brain regions including the insula has not been excluded.

Recent understandings of the wide-ranging connectivities of the ARAS and its diverse neurochemistries only affirm its critical importance as a foundation for all of consciousness as it controls higher brain cognitive processing through the reticular intralaminar fields of the thalamus that sustain cognitive consciousness, as well as the emotional-affective processing, which arise more via the reticular fields of the hypothalamus [50]. Perhaps the most important empirical-functional findings have been the discoveries that a very large number of sites within this later trajectory are rewarding or punishing during localized brain stimulation of pathways, whether via electrical and neurochemical DBS (for extensive summaries, see reference [27]), now being extended with optogenetic and DREADD (Designer Receptors Exclusively Activated by Designer Drugs) methods.

One of the most prominent and well-studied systems for rewarding states (which can diminish feelings of pain) is a massive trans-diencephalic conglomeration of pathways known as the medial forebrain bundle (for modern human anatomy, see reference [4]). Although this was traditionally called "the brain reward system", in the ensuing 60 years there has emerged remarkably little agreement about what those DBS-evoked rewards feel like (for extensive discussion, see reference [51]). Most agree that it is certainly not like any sensory pleasure we experience, and many alternatives have been proposed [37]. The most reasonable conclusion is that the feeling is akin to *enthusiasm* or *exuberance,* which is an essential part of all energized exploratory and goal-direct behaviors (see reference [35]). Indeed, it is a common experience that when one is pursuing sports enthusiastically (in the "flow" so to speak), minor injuries are hardly noticed.

Also, the brain has many negatively valenced zones and pathways, perhaps none as intensely aversive as stimulation of the dorsal periaqueductal central gray (PAG). For instance, one person stimulated there went from a nonemotional state rapidly to exclaiming "I'm scared to death" soon after onset of PAG stimulation [22]. Also, the PAG has strong pain- and distress-modulatory areas some of which project to dorsomedial thalamic areas to regulate feeling of separation distress [12], with abundant implications for understanding empathy [49].

Parenthetically, based on the famous James–Lange theory of emotions, there are still schools of thought in academic psychology that believe affective experiences are completely dependent on higher neocortical expansions. There is no consistent stream of data to support that hypothesis. Granted, there are studies where surgical damage to higher cortical regions, such as anterior cingulate, provided pain relief [10], but that may reflect decreased worrying about one's chronic pain. There is also data that such higher brain damage reduces pain responses in rats [13]. Still, currently there is more abundant data that raw (nonreflective) affective experience are critically dependent on subcortical brain systems, as highlighted by the "rewarding" and "punishing" properties of DBS of many subcortical regions but essentially no neocortial regions in preclinical (animal) models; indeed, it has long been known that such measures of affect in animals survive radical neodecortication [27]. Higher forms of cognitive/reflective consciousness surely can contextualize and regulate primary-process affective states, including pain, but the primal affects can be envisioned as the original experiential survival "gifts" of evolution, that emerged long before our capacity to think about our feelings (Fig. 15-1).

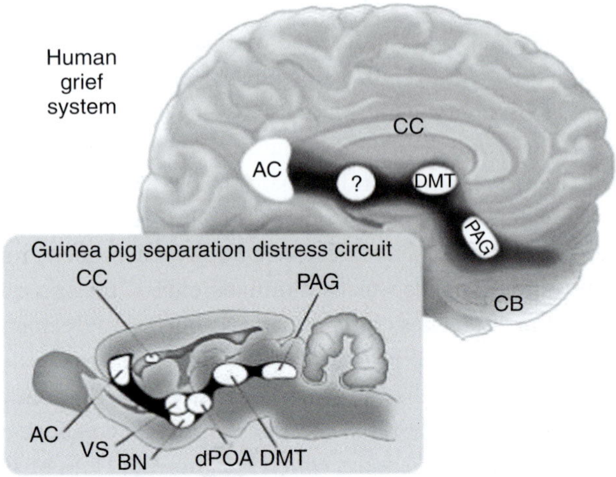

FIGURE 15-1 A schematic summary of guinea pig brain regions where one can readily evoke social separation–induced vocalizations in young guinea pigs (as mapped in Barbara Herman's PhD dissertation, Bowling Green State University, 1980). Very similar anatomies were observed in domestic chicks (Paul Bishop's PhD dissertation, BGSU, 1984). In 1980 when Antonio Damasio et al. [5] published PET scan images of human beings feeling very sad, a very similar anatomy was evident, suggesting that all warm-blooded vertebrates share this social cohesions mediating PANIC/GRIEF system. The areas that lit up are anterior cingulate (AC), the dorsomedial thalamus (DMT) and the periaqueductal gray (PAG), and also regions in the most ancient parts of the cerebellum (CB). Animals showed remarkably similar anatomies including ventral septal area (VS), dorsal preoptic areas (dPOA), and the bed nucleus of the stria terminalis (BN), which are too small to be accurately identified on human PET images, thus the question mark there in the human depiction.

THE PANIC SYSTEM—SEPARATION DISTRESS AND THE PAIN OF SOCIAL LOSS

One of the most intense forms of emotional "pain" that we humans experience is the death of loved ones, especially when we are young. Abundant data indicate that all other mammals, indeed birds born precocious (e.g., chickens, ducks, geese) also, exhibit pain-like crying when socially isolated from mothers. That is the kind of "psychological pain" that reflects the dynamics of social bonding—namely, the crying of separation-induced distress vocalizations (DVs). DVs primarily arise from social loss and probably at latter ages from ostracism (social marginalization). We have studied such emotional pains for 40 years [30, 31]. Why would we distinguish this from fearful anxiety? The key finding is that the behaviors, anatomies, and many chemistries of separation distress are quite distinct from fear-type anxiety responses [27, 39]. Such knowledge has abundant implications for the way we handle diverse medical problems, especially psychiatric ones such as depression and panic attacks.

While feeling of physical pain most probably emerged before the "psychological pain" of social loss, major regulatory features such as neurochemical controls were probably conserved. For instance, once primal physical pain had evolved, it could have been used as a foundation for various homeostatic and emotional pain (hunger pangs and separation distress). We initiated our work in the area with the hypothesis that "painful" feelings of social loss—the profound internal "ache" resulting from the loss of social support, whether by death or abandonment by a loved one—achieves part of its affective intensity from the same brain chemistries that emerged earlier to regulate physical pain, especially brain opioids, and the addictive qualities of opiates may reflect their capacity to mediate social bonding. Our research on the separation-distress (so-called PANIC) systems in socially bonded animals was guided by this evolutionary relationship [27]. In a sense, feelings engendered by social loss were comparable to the ache of bodily injury. One straightforward prediction was that brain opioid system also regulated the pain of social loss, and that relationship was abundantly supported; indeed, the reduction of separation-induced crying was reduced at the lowest dose of opioids ever used in the animal research (for earliest review, see reference [24]).

Considering how survival of mammalian young is critically depended on maternal care, it is easy to understand the strong survival value conferred by neurochemistries that elaborated both the affective intensity of physical pain and social bonds. In other words, once physically painful affect had evolved, it may have been relatively easy to use this solution for social cohesion purposes. There are many implications of this finding for clinical management of physical pain, for instance the power of placebos, as well as social influence, on the felt intensity of physical pain and psychological grief. One of the biggest impediments for scholars pursuing such ideas experimentally has been the long-standing controversy whether other animals (indeed infants who cannot yet speak) actually experience pain (also see Chapter 11) as opposed to just exhibiting nociceptive reflexes (e.g., see reference [45]). Indeed, animal models of physical pain have long been used in medicinal discoveries, and probably that will also apply for psychological pains that are of psychiatric significance, such as in the dysphoria of depression [42]. But first, let us consider possible linkages between emerging knowledge of psychological and physical pain.

HOW DOES THE BRAIN FEEL THE ACHE OF SOCIAL EXCLUSION AND A "Broken Heart"?

Evidence for evolutionary relationships between physical and social pain come from several lines of animal brain research: Localized DBS of various subcortical brain systems, long implicated in the regulation of physical pain, evoke separation cries which are auditorialy and sonographically similar to natural separation calls [12, 27, 32, 39]. Among the most prominent subcortical areas where DBS can evoke separation cries, even in adult animals, are dorsomedial thalamus, bed nuclei of the stria terminalis, ventral septal and dorsal preoptic regions, and most intensely and at the lowest current levels from midbrain PAG, where some of the evoked sounds are sonographically closer to pain squeals while at other nearby sites they more closely resemble separation cries. Indeed, the most intense emotional distress with the lowest current intensities is obtained from the dorsal PAG. Of course opiates are among the best medications for somatic pain, and the shared neurochemistries, highlighted most by endogenous opioids, suggest an evolutionary relationship between somatic and emotional pain [12, 53]. Indeed, it has been found that safe opioids such as buprenorphine at very low doses might be effective in reducing both depression and suicidal urges (for discussion, see reference [42, 52]).

Thus, once again, the psychological pain of social loss (grief and loneliness) may have arisen as evolutionary explanation from physical pain processes. Indeed, there is abundant evidence indicating that social support reduces affective pain intensity [3, 20], which is coded in part by anterior cingulate processes that are also highly responsive to being socially ostracized, as originally evaluated through the use of a video "cyberostracism game," while emotional regulatory areas of prefrontal cortex exhibited diminished arousal [8]. These brain regions are well connected to other separation distress–mediating brain areas, especially PAG and dorsomedial thalamus, from where DVs can be evoked with DBS [39]. Indeed, such brain regions have exhibited strong arousals during PET imaging of human sadness [5, 18]. In this context several other brain chemistries have been identified that powerfully and specifically regulate separation distress, especially oxytocin [26], a neuropeptide that can also attenuate physical pain [44].

PLACEBO EFFECTS AND EMPATHY

With the discovery that the affective sting of social loss shares evolutionary relations to physical pain, novel avenues for understanding related phenomena such as empathy, as well as novel clinically intervention in psychiatric disorders related to social loss, such as depression, have opened up. Indeed, it has long been recognized that the quality of social environments may contribute much to our ability to cope with pain [11]. For instance the pain of childbirth can be substantially eased with social support [16], as can postoperative pain (see more extensive discussion in reference [30]). Indeed, these effects may have underlying similarities to how placebos control pain.

Might placebo effect be evolutionarily conceptualized as cerebral manifestations of the "healing touch" based in part on opioid release within the brain. Contact comfort in animals can release opioids [15, 32] as can joyful social play [34, 41]. Likewise, placebo analgesia in humans operates partly through opioid release [43].

Indeed, placebos may reduce arousal of anterior cingulate brain regions that are commonly overactive in depression and psychological distress [21], and participate in empathy-related brain responses [46]. For an extensive review of the preclinical (animal) findings in this area, see reference [40].

In this context it may be worth considering how very low doses of opioid analgesics may be used in psychiatry. Many people contemplate suicide because they simply have too much psychological pain resulting from social losses [34, 41]. Might we be able to use safe opioids (e.g., buprenorphine, which are *partial agonists* at μ-opioid receptors, meaning that they promote μ-opioid dynamics at low doses but begin block receptors at high doses, which minimizes their suicide potential). Indeed, at such higher doses buprenorphine blocks κ-opioid receptors, reducing activity in a stress-promoting opioid (dynorphin) system of the brain. Indeed, we have completed such a trial, which suggests good results for both treatment-resistant depression and suicidality (for pilot data, see reference [42]). Of course, this promising finding needs abundant further testing. In this vein it may be useful to note that Emil Kraepelin, the father of biological psychiatry, described in the first modern *Textbook of Psychiatry* how he was able to treat the psychological pain of depression with small doses of morphine that he tapered off gradually to minimize the return of depression that he supposed would happen with rapid withdrawal of the medication. Whether recent findings indicating that acetaminophen can blunt positive and negative emotions [7], and hence also reduce social pain [6], have comparable psychiatric implications needs to be further explored.

CONCLUSION

The overall message seems obvious. There is still abundant room for human empathy and the healing touch in the management of pain and distress. This can include music, which often quintessentially captures social feelings [33]. Since self-selected music can readily enhance prosocial feelings, it is understandable why music therapy is being proposed to reduce feelings of pain [2]. With an understanding of how positive social interactions, as well as symbolic ones activated by placebos recruit endogenous brain opioid system [48], such psychosocial approaches need to be studied further and considered as a potential addition to effective pain management. This brings us to how the empathy and placebo effects may be organized in the brain. Accumulating data indicate that partly we are relieved by such social and medical maneuvers because they also influence brain opioids and oxytocin systems.

In sum, these various therapeutic effects may reflect how certain prosocial processes of the brain/mind control opioid release within the brain. For instance, many years ago we found that when young chicks are socially isolated, and exhibiting strong separation distress, they are promptly comforted when held in human hands, an effect that is counteracted by opioid antagonists [32]. We have found similar effects in young rats. Perhaps opioids are so commonly used to treat pain in terminal patients (as well as assisted suicides) not just for attenuation of physical pain, but also attenuation of the emotional distress of dying. This is both humane and appropriate. However, it would be a shame if humans did not continue to be the ultimate carriers of the healing touch. Indeed, there is now abundant room for evaluating whether analgesics and other psychotropics could be used at lower doses in more empathic and supportive psychosocial contexts (see reference [36]).

Overall, the experienced affective intensity of "painful" emotional arousal arise largely from subcortical neurodynamics—from ancient brain regions shared homologously, because of common descent, by all mammals and other vertebrates. Higher neocortically mediated forms of cognitive consciousness can regulate lower brain/mind regions. The neocortex, especially frontal regulatory regions, can reduce feelings of pain in certain situations and promote suffering under others. However, fundamental forms of pain emerged with the earliest glimmers of primary process consciousness, not from our developmentally acquired abilities to have episodic memories and to cognitively reflect on our life experiences. Being couriers of urgent survival concerns, the primal emotional feelings, including our ability to experience emotional pains (e.g., separation distress), reflect subcortical brain functions that created useful forms of "simple-minded" primary-process affective consciousness, early in brain evolution. These foundations of consciousness are still necessary for higher forms of consciousness (e.g., awareness—namely, knowing one is experiencing) to operate [29].

Although the psychological functional analysis of these ancient brain systems is understandably slow, there are fascinating questions to be pursued: For instance, (i) Do activations of separation distress networks in relatively helpless young animals evoke resonant activity in homologous pain circuits of nearby adults? Indeed, Lorberbuam and colleagues [19] provided fMRI analyses of mother listening to the cries of their babies, and brain arousals were seen in many brain regions implicated in separation distress in animal studies. (ii) That naturally leads to the question whether perceptually induced resonances emerge more readily between individuals who are socially bonded than those who are strangers. This may well be the case, since the so-called brain reward system, which probably mediates feeling of enthusiasm, are recruited more when one is viewing one's own child than strangers' infants [1]. Indeed, there are relevant studies asking whether resonant brain arousals are more prominent among those who share the same ethnic background in caregiving in adults [14]. Still it is hard to conduct the needed *causal* studies in human, while brain *correlational* studies are easy to do with modern human brain imaging, highlighting racial sensitivities in humans. Of course, the required causal studies do not require lesioning parts of the human brain that have so far been implicated by brain imaging of such processes (see reference [17]); they could be studied with virtual lesions through stimulation techniques such as transcranial magnetic stimulation (TMS) and other less invasive modalities. Thus, detailed invasive causal studies can only be readily pursued in animal models, but detailed neuroscientific work on such topics in other animals has barely begun.

Why is that? There is still considerable resistance to granting other animals the capacity to have experiences. That is an unfortunate residue of the history of rigid forms of behaviorism in psychology [25] that are still robust in behavioral neuroscience. For anyone who may still wish to argue that animals do not experience pain (i.e., do not have consciousness), please explain the following: Why would animals that have been obviously "hurt" by experimental procedures begin to spontaneously consume drugs that are analgesic in humans (see reference [23]). Of course, data-based conclusions for the existence of phenomenal affective consciousness in animals does not imply that they are *"self-conscious"* as is commonly implied by the term "awareness." Our study demonstrating that low doses of sublingual buprenorphine can significantly reduce depression and suicidality has just been published (see reference [52]).

REFERENCES

1. Bartels A, Zeki S. The neural correlates of maternal and romantic love. Neuroimage 2004;21:1155–66.
2. Bernatzky G, Presch M, Anderson M, Panksepp J. Emotional foundations of music as a non-pharmacological pain management tool in modern medicine. Neurosci Biobehav Rev 2011;359:1989–99.
3. Brown JL, Sheffield D, Leary MR, Robinson ME. Social support and experimental pain. Psychosom Med 2012;65:276–83.
4. Coenen VA, Panksepp J, Hurwitz TA, Urbach H, Mädler B. Human medial forebrain bundle (MFB) and anterior thalamic radiation (ATR): diffusion tensor imaging of two major subcortical pathways that may promote a dynamic balance of opposite affects relevant for understanding depression. J Neuropsychiatry Clin Neurosci 2012;24:223–36.
5. Damasio AR, Grabowski TJ, Bechara A, Damasio H, Ponto LLB, Parvizi J, Hichwa RD. Subcortical and cortical brain activity during the feeling of self-generated emotions. Nat Neurosci 2000;3:1049–56.
6. Dewall CN, Macdonald G, Webster GD, Masten CL, Baumeister RF, Powell C, Combs D, Schurtz DR, Stillman TF, Tice DM, Eisenberger NI. Acetaminophen reduces social pain: behavioral and neural evidence. Psychol Sci 2010;21:931–7.
7. Durso GR, Luttrell A, Way BM. Over-the-counter relief from pains and pleasures alike: acetaminophen blunts evaluation sensitivity to both negative and positive stimuli. Psychol Sci 2015;26(6):750–8.

8. Eisenberger NI, Lieberman MD. Why rejection hurts: a common neural alarm system for physical and social pain. Trends Cogn Sci 2004;8:294–300.
9. Feinstein JS, Khalsa SS, Salomons TV, Prkachin KM, Frey-Law LA, Lee JE, Tranel D, Rudrauf D. Preserved emotional awareness of pain in a patient with extensive bilateral damage to the insula, anterior cingulate, and amygdala. Brain Struct Funct 2015: Epub Jan 11.
10. Folt EL, White LE. Pain relief by frontal cingulotomy. J Neurosurg 1962;19:89–100.
11. Gatchel R, Turk D, editors. Psychosocial factors in pain: critical perspectives. New York, NY: The Guilford Press; 2000.
12. Herman BH, Panksepp J. Ascending endorphinergic inhibition of distress vocalization. Science 1981;211:1060.
13. Johansen JP, Fields HL, Manning BH. The affective component of pain in rodents: direct evidence for a contribution of the anterior cingulate cortex. Proc Natl Acad Sci U S A 2001;98:8077–82.
14. Kaseweter KA, Drwecki BB, Prkachin KM. Racial differences in pain treatment and empathy in a Canadian sample. Pain Res Manag 2012;17:381–4.
15. Keverne EB, Martenz N, Tuite B. B-endorphin concentrations in CSF of monkeys are influenced by grooming relationships. Psychoneuroendocrinology 1989;14:155–61.
16. Klaus M, Kennel J, Robertson S, Rosa R. Effects of social support during parturition on maternal and infant mortality. BMJ 1986;293:585–97.
17. Leigh R, Oishi K, Hsu J, Lindquist M, Gottesman RF, Jarso S, Crainiceanu C, Mori S, Hillis AE. Acute lesions that impair affective empathy. Brain 2013;136:2539–49.
18. Liotti M, Panksepp J. On the neural nature of human emotions and implications for biological psychiatry. In: Panksepp J, editor. Textbook of biological psychiatry. New York, NY: Wiley; 2004. pp. 33–74.
19. Lorberbaum JP, Newman JD, Horwitz AR, Dubno JR, Lydiard RB, Hamner MB, Bohning DE, George MS. A potential role for thalamocingulate circuitry in human maternal behavior. Biol Psychiatry 2002;51:431–45.
20. MacDonald G, Leary MR. Why does social exclusion hurt? The relationship between social and somatic pain. Psychol Bull 2005;131:202–23.
21. Mayberg HS, Silva JA, Brannan SK, Tekell JL, Mahurin RK, McGinnis S, Jerabek PA. The functional neuroanatomy of the placebo effect. Am J Psychiatry 2002;159:728–37.
22. Nashold BS, Wilson WP, Slaughter G. Sensations evoked by stimulation of the midbrain of man. J Neurosurg 1969;30:14–24.
23. Navratilova E, Porreca F. Reward and motivation in pain and pain relief. Nat Neurosci 2014;17:1304–12.

24. Panksepp J. Brain opioids: a neurochemical substrate for narcotic and social dependence. In: Cooper S, editor. Progress in theory in psychopharmacology. London: Academic Press; 1981. pp. 149–75.

25. Panksepp J. Can "mind" and behavior be understood without understanding the brain?: a response to Bunge. New Ideas Psychol 1990;8:139–49.

26. Panksepp J. Oxytocin effects on emotional processes: separation distress, social bonding, and relationships to psychiatric disorders. Ann N Y Acad Sci 1992;652:243–52.

27. Panksepp J. Affective neuroscience: the foundations of human and animal emotions. London: Oxford University Press; 1998.

28. Panksepp J. Can anthropomorphic analyses of separation cries in other animals inform us about the emotional nature of social loss in humans? Comment on Blumberg and Sokoloff (2001). Psychol Rev 2003;110:376–8.

29. Panksepp J. On the embodied neural nature of core emotional affects. J Conscious Stud 2005;12:158–84.

30. Panksepp J. On the neuro-evolutionary nature of social pain, support, and empathy. In: Aydede M, editor. Pain: new essays on its nature & the methodology of its study. Cambridge, MA: The MIT Press; 2006. pp. 367–87.

31. Panksepp J. Affective consciousness. In: Velmans M, Schneider S, editors. The Blackwell companion to consciousness. Malden, MA: Blackwell Publishing; 2007. pp. 114–29.

32. Panksepp J, Bean NJ, Bishop P, Vilberg T, Sahley TL. Opioid blockade and social comfort in chicks. Pharmacol Biochem Behav 1980;13:673–83.

33. Panksepp J, Bernatzky G. Emotional sounds and the brain: the neuro-affective foundations of musical appreciation. Behav Processes 2002;60:133–55.

34. Panksepp J, Bishop P. An autoradiographic map of (3H)diprenorphine binding in the rat brain: effects of social interaction. Brain Res Bull 1981;7:405–10.

35. Panksepp J, Biven L. The archaeology of mind: neuroevolutionary origins of human emotions. New York, NY: Norton; 2012.

36. Panksepp J, Harro J. The future of neuropeptides in biological psychiatry and emotional psychopharmacology: goals and strategies. In: Panksepp J, editor. Textbook of biological psychiatry. New York, NY: Wiley; 2004. pp. 627–60.

37. Panksepp J, Moskal J. Dopamine and SEEKING: subcortical "reward" systems and appetitive urges. In: Elliot A, editor. Handbook of approach and avoidance motivation, New York, NY: Taylor & Francis Group, LLC; 2008. pp. 67–87.

38. Panksepp J, Newman JD, Insel TR. Critical conceptual issues in the analysis of separation-distress systems of the brain. In: Strongman KT, editor. International review of studies on emotion, Vol. 2. Chichester, England: Wiley; 1992. pp. 51–72.

39. Panksepp J, Normansell LA, Herman B, Bishop P, Crepeau L. Neural and neurochemical control of the separation distress call. In: Newman JD, editor. The physiological control of mammalian vocalizations. New York, NY: Plenum; 1988. pp. 263–300.
40. Panksepp J, Panksepp JB. Toward a cross-species understanding of empathy. Trends Neurosci 2013;36:489–96.
41. Panksepp J, Wright JS, Döbrössy MD, Schlaepfer TE, Coenen VA. Affective neuroscience strategies for understanding and treating depressions: from preclinical models to novel therapeutics. Clin Psychol Sci 2014;2:472–94.
42. Panksepp J, Yovell Y. Preclinical modeling of primal emotional affects seeking, panic and play: gateways to the development of new treatments for depression. Psychopathology 2014;476:383–93.
43. Petrovic P, Kalso E, Petersson KM, Ingvar M. Placebo and opioid analgesia: imaging a shared neuronal network. Science 2002;295:1737–40.
44. Rash JA, Aguirre-Camacho A, Campbell TS. Oxytocin and pain: a systematic review and synthesis of findings. Clin J Pain 2014;305:453–62.
45. Rose JD. The neurobehavioral nature of fishes and the questions of awareness and pain. Rev Fisheries Sci 2002;10:1–38.
46. Singer T, Seymour B, O'Doherty J, Kaube H, Dolan RJ, Frith CD. Empathy for pain involves the affective but not sensory components of pain. Science 2004;303:1157–62.
47. Solms M, Panksepp J. The "Id" knows more than the "Ego" admits: neuropsychoanalytic and primal consciousness perspectives on the interface between affective and cognitive neuroscience. Brain Sci 2012;2:147–75.
48. Wager TD, Scott DJ, Zubieta JK. Placebo effects on human mu-opioid activity during pain. Proc Natl Acad Sci U S A 2007;104(26):11056–61.
49. Watt DF. Toward a neuroscience of empathy. Neuropsychoanalysis 2007;9:119–72.
50. Watt DF, Pincus DI. Neural substrates of consciousness: implications for clinical psychiatry. In: Panksepp J, editor. Textbook of biological psychiatry. New York, NY: Wiley; 2004. pp. 75–110.
51. Wright JS, Panksepp J. An evolutionary framework to understand foraging, wanting, and desire: the neuropsychology of the SEEKING system. Neuropsychoanalysis 2012;14:5–39.
52. Yovell Y, Bar G, Mashiah M, Baruch Y, Briskman I, Asherov J, Lotan A, Rigbi A, Panksepp J. Ultra-low-dose buprenorphine as a time-limited treatment for severe suicidal ideation: a randomized, controlled trial. Am J Psychiatry 2015. doi: 10.1176/appi.ajp.2015.15040535
53. Zubieta JK, Stohler CS. Neurobiological mechanisms of placebo responses. Ann N Y Acad Sci 2009;1156:198–210.

CHAPTER 16

Robot Pain: A Speculative Review of Its Functions

Carme Torras

"There are no gains, without pains..."
—Benjamin Franklin, *The Way to Wealth* (1758)

"Their minds are so narrow that they cannot hold the slightest doubt"
—Emil Cioran

Nowadays robots exhibit a wide variety of cognitive abilities, among them that of learning from bad experiences. Does this mean that robots may have doubts about what course of action to take and ultimately be able to experience pain?

Before trying to answer this question, let me quote the Nobel Prize-winner Herbert A. Simon [19], who in the late 1960s claimed that we should not push biological inspiration too far when designing artificial creatures, since the best natural mechanisms may not be the best artificial ones. Wheels, airplanes' nonflapping wings, and calculators have often been mentioned as examples of artificial solutions considerably different from their natural equivalents, and more performant according to certain criteria. The resources available to engineering design depart a lot from those in nature, and not just when it comes to materials, but also in the number of instances and spendable time. Robots have been incrementally designed along 60 years of technological research, instead of being the outcome of thousands of years of evolution.

Thus, in case of existence, *robot pain* and *robot cognition* must be of a different nature than human ones, and if these labels are used, it is because the underlying functions play a similar role as those of their human counterparts.

With this note of caution in mind and accepting that biological plausibility adds no special value from an engineering viewpoint, human biology constitutes a great source of inspiration for robotics researchers, since it provides existence proofs of many useful physical and cognitive mechanisms. Thus, robots often have an anthropomorphic anatomy with legs, arms, and hands having as many degrees of freedom as the human ones, their actuators mimicking the flexibility and power of biological muscles, with visual, auditive, tactile, as well as proprioceptive sensors, and with a hierarchical control system whose uppermost layer is a symbolic decision-maker that governs lower layers, often in the form of neural networks encoding sensorimotor mappings.

In trying to unravel the roles pain may play at all these levels, we adopt the distinctions between types of pain made by de Vignemont (Chapter 3). A first distinction is between chronic pains, occurrent pains, and pain expertise based on prior experiences of pain. Since chronic pains do not have adaptive value and thus cannot fulfill a function in robot development, we will not consider them further. *Occurrent pains* can be used as punishment within reinforcement learning (RL) schemes, as described in "Occurrent Pain As Punishment in Reinforcement Learning," whereas *pain expertise* can be incorporated in a motivational/cognitive system modulating reactions to stimuli, as elaborated in "Pain Expertise As a Form of Emotion and Knowledge." One can further distinguish between merely unpleasant and excruciating pains, upon which the motivational modulation will act differently.

Another useful distinction is between *exogenous* and *endogenous* pains. Although the underlying criterion is whether the cause is external or internal to the organism, in order to provide concrete examples of each we need to enter the slippery terrain of defining what we mean by robot pain. A short digression may help. This is an excerpt of a fictional dialogue [4] in which "Russell" argues for the importance of a clear definition of pain to make scientific progress, while "Edison" takes the pragmatic view of the inventor who just wants to build robots whose pain serves a function:

> RUSSELL: How do we define self and pain in ways that even begin to be meaningful for a machine? For example, a machine may overheat and have a sensor that measures temperature as part of a feedback loop to reduce overheating, but a high temperature reading has nothing to do with pain.

We agree: this would correspond to nociception, not pain, at least in humans.

> EDISON: I disagree! Overheating is not human pain for sure but certainly "machine" pain! I see no problem in defining self and pain for a robot. The self could be (at least in part) machine integrity with all functions operational within nominal parameters. And pain occurs with input from sensors that are tuned to detect non-nominal parameter changes (excessive force exerted by the weight at the end of a robot arm).

Paradoxically, we agree with this view too. A percept that compromises the normal functioning of the robot could be interpreted as robot pain.

> RUSSELL: [...] my earlier examples were to make clear that "pain" and detection of parameter changes are quite different. If I have a perfect local anesthetic but smell my skin burning, then I feel no pain but have

sensed a crucial parameter change. True, we cannot expect all aspects of human pain to be useful for the analysis of robots, but it does no good to throw away crucial distinctions we have learned from the studies of humans or other animals.

Of course, we intend to keep crucial distinctions, and we note that the word "crucial" has a self-referential meaning in the paragraph above, as it provides the key to our pragmatic definition of robot pain: a crucial parameter change that diminishes robot competence and degrades its performance.

EDISON: [...] Inspired by what was learned with fear in rats, a roboticist would say "OK! My walking robot has analogous problems: encountering a predator—for a mobile robot, a car or truck in the street—and reacting to a low battery state, which signals the robot to prepare itself for functioning in a different mode, where energy needs to be saved." Those two robot behaviors are very similar to the rat behaviors in the operational sense that they serve the same kind of purpose. I think we might just as well call them "fear" and "pain." I would argue that it does not matter what I call them—the roboticist can still be inspired by their neural implementations and design the robotic system accordingly.

We will follow this biologically inspired, operational approach here and, adhering to our above-mentioned pragmatic definition of robot pain, colliding with an obstacle or getting too close to a light source so that the camera saturates would be examples of exogenous pain, while an endogenous pain would involve proprioceptive sensors detecting, for instance, that a robot arm is at a singular configuration, thus lacking one degree of freedom, or simply that a joint has reached its limit, thus losing manipulability. All these situations have in common that robot competence decreases and performance degrades.

Endogenous pains can contribute to the acquisition of a body schema by the robot (a kinematic model of its mobility), which is loosely reminiscent of the development of a sense of bodily ownership in humans, as described in "Acquisition of a Body Schema." Although some authors relate the discovery of the body boundaries to the distinction between self and others, and ultimately to the emergence of a conscious self, we share the view of Hoffmann et al. [6] that robots have not yet reached the level of competence where notions like conscious representations can be investigated in a grounded fashion.

Going back to the initial question, in this chapter we will try to unravel the role pain (and choice) may play in developing robot competences. We can pinpoint at least three adaptive functions where pain plays a role in the biological world and which have been incorporated into robots, namely learning through reward/punishment (both at the sensorimotor and cognitive levels), providing intrinsic motivation, and engaging in empathized interaction. While in punishment and aversive motivation the robot can be said to "experience" pain, although in its own artificial way, the interaction context entails perceiving pain in humans and (up to now) faking empathy so as to give them comfort, thus being of a very different nature. In what follows we will concentrate on the former contexts in which robots "experience" pain, which can all be formulated in the common framework of RL.

OCCURRENT PAIN AS PUNISHMENT IN REINFORCEMENT LEARNING

In the biological world, occurrent pain clearly serves an adaptive purpose by eliciting escape responses and thus protecting organisms from further danger. Taking a design perspective, adaptivity could be dispensable for robots that perform repetitive tasks in predefined environments (such as production lines), but it is a sine qua non if they are to work and survive in human, dynamic scenarios, where there is no expert programmer at hand. Among the repertoire of artificial adaptive mechanisms ranging from unsupervised to supervised ones [23], RL algorithms are the most appropriate in the aforementioned scenarios, where evaluating the performance of a behavior is possible but the optimal behavior is unknown.

RL refers to the process of improving performance through trial and error. The simplest RL algorithms rely on the intuitive idea that if an action is followed by an improvement in the robot's state, then the tendency to produce such action should be strengthened in that situation, whereas it should be weakened if a negative effect like pain occurs. This is the classic mechanism of reward/punishment. More formally, RL algorithms entail progressively building a mapping from situations to actions so as to maximize a scalar reward or reinforcement signal. The robot is not told which action to take, as in supervised learning, but instead must discover which actions yield the highest reward by trying them. In more complex cases, actions may affect not only the immediate reward, but also the next situation, and through that all subsequent rewards. These two characteristics—trial-and-error search and delayed reward—are the two most important distinguishing features of RL [21].

Fig. 16-1A shows the classic diagram of an RL agent (e.g., a robot controller) interacting with its environment. The agent generates actions in the context of sensed states of this environment, and its actions influence how the environment's states change over time. The environment contains a "critic" component that, at each time step, provides the agent with a numeric evaluation of its ongoing behavior. The term critic is used, instead of "teacher," because in supervised learning algorithms a teacher provides more informative instructional information, such as directly telling the agent what its actions *should have been* instead of merely scoring them.

In the biological world, the critic's evaluation corresponds to what behavioral psychologists call *primary reward,* namely that encouraging behavior directly related to survival and reproductive success, such as eating, drinking, and escaping. The mapping from states to rewards is called a *reward function,* which is an essential

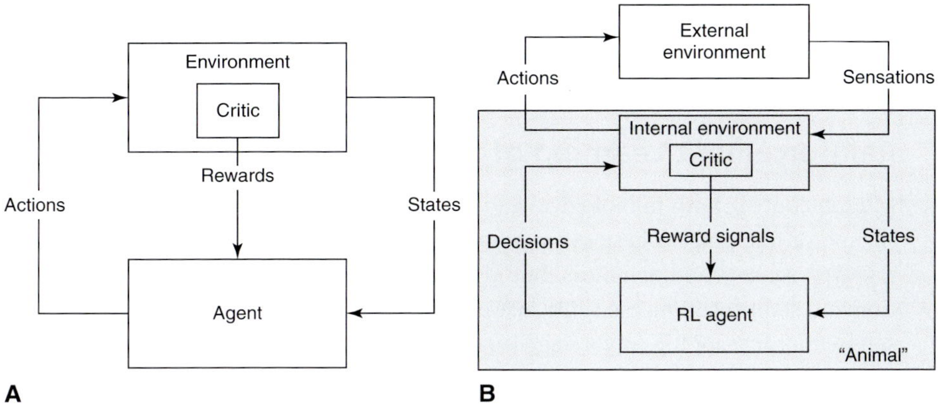

FIGURE 16-1 Agent–environment interaction in reinforcement learning [2]. **A:** Primary reward signals are supplied to the agent from a "critic" in its environment. **B:** A refinement in which the environment is divided into an internal and an external environment, with all reward signals coming from the former. The shaded box corresponds to what we would think of as the animal or robot.

component of RL algorithms since it implicitly encodes the problem the agent must learn to solve. Pain takes the form of negative reward.

As mentioned above, the objective of a complex agent is to act at each time step so as to maximize not the immediate reward, but the total reward it expects to receive over the future (called the *expected return),* which is usually a weighted sum in which later rewards are weighted less than earlier ones. Because the agent's actions influence the environment's state over time, maximizing expected return requires the agent to control the evolution of its environment. This is very challenging, since the agent might have to sacrifice short-term reward in order to achieve more reward over the long term. Some pains are bearable if the expected return is high enough.

The simplest RL agents attempt to achieve this objective by adjusting a *policy,* which is a rule that associates actions to observed environment states. A policy corresponds to a stimulus–response (S-R) rule of animal learning theory. But RL is not restricted to simple S-R agents: more complex RL agents learn models of their environments that they can use to make plans about how to act appropriately. This entails the capacity to predict and choose between alternative courses of action.

Analogously, RL in robotics is applied in two rather different forms depending on whether it takes place at the sensorimotor or cognitive levels. Sensorimotor adaptation is implemented by building mappings from stimuli to proper movements, while cognitive learning entails constructing symbolic representations to guide decision making. In the following two subsections, we will describe how associative S-R agents have been used to learn robot sensorimotor mappings and a body schema, respectively, whereas symbolic RL agents for learning to plan will be described in

"Reinforcement Learning to Plan." A detailed survey of the challenges and successes in the application of RL to robotics is provided in [8].

Reinforcement Learning of Sensorimotor Mappings

Motion control, both in biological and technological systems, relies strongly on sensorimotor mappings. These mappings vary depending not only on the nature of the involved sensors and actuators, but also on the goal pursued. Hand–eye coordination and stable walking are skills that may be acquired through RL, their underlying sensorimotor mappings involving visual and proprioceptive signals, respectively, and their reward functions relying on somewhat delayed reinforcement in the form of success (object grasped) or pain (falling down).

Despite their apparent disparity, these mappings have in common an underlying highly nonlinear relation between a continuous (often hard to interpret) input domain and a continuous motor domain; a relation that in most cases would be impossible to derive analytically. Thus, such relation needs to be approximated through associative learning. Neural network architectures have the versatility to encode a large range of nonlinear mappings, and, through RL, they have proven adequate to handle the massively parallel task of relating perception patterns to motor commands.

For further details, the reader is referred to a review of neural learning algorithms used to approximate sensorimotor mappings for the control of articulated robots [24]. Similar procedures apply to wheeled robot navigation [13], where a mapping from proximity sensor readings to obstacle avoidance motions is learned by using as reward function the pain (or punishment) derived from collisions with environmental obstacles.

Acquisition of a Body Schema

In this volume, de Vignemont (Chapter 3) relates pain to the learning of the body boundaries and ultimately to the development of a bodily self. Along the same line but without referring to pain, Haselager et al. [5] highlight the importance of sensing one's own movements for the development of a nonconceptual sense of self. These authors claim that proprioception and kinesthesis are essential in this development, and make a plea for robots to be equipped with a richer sense of proprioception, so as to advance in the understanding of creatures acting in the world with a sense of themselves.

In neurosciences, the correlation of proprioceptive sensory information, for example, joint configurations, with the visible shape of the body has been termed "body schema" and is assumed to provide an unconscious awareness of the current body state. Experiments with both macaque monkeys and humans have shown that the body schema is not congenital but learnable [10], and may not be a localized pattern but rather be distributed across several groups of connected neurons that represent opportunistically learned manifolds spanning several brain regions [20].

Hoffmann et al. [6] provide a detailed review of robotics works tackling the learning of a body schema, which they define to be a sensorimotor representation of the body used for action. As an example, for arm robots such representation is usually restricted to an inverse kinematics/dynamics mapping relating the gripper's pose (position and orientation) and velocity to the arm's joint angles and torques. Then, according to this definition, the body schema can be learned in the same way as the sensorimotor mappings in the previous subsection by using pose/velocity as input and the robot kinematic parameters as output.

Besides this parameter adjustment of phylogenetic skills through learning, biological creatures show an impressive capacity to adapt their body scheme to newly acquired abilities (e.g., tool usage), as well as to abrupt changes in their bodies (e.g., limb loss). For instance, a monkey's proximal visual receptive field was enlarged by the length of a tool after being trained to use it [10]. This led to hypothesize that the tool itself became incorporated into the monkey's own body schema [3]. Similar conclusions were drawn from experiments with human patients who suffered from phantom pain after having lost a limb.

Not surprisingly, replicating this capacity has raised a lot of interest in the robotics community, since making robots adaptive to changes in their own geometry due to damage, wear and tear or tool replacement increases their robustness and widens their range of application. Hence, neural learning algorithms have been used to learn not the whole kinematics mapping from scratch, as previously done, but only the deviations from the nominal kinematics embedded in the original robot controller [17], resulting in a significant speed-up that permits online adaptation of the body schema, a crucial feature for autonomous robots that need to operate for a long time without assistance (e.g., in space). Likewise, the body schema of humanoid robots has been extended to encompass a tool through training [25] and RL algorithms relying on a self-model have been implemented on a hexapod robot that needed to adapt to leg removal, broken legs, and motor failures [9].

As a final note, let us mention that hand in hand with the development of the body representation, infants acquire a notion of body ownership and agency, which at the present time goes beyond the scope of the functional approach to robot pain adopted in this chapter.

PAIN EXPERTISE AS A FORM OF EMOTION AND KNOWLEDGE

Animal behavior is the joint effect of environmental sensory impingement and the animal's emotions and knowledge of the situation. In Rolls's evolutionary theory [16], the *flexibility* of behavioral responses to reinforcing stimuli is the crucial function that explains why emotion and knowledge are so important. The essential idea is that reward and punishment specify behavioral goals, instead of particular actions, thus defining flexible routes to action. This is in contrast to S-R learning in which a particular response to a particular stimulus is learned, as described in the preceding section.

Notably, this modulation of behavior can be formulated in the same framework of RL, and in the next two subsections we will show that pain expertise (i.e., that based on prior experiences of pain) can be a source of emotions and knowledge effectively exerting such modulation.

Emotion Provides Intrinsic Motivation in Reinforcement Learning

The RL framework is particularly appropriate for bringing learning together with what in animals one would call intrinsic motivation [2]. Despite the common perception that an RL agent's reward has to be extrinsic because the agent has a distinct input channel for reward signals, reward functions can depend on the state of the robot's internal environment, which includes remembered and learned information (see Fig. 16-1B).

The dominant animal's motivation at any given time influences the arousal, strength, and direction of behavior. Similarly, each robot motivation may have a quantitative intensity and the motivation with the current highest intensity will modulate the robot reaction to stimuli. Where could robot motivation come from? Emotions are certainly motivating; for example, fear learned by stimulus-pain association provides the motivation to avoid noxious stimuli.

Rumbell et al. [18] review emotion mechanisms that have been used in artificial agents to improve action selection. Many include arousal and pleasure/pain components, to which the synthetic forces approach add a clarity/confusion one. Emotion modulates behavior by using arousal to focus attention and associating pleasure/pain to goals, that is, courses of action that should be pursued or avoided. Confusion tends to increase pain, and clarity tends to increase pleasure, ensuring that the agent will seek situations where its expectations are confirmed.

But is robot emotion (e.g., fear of pain) possible? Currently, two main programs of scientific research investigate this question: psychological behaviorism and role functionalism. Psychological behaviorism assumes that emotion behavior can be explained in a robot without reference to subjective or mental states. On the contrary, a role functionalist defines pain as "a subjective qualitative state that is reliably caused by noxious stimulation, to cause the desire to make it stop, to cause distraction regarding concurrent projects or plans and their completion, and to cause changes in preferences among alternative states of affairs" [26]. According to role functionalism, only beings with subjective qualitative states that fulfill these causal roles can be in pain.

Following this view, Parisi and Petrosino [15] equipped robots with an emotional circuit and devised five experiments, one of them exploring robot pain. Their claim was that, for robots to "experience" pain, they need to have more than one dispositional motivation; and competition between the motivations must result in an overriding aversion, or some disposition to avoid if the result is to be painfulness. In the experiment, the emotional circuit succeeded in arousing a compelling aversion, despite concurrent hunger. Thus, in the terms of role functionalism, Parisi and Petrosino's robots are considered to be in pain because it is possible to describe the functional role that pain states have in their behavior and to identify the specific part of the neural network causing their behavior that makes pain states possible.

Reinforcement Learning to Plan

To go beyond sensorimotor adaptation and emotionally modulated reactive behavior, planning capabilities are needed and, in order to develop them, a cognitive architecture [27] should be able to progressively learn an action model from experiences and rehearse hypothetical future scenarios on that model so as to determine the best course of action. Moreover, such action model must be probabilistic to account for noise in perceptions and uncertainties in action outcomes.

Relational RL [2] has been developed toward this aim. By enhancing RL with relational representations of states and actions (i.e., explicitly encoding relations in a symbolic data structure), the knowledge acquired by the RL agent can be generalized across states and transferred across tasks [12].

Some robot actions may be irreversible leading to unrecoverable failures (e.g., damaging some robot element, breaking an object, or losing a tool). On the contrary, a planner can always backtrack from a dead-end so as to try to find an alternative sequence of actions to reach the goal. Thus, prior experiences of pain can be very helpful for safety-aware planning, that is, to generate plans that preserve robot integrity while pursuing task accomplishment.

We have proposed a relational RL method that allows a robot to reason about dead-ends and their causes. If a plan might lead to a dead-end (e.g., one that potentially includes a painful action effect), the robot tries to find an alternative safe plan and, if not found, it asks a teacher whether the risky action should be executed. This method permits learning safe policies as well as minimizing unrecoverable errors during the learning process, and it has been validated on a robot learning to clear a table [11].

CONCLUSIONS AND FUTURE PROSPECTS

Given the scarce bibliography dealing explicitly with robot pain, this chapter has tried to enrich its review with related research works about robot behaviors and capacities in which pain could play a role. All such roles—ranging from punishment to intrinsic motivation and planning knowledge—can be formulated within the unified framework of reinforcement learning.

We foresee that *self-knowledge* will be the key ingredient to significantly increase robot autonomy in the years to come and that pain could serve to acquire such knowledge. Several degrees of self-knowledge could be distinguished progressively, leading to more complex functionalities. The simplest body schema consisting of a parameterized kinematic/dynamic model has already been incorporated into robots through sensorimotor learning. More elaborate self-models would include a body image precisely delimiting the robot boundaries acquired through exploratory actions, leading to the distinction between a body self and others [14], from which the notions of body ownership and agency could develop. These would ground the foundations for robots to construct a model of their own physical/cognitive abilities which, for instance, could allow them to ask for help whenever a task goes beyond their capabilities or explore new actions [1] and try to acquire the required skills if no helper is around. Finally, some authors hypothesize that the most sophisticated internal models would lead to consciousness [7]. Whether this intriguing, largely unknown feature of the human brain could serve a functional purpose in robots constitutes an amazing challenge for future technological research, while at the same time posing decisive questions that promise to ignite an exciting moral and ethical debate.

REFERENCES

1. Agostini A, Torras C, Wörgötter F. An efficient and interactive decision-making framework for robotic applications. Artifi Intell 2015;special issue 'AI and Robotics', to appear. Available at: http://dx.doi.org/10.1016/j.artint.2015.04.004
2. Barto AG. Intrinsic motivation in reinforcement learning. In: Baldassarre G, Mirolli M, editors. Intrinsically motivated learning in natural and artificial systems. Heidelberg/Berlin: Springer-Verlag; 2013. pp. 17–47.
3. Cardinali L, Frassinetti F, Brozzoli C, Urquizar C, Roy AC, Fame A. Tool-use induces morphological updating of the body schema. Curr Biol 2009;19(12): R478–R479.
4. Fellous JM, Arbib MA, editors. Who needs emotions? The brain meets the robot. Oxford: Oxford University Press; 2005.
5. Haselager WFG, Broens M, Gonzalez MEQ. The importance of sensing one's movements in the world for the sense of personal identity. Rivista Internazionale di Filosofia e Psicologia 2011;3(1):1–11.
6. Hoffmann M, Gravato H, Hernandez A, Sumioka H, Lungarella M, Pfeifer R. Body schema in robotics: a review. IEEE Trans Auton Mental Develop 2010;2(4): 304–24.

7. Holland O, Goodman R. Robots with internal models: a route to machine consciousness? J Conscious Stud 2003;10(4–5):77–109.
8. Kober J, Bagnell D, Peters J. Reinforcement learning in robotics: a survey. Int J Robot Res 2013;32(11):1238–74.
9. Koos S, Cully A, Mouret JB. Fast damage recovery in robotics with the t-resilience algorithm. Int J Robot Res 2013;32(14):1700–23.
10. Maravita A, Iriki A. Tools for the body (schema). Trends Cogn Sci 2004;8(2):79–86.
11. Martinez D, Alenyà G, Torras C. Finding safe policies in model-based active learning. IROS Workshop on Machine Learning in Planning and Control of Robot Motion. Chicago; 2014. pp. 1–6.
12. Martinez D, Alenyà G, Torras C. Relational reinforcement learning with guided demonstrations. Artif Intell 2015;special issue 'AI and Robotics', to appear. Available at: http://dx.doi.org/10.1016/j.artint.2015.02.006
13. Millân JR, Torras C. Learning sensor-based navigation. In: Morik K, Kaiser M, Klingspor V, editors. Making robots smarter: combining sensing and action through robot learning. Boston, MA: Kluwer Academic Publishers; 1999. pp. 85–108.
14. Oudeyer P-Y, Kaplan F, Hafner VV. Intrinsic motivation systems for autonomous mental development. IEEE Trans Evol Comput 2007;11(2):265–86.
15. Parisi D, Petrosino G. Robots that have emotions. Adapt Behav 2010;18(6):453–69.
16. Rolls ET. Emotion and decision-making explained. Oxford: Oxford University Press; 2013.
17. Ruiz de Angulo V, Torras C. Self-calibration of a space robot. IEEE Trans Neural Networks 1997;8(4):951–63.
18. Rumbell T, Barnden J, Denham S, Wennekers T. Emotions in autonomous agents: comparative analysis of mechanisms and functions. Auton Agent Multi-Agent Syst 2012;25(1):1–45.
19. Simon HA. The sciences of the artificial. Cambridge, MA: MIT Press; 1969.
20. Stamenov MI. Body schema, body image, and mirror neurons. In: De Preester H, Knockaert V, editors. Body image and body schema: interdisciplinary perspectives on the body, Vol. 62. Amsterdam: John Benjamins Publishing; 2005. pp. 21–43.
21. Sutton RS, Barto AG. Reinforcement learning: an introduction. Cambridge, MA: MIT Press; 1998. Available at: https://www.dropbox.com/s/b3psxv2r0ccmf80/book2015oct.pdf (2nd ed.).
22. Tadepalli P, Givan R, Driessens K. Relational reinforcement learning: an overview. Proceedings of the ICML Workshop on Relational Reinforcement Learning. Banff; 2004. pp. 1–9.

23. Torras C. Robot adaptivity. In: Steels L, editor. The biology and technology of intelligent autonomous agents. Berlin/Heidelberg: Springer-Verlag; 1995. pp. 53–71.

24. Torras C. Robot arm control. In: Arbib MA, editor. Handbook of brain theory and neural networks. 2nd ed. Cambridge, MA: MIT Press; 2003. pp. 979–83.

25. Ulbrich S, Ruiz de Angulo V, Asfour T, Torras C, Dillmann R. Rapid learning of humanoid body schemas with kinematic Bézier maps. 9th IEEE-RAS International Conference on Humanoid Robots. Paris; 2009. pp. 431–38.

26. van Rysewyk S. Robot pain. Int J Synth Emot 2013;4(2):22–33.

27. Vernon D, Metta G, Sandini G. A survey of artificial cognitive systems: implications for the autonomous development of mental capabilities in computational agents. IEEE Trans Evol Comput 2007;11(2):151–80.

INDEX

Note: Page numbers followed by *f* indicate figures; those followed by *t* indicate tables.

D

E

F

M

N